MW01532975

Ciguatera Seafood Toxins

Editor

Donald M. Miller, Ph. D.
Professor
Department of Physiology
School of Medicine
Southern Illinois University
Carbondale, Illinois

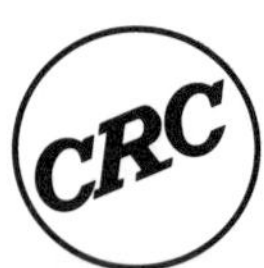

CRC Press
Boca Raton Ann Arbor Boston

Library of Congress Cataloging-in-Publication Data

Ciguatera seafood toxins / editor, Donald M. Miller.
p. cm.
Includes bibliographical references.
Includes index.
ISBN 0-8493-6073-0
1. Marine toxins—Analysis. 2. Poisonous fishes—Toxicology. I. Miller, Donald M., 1930—
[DNLM: 1. Marine Toxins—analysis. 2. Marine Toxins—poisoning.
QW 630 C571]
QP632.M37C54 1991
615.9′45—dc20
DNLM/DLC 90-2606
for Library of Congress CIP

Direct all inquiries to CRC Press, Inc., 2000 Corporate Blvd., N.W., Boca Raton, Florida, 33431.

International Standard Book Number 0-8493-6073-0

Library of Congress Card Number 90-2606
Printed in the United States

PREFACE

This book began a long time ago when three former mentors, John Denton Anderson, Bernard C. Abbott, and Theodore L. Jahn sparked my interest in the flagellates. John Anderson began my career acting as my advisor for a Master's Degree in Physiology. Bud Abbott took me on for a Doctoral program, and Ted Jahn provided postdoctoral schooling in high-speed photography of flagellates and ciliates. I can remember laughing at a fellow graduate student John Sassner, when he would admonish Yoromi Matsumoto, Father Cappell, Hiroshi Mizukami, and myself to walk softly in the laboratory because the dinflagellates he was trying to grow were very delicate.

Little did I realize then that some 30 years later I would be involved in producing this volume on *Ciguatera Seafood Toxins*. Ciguatera recorded history, as indicated by Mike Capra in his chapter, dates back to the voyages of Captain Cook. In more recent history, the number of reported cases and the public awareness of ciguatera has dramatically increased. Several factors have perhaps contributed to this increase, including growth of the seafood industry, more frequent travel by tourists, recent accent on the consumption of seafood, and better diagnosis of the ciguatera syndrome. This volume attempts to bring together a summary of some medical, legal, and scientific aspects of this enigmatic disease, ciguatera. As such, it should be useful to the doctor, lawyer, and researcher and provide not only a brief encapsulation of what is known, but also stimulate new ideas.

The majority of the credit for this volume belongs to the several authors who labored on their chapters and also to the U.S. Army Research Institute of Infectious Diseases, Fort Detriek, MD, whose funding made some of the research and writing of the entire volume a reality. I thank them for their interest and support of what I feel is a worthwhile endeavor.

Finally, a significant amount of credit goes to Linda Sikora, who did a lot of typing and the laboratory boffins (a term I learned from Seymour Hutner), who looked up references, and otherwise freed up my time.

Donald Miller

THE EDITOR

Donald M. Miller, Ph.D., is a Professor in the Department of Physiology, School of Medicine, Southern Illinois University, Carbondale.

Professor Miller received his B.A. degree in 1960, his M.S. degree in 1962, and his Ph.D. degree in 1965 from the University of Illinois, Champaign. He did NIH postdoctoral work at the University of California, Los Angeles in 1966. He was appointed Assistant Professor in the Department of Physiology, Southern Illinois University in 1966, Associate Professor in 1972 and Professor in 1976.

Professor Miller is a member of Sigma Xi, the American Physiological Society, the American Society of Photobiology, the American Trauma Society, the Association of Official Analytical Chemists, the Biophysics Society, the International Society for Magnetic Resonance, and the International Society of Toxicology and Toxinology.

Professor Miller has worked on ciguatera toxins for 12 years, and 30 of his 200 publications are on some aspects of ciguatera. The current focus of his research is on isolation of toxins and determination of their structure.

CONTRIBUTORS

Jeff W. Bomber, Ph.D.
Student Doctor
University of Osteopathic Medicine and Health Sciences
Des Moines, Iowa

Geoffrey M. Calvert, M.D.
Assistant Clinical Professor
Department of Community Medicine
Wright State University School of Medicine
Dayton, Ohio

John Cameron, M.D., Ph.D.
Doctor
Department of Neurology
Princess Alexandra Hospital
Brisbane, Australia

Michael F. Capra, Ph.D.
Professor
Public Health and Nutrition
Queensland University of Technology
Brisbane, Australia

Faiqa Hassan, Ph.D.
Doctor
Department of Physiology
Southern Illinois University
Carbondale, Illinois

Mark Jacyno, M.S.
Graduate Student
Department of Physiology
Southern Illinois University
Carbondale, Illinois

Joe Maran, LLB
Certified Civil Trial Attorney
Partner
Maran and Maran
Newark, New Jersey

Donald M. Miller, Ph.D.
Professor of Physiology
Department of Physiology
Southern Illinois University
Carbondale, Illinois

Claude A. Rakotoniaina, D.V.M.
Researcher
Department of Physiology
School of Medicine
Carbondale, Illinois

Donald R. Tindall, Ph.D.
Professor
Department of Botany
Southern Illinois University
Carbondale, Illinois

Charles W. Venable, Ph.D.
Research Associate
Department of Botany
Southern Illinois University
Carbondale, Illinois

TABLE OF CONTENTS

Chapter 1

THE RECOGNITION AND MANAGEMENT OF CIGUATERA FISH POISONING

Geoffrey M. Calvert

TABLE OF CONTENTS

I. SIGNS AND SYMPTOMS

A. SYMPTOMS

The onset of symptoms is highly variable, even among individuals consuming the same fish.[1] Symptoms usually begin 2 to 12 h after ingestion of fish contaminated with ciguatera toxin.[1,2] However, onset of symptoms as early as 30 min after ingestion[3] or as late as 48 h after ingestion have been reported.[4]

Symptoms primarily involve three organ systems: the gastrointestinal, cardiovascular, and neurologic systems.

The gastrointestinal symptoms are usually the first to appear[5,6] and usually resolve in 24 h.[1,2,5] These can consist of watery, nonbloody diarrhea, abdominal pain, nausea, and vomiting.[2,4,5]

The cardiovascular symptoms usually consist of bradycardia and hypotension.[1,7] However, a biphasic course consisting of initial bradycardia and hypotension, followed by tachycardia and hypertension, has been reported.[8] Nonspecific electrocardiographic changes can occur.[2,9] Although the cardiovascular symptoms usually resolve within 24 to 48 h,[2] they can persist for weeks.[3]

The neurologic symptoms consist of extremity and perioral dysesthesia, ataxia, pruritis, cranial nerve palsy, vertigo, tremor, dizziness, headache, superficial hyperesthesia, weakness, myalgias, arthralgias, temperature reversal, hyporeflexia, and dental pain.[1,2,5-7,10] Shock, seizures, coma, and respiratory depression have been reported rarely.[2,11,12] Some investigators report that patients found myalgia to be the most discomforting symptom.[6] Temperature reversal, a symptom in which warm objects feel cold and cold objects feel warm, is highly suggestive of ciguatera fish poisoning. This symptom has been observed in 23%[4] to 87.6%[2] of individuals with ciguatera fish poisoning. Although probably rare, temperature reversal can also be observed in individuals with chronic peripheral neuropathy.[13] The neurologic symptoms usually resolve in 3 to 4 weeks,[5] however, they can persist for months or years.[1,6]

Rarely, skin rashes have been reported by investigators.[1,6]

B. FREQUENCY OF SYMPTOMS

Table 1 presents the frequency of symptoms observed in three different surveys. Individuals most commonly complain of symptoms involving the gastrointestinal and neurologic systems.[1,2,4-6] Cardiovascular symptoms are less frequently observed.[2,4,11,14] The type and severity of symptoms vary widely among individuals, even among those eating from the same toxic fish.[1,2,4]

The proportion of individuals complaining of any specific symptom varies by geographic location (Table 1).[1,2,4] This may reflect the different criteria used to define a case by investigators in different geographic locations. Alternatively, these geographic differences may be due to regional variability in the types and concentrations of toxin in the fish.[5] The ciguatera toxin-producing dinoflagellate, *Gambierdiscus toxicus*, is known to produce at least two toxins: ciguatoxin and maitotoxin.[15] The two toxins have different modes of action (see Pathophysiology, Section II). The toxins may give rise to different symptoms due to this difference in the mode of action. The variability in the amount and type of toxins present in fish may also explain the variability in symptoms experienced by different individuals in the same geographic region.[5]

Gender also appears to affect the type of symptoms observed.[2] Compared to men, Bagnis et al.[2] found a significantly higher proportion of women with arthralgias and myalgias ($p < 0.01$). Compared to women, he found a significantly higher proportion of men with diarrhea and abdominal pain ($p < 0.01$). These investigators also found that, among those complaining of ciguatera fish poisoning, men accounted for 1.5 times more cases than women (men = 59.3%, women = 40.7%). However, other investigators found that gender did not affect the risk of developing ciguatera fish poisoning.[5,6]

TABLE 1
Frequency of Symptoms from Three Different Geographic Areas

Symptom	U. S. Virgin Islands[4] (%)	Queensland Australia[1] (%)	South Pacific Islands[2] (%)
	Gastrointestinal		
Diarrhea	81	64	71
Nausea	—	55	43
Vomiting	40	35	37
Abdominal pain	64	52	46
	Neurologic		
Perioral dysesthesia	38	66	89
Extremity dysesthesia	40	—	89
Temperature reversal	23	76	88
Pruritus	66	76	45
Headache	45	62	59
Myalgia or arthralgia	34	>79	>80

While some studies have found differences in the incidence rate among different ethnic groups,[2] other studies have not.[5,6] In addition, age does not appear to be a risk factor.[5,6]

C. SIGNS

Unless the patient is severely ill with shock, convulsions, coma, respiratory depression, or other extensive neurologic involvement, a physical exam is not contributory. There are no findings on a physical exam that are specific for ciguatera fish poisoning. In one survey, approximately 15% had systolic blood pressures less than 100, 13.6% had a heart rate less than 60 bpm, and 21% had neck stiffness.[2] Paresthesias are ill defined and follow no apparent dermatome distribution.[2,14]

1. Need for Better Assessment of the Frequency of Signs and Symptoms

In most studies, the methods used to define cases may have resulted in some inaccuracies in the determination of symptom frequency.[1,2,5] This is because case definitions for ciguatera fish poisoning are vague and are based on the presence of characteristic symptoms beginning after recent ingestion of a fish species known to be potentially ciguateric. A bias arises since the same symptoms used to identify the affected individuals will also be found to have a high frequency of occurrence. For instance, several surveys used the presence of gastrointestinal and neurologic symptoms to identify affected individuals and found a high frequency of occurrence of these same symptoms.[5,6]

To accurately define the frequency of symptoms and signs arising from ciguatera, confirmation of the presence of ciguatera toxins in fish consumed by individuals with symptoms suggestive of ciguatera fish poisoning is needed. Then, by documenting the symptoms of all who consumed the contaminated fish, the frequency of symptoms in both severely and mildly affected individuals can be determined.

The closest any study has come to using this method involved an outbreak investigation on St. Croix in 1981.[4] The outbreak of ciguatera fish poisoning was traced to two large fish catches delivered to the island on February 25 and March 5. Twenty kilograms of fish caught on March 5 were tested for the presence of ciguatera toxin using the mouse bioassay detection method.

Fifty-five percent of the sampled fish were found "to be toxic". It is not clear how representative the samples of fish tested were to the fish ingested by individuals who developed the illness. That is, it is not clear if the fish tested were the ones responsible for the illness. Although the testing demonstrated that a large proportion of fish caught on March 5 were toxic, the testing played no role in defining cases in the epidemiologic study. Cases were defined as having had a history of symptoms consistent with ciguatera fish poisoning that developed within 48 h of fish ingestion and persisted for at least 1 h. Initially, emergency room records from February 25 to March 20 were used to identify cases. In order to maximize case ascertainment, a visit was made to the home of each case detected from emergency room records, and all household members who had eaten a portion of the implicated fish were interviewed. The most surprising finding from the investigation was that 6% of the cases had neither gastrointestinal nor neurologic symptoms. They also found that 94% had some type of gastrointestinal symptom, 53% had both gastrointestinal and neurologic symptoms, 11% had only gastrointestinal symptoms, and none of the cases had only neurologic symptoms (Table 1).

Further study is needed to better assess the frequency of symptoms in ciguatera fish poisoning. Specifically, a study is needed that will confirm the presence of ciguatera toxins in the suspected fish consumed by every individual with symptoms suggestive of ciguatera fish poisoning.

II. PATHOPHYSIOLOGY

Little is known about the pathophysiology or the pathology of ciguatera fish poisoning in humans. There are no consistently abnormal laboratory tests. Edema of the Schwann cells in peripheral nerves has been reported.[16]

Ciguatoxin has been shown to increase sodium permeability in excitable membranes, causing depolarization.[17,18] Maitotoxin appears to have two actions: it stimulates cellular uptake of calcium by activating calcium channels[19] and inhibits the guinea-pig ileum response to histamine.[20]

There are few animal studies describing the pathologic effects of ciguatoxin and maitotoxin. In mice, intraperitoneal administration of ciguatoxin has lead to epithelial damage in both the small and large intestine.[21] After intraperitoneal administration of maitotoxin in mice and rats, histopathologic changes in the stomach, heart, and thymus were observed.[22]

III. DIAGNOSIS

The diagnosis of ciguatera fish poisoning is based on clinical findings. One should suspect the diagnosis if the patient complains of suggestive symptoms within minutes to hours after consuming a species of fish that has been known to harbor ciguatera toxin.

There are no confirmatory laboratory tests. Laboratory testing is only useful for ruling out other diagnoses and for assessing the need for supportive therapy.

Computerized tomogram (CT) of the brain, lumbar puncture with oligoclonal banding, nerve conduction velocity (NCV), and electromyogram were described as normal when obtained 7 d after the onset of illness in an individual who developed severe lower extremity ataxia and paresthesias after consuming a meal of grouper.[23] No other investigators have reported performing these tests.

Additional diagnostic evidence can be obtained by performing an assay to detect ciguatera toxins in the uneaten portions of the culpable fish. There are several different assays available for detecting ciguatera in fish. These include bioassays,[24] radioimmunoassays (RIA),[25] enzyme immunoassays (EIA),[26] and counterimmunoelectrophoresis techniques (CIEP).[27]

The enzyme immunoassay stick test, an adaptation of the enzyme immunoassay, is a rapid, simple, inexpensive, and sensitive assay.[28] A fish is assessed with six sticks. Each stick is 21 cm long and 3 mm wide. A stick is inserted into a fish five times, about 1 s per insertion. The stick is then immersed into a series of solutions, including purified sheep anti-ciguatoxin-human serum albumin. This process requires approximately 2 min. After waiting 10 min, the stick is read. If the stick turns moderately to intensely bluish-purple, the fish is considered to be contaminated with ciguatera toxin. The readings from the six sticks are averaged to arrive at a final determination on the toxicity of the fish. The color intensity can be read by either the unaided eye, an immunoassay reader, or a colorimeter. This test is not specific for ciguatera toxins, since it also reacts with similar polyether toxins, such as okadaic acid and brevetoxin.

The other assays for detecting the presence of ciguatera toxins have several disadvantages. The RIA is expensive, time consuming, and requires elaborate instrumentation.[25,26] The bioassay, in addition to being expensive and time consuming, requires the presence of high levels of toxin.[29] Additional testing of the CIEP is needed before conclusions can be made about its usefulness.

IV. DIFFERENTIAL DIAGNOSIS

Ciguatera fish poisoning needs to be distinguished from neurotoxic and paralytic shellfish poisoning, scromboid fish poisoning, type E botulism, eosinophilic meningitis, organophosphate pesticide poisoning, monosodium glutamate poisoning, bacterial food poisoning, and malingering.

Neurotoxic shellfish poisoning is caused by the ingestion of shellfish contaminated with toxins elaborated by *Ptychodiscus brevis*, a dinoflagellate responsible for producing red tides.[30,31] Although the toxins, called brevetoxins, are harmless to shellfish (clams and oysters), they are lethal to other fish.[30] Shellfish are not known to concentrate ciguatera toxins. Therefore, the two poisonings can be distinguished by determining the fish eaten. The symptoms begin within 3 h of eating toxic shellfish and can involve the gastrointestinal and neurologic systems. The gastrointestinal symptoms include nausea, vomiting, diarrhea, and abdominal pain. The neurologic symptoms include ataxia, temperature reversal, and paresthesias of the mouth, pharynx, trunk, and extremities. Symptoms resolve within days and no fatalities have been reported. Brevetoxin, like ciguatoxin, appears to act by increasing sodium permeability in excitable membranes.[32,33]

Paralytic shellfish poisoning is a more severe disease than neurotoxic shellfish poisoning.[30,31] It is caused by the ingestion of bivalve mollusks (mussels, clams, oysters, and scallops) contaminated with toxins produced by the *Protogonyaulax* species. Symptoms begin 30 min after ingestion and primarily involve the neurologic system. The gastrointestinal system is less commonly involved. Neurologic symptoms can include circumoral and extremity paresthesias, ataxis, paresis or paralysis, and respiratory depression. Gastrointestinal symptoms include nausea, vomiting, and diarrhea. Fatal cases are rare, usually occurring within 12 h after the onset of symptoms and commonly are due to respiratory failure. In most cases, symptoms resolve in 1 week. As with neurotoxic shellfish poisoning, this poisoning can be distinguished from ciguatera by determining the type of fish eaten.

Scromboid fish poisoning is caused by the ingestion of scromboid species (tuna, bonito, and mackerel) and selected other dark-meat fish (mahi mahi) that contain high levels of histamine.[31,34,35] When the fresh fish are not continuously refrigerated, bacteria may convert histidine, an amino acid found in fish muscle, to histamine. The symptoms are consistent with a histamine reaction: flushing, fever, headache, oral paresthesias (likened to a peppery taste), nausea, vomiting, abdominal pain, diarrhea, and occasionally urticaria and generalized pruritis. Symptoms begin within minutes to hours after eating the contaminated fish and resolve within hours. The disease can be effectively treated with antihistamines. Scromboid can be distinguished from ciguatera by its rapid onset and resolution, and by detecting high levels of histamine in unconsumed samples of the fish.

Type E botulism is associated almost exclusively with ingestion of inadequately cooked fish, fish products, or sea mammals.[36,37] The type E toxin is produced by *Clostridium botulinum* and acts by irreversibly binding to peripheral cholinergic synapses, thereby blocking acetylcholine release. Signs and symptoms include nausea, vomiting, weakness, dilated nonreactive pupils, hypotension, respiratory difficulty, and urinary retention. Symptoms begin about 2 h after toxic fish are ingested. Death can occur if the disease is not recognized early. Because the toxin is very heat labile, the illness can be prevented by cooking the fish at 60°C for several minutes. The disease can be distinguished from ciguatera by the presence of type E botulism toxin in the patient's serum and characteristic electromyographic findings in affected limbs. The ingestion of properly cooked fish rules out type E botulism.

Eosinophilic meningitis is a helminthic infection caused by *Angiostrongylus cantonensis*.[38,39] The infection is acquired by ingestion of raw mollusks (snails and slugs), fresh water shrimp, amphibious and aquatic crabs, and certain fish (skipjack tuna, yellow fin tuna, and bigeye scad). The incubation period is between 2 and 4 weeks. Signs and symptoms include frontal or bitemporal headache, neck stiffness, vomiting, and paresthesias. The disease usually resolves spontaneously and is rarely fatal. The paresthesias can persist for months. Although there are no diagnostic tests, this disease can be distinguished from ciguatera by its long incubation period and by the presence of peripheral and cerebrospinal fluid eosinophilia.

Some of the symptoms observed in organophosphate pesticide poisoning are similar to those observed in ciguatera.[40] These include nausea, vomiting, diarrhea, weakness, and in severe cases, bradycardia, hypotension, and respiratory depression. Organophosphate pesticides act by inhibiting the enzyme cholinesterase, resulting in the accumulation of acetylcholine at synaptic sites. This poisoning can be distinguished from ciguatera by obtaining a history of recent and significant exposure to organophosphate pesticides.

The symptoms of both monosodium glutamate poisoning[41] and bacterial food poisoning[42] can be similar to ciguatera. Distinguishing these poisonings from ciguatera requires a careful solicitation of recent food ingestion.

In areas where it is not endemic, awareness of ciguatera among physicians is probably low. In these areas, ciguatera may be misdiagnosed as malingering, depression, or neurosis. Therefore it is important to be aware of ciguatera fish poisoning so that when a patient presents with consistent symptoms, ciguatera can be distinguished from these psychiatric disorders.[1]

V. TREATMENT

Treatment generally involves supportive care and reassurance. No treatment has been shown to be an effective cure in randomized, double-blind, controlled clinical trials. Fortunately, in most cases the disease is mild and brief.

Because appropriate selection of supportive care is contingent on the severity of the intoxication, severity can be used to classify treatment into two broad categories. The first category involves the treatment of mild intoxication and chronic neurologic effects, and the second category involves the treatment of severe intoxication.

A. TREATMENT OF MILD CIGUATERA INTOXICATION AND CHRONIC NEUROLOGIC EFFECTS

Vomiting and diarrhea in the early stages should not be suppressed, since it may help rid the body of unabsorbed toxin. In the absence of these symptoms, emetics and cathartics should be administered.[1,14,43] Activated charcoal, 1 mg/kg in a 1:3 slurry with water, may also be useful in removing ciguatera toxin.[44] Acetomenophen has been recommended for relief of headache.[45] Indomethacin has been reported to relieve myalgias and arthralgias.[14,45] Antihistamines, such as diphenhydramine or cyproheptadine, have been reported to relieve pruritis.[10,14,45] Cool showers have also been recommended to relieve pruritus.[10,14,43]

Since ciguatoxin causes increased sodium permeability in excitable membranes, Gillespie et al.[1] have proposed that a drug that selectively blocks sodium channels may be an effective treatment. Local anesthetic agents may be useful since they selectively block sodium channels.[46] However, there are differences in the sodium-channel binding affinities of the various local anesthetics. The binding affinity depends on the position of the sodium-channel gates, that is, whether the activation and inactivation gates are open and conducting, or closed and not conducting.[1] The most effective anesthetic agent would be one that has selective affinity for sodium channels altered by ciguatoxin. However, before the most effective anesthetic agent can be selected, further study to better define the sodium channel alterations caused by local anesthetics and ciguatoxin is needed.

Tocainide is an orally administered lidocaine analog that acts by blocking sodium channels. It has been reported to provide long-lasting improvement of neurologic symptoms in three individuals with ciguatera fish poisoning.[47] It appears to be effective, even when first administered 4 years after the onset of symptoms. The investigators did not report the dose that was administered, but found that a 2-week trial was effective. It is possible that tocainide acts by selectively blocking sodium channels that have been altered by ciguatoxin. Because the investigators reported a case series and did not conduct a randomized, double-blind, controlled clinical trial, further study of tocainide is needed before routine use in the treatment of ciguatera fish poisoning can be recommended.

Amitriptyline acts as a membrane stabilizer by blocking sodium channels in excitable membranes.[48] Two reports demonstrated effective relief of neurologic symptoms with amitriptyline at a dose of 25 mg once to twice daily for 3 weeks.[49,50] In another report, amitriptyline relieved some neurologic symptoms, but not temperature reversal.[51] Further study of this agent is needed.

Maitotoxin, another toxin elaborated by *Gambierdiscus toxicus*, can act by stimulating cellular uptake of calcium. Calcium-channel blockers have been shown in guinea-pig ileum preparations to block the action of maitotoxin.[20] In the only report of its use in humans, investigators found that it relieved headache but had no effect on temperature reversal, myalgias, or pruritis.[51] Further study with this agent is warranted. In contrast, other investigators have advocated the use of 10% calcium gluconate infusions,[43,52] based on evidence that ciguatoxin competitively inhibits the membrane-polarizing action of calcium.[53] However, calcium gluconate has not yielded consistent success and cannot be routinely recommended.

Home remedies used in the South Pacific include the ingestion of the green fruits of some cultivated and wild plants that have emetic properties and eating *Duboisia myoporides*, an atropine-containing herb found in New Caledonia.[54]

Russell[7] found that administration of intravenous electrolytes, vitamin B complex, and calcium gluconate, combined with a high-protein diet and vitamin C supplementation, shortened the duration of disease. Gelb[10] documented one individual that reported improvement after ingestion of large doses of vitamins B complex, B_{12}, and C in conjunction with one B_{12} injection; however, he did not specify which symptoms improved. These therapeutic regimens cannot be recommended until their effectiveness has been demonstrated in randomized, double-blind controlled clinical trials.

Medications found to be ineffective in the treatment of ciguatera include corticosteroids,[7] pralidoxime,[5,7] neostigmine,[7] and chlorpromazine.[7]

B. TREATMENT OF SEVERE CIGUATERA INTOXICATION

One recent report of 24 patients with severe ciguatera fish poisoning found that mannitol reversed coma, severe diarrhea, hypotension, weakness, and other neurologic symptoms (i.e., mouth, facial, and extremity paresthesias and temperature reversal) within hours.[12] The mannitol (20%) was administered intravenously in a piggyback manner up to a maximum dose of 1 mg/kg. The report should be cautiously interpreted, since it was not a double-blind, randomized clinical trial. The authors speculate that the mechanism of action of mannitol is either through competitive inhibition at the cell membrane or inactivation of the ciguatera toxin. Mannitol is used to treat poisonings due to several other agents, including phenobarbital and salicylates, because it helps to promote their excretion.[55] Conceivably, mannitol may be acting by promoting ciguatera toxin excretion. Additional study of mannitol is needed before its routine use in severe ciguatera poisoning can be recommended.

Supportive therapy of severe ciguatera has successfully kept mortality to a minimum. Fluids and atropine are reported to be useful for controlling severe vomiting and diarrhea,[7] and for treating bradycardia and hypotension.[5,7,14] Phenytoin, phenobarbitol, or thiopental sodium, given intravenously, have been recommended for the treatment of convulsions.[56] Mechanical ventilation is required for severe respiratory depression.[31]

VI. PROGNOSIS

Although signs and symptoms usually resolve in days or weeks, neurologic symptoms can persist for months or years.[1,6]

Immunity is not conferred on those with previous exposure to ciguatera toxins.[3] In fact, sensitization to ciguatera toxin is known to occur. After an initial case of ciguatera, subsequent exposures are associated with a more rapid onset[1] and more severe illness.[2] Individuals suffering repeat episodes are more likely to experience paresthesias of the extremities and mouth, temperature reversal, diarrhea, asthenia, arthralgias, headache, and chills.[2] Individuals previously afflicted with ciguatera have been reported to have a recurrence of symptoms after ingestion of chicken, alcohol, and fish species not normally considered ciguateric.[1]

In the past, case fatality rates have been reported to be as high as 12%.[57] More recently mortality has been found to be rare,[1,5,6] with one report citing a case fatality rate of 0.1%.[2] No fatalities have been reported in the U.S.

VII. PREVENTION

The best way to prevent ciguatera fish poisoning is to avoid eating contaminated fish. However, it is difficult to identify contaminated fish because the toxins do not affect the odor, color, or taste of the fish. Tropical islanders have used several different tests to detect the presence of ciguatera toxin. These have included cooking the fish with a silver object to see if the silver becomes discolored, determining if the fish repels ants or flies, avoiding sliced fish that fails to reflect a rainbow when held up to the sun, rubbing one's gums with the liver to see if it produces tingling, or using a primitive bioassay that involves feeding portions of the fish to a cat or dog and watching for the onset of vomiting or other peculiar behavior.[8,54,58,59] Rubbing the gums and feeding the fish to a pet are probably the most reliable of these methods.[54]

There is no effective method for detoxifying fish. Because the toxins are heat, cold, and gastric-acid stable, no amount of preparation or storage will detoxify the fish. Islanders have been reported to soak the fish in water in an effort to leach toxin from the fish.[54] This may be useful for removing maitotoxin, a water-soluble toxin, but not ciguatoxin, a lipid-soluble toxin.

Avoidance is commonly used to prevent ciguatera. In some areas, large members of fish species commonly contaminated with ciguatoxins are not eaten.[1,54] In other areas, certain fish species are avoided all together. Miami, Florida has a city ordinance banning the sale of barracuda.[60] Avoidance of viscera in suspect fish, especially the liver, has also been recommended.[54,58] The viscera can contain up to 50 times more toxin per unit weight than the flesh.[61]

By avoiding fish in the diet, island populations are deprived of an important source of protein. Often, these economically disadvantaged areas are forced to rely on expensive, imported sources of protein or go without.[54] These problems could be solved if a simple and affordable method existed to distinguish contaminated from uncontaminated fish. However, at present an affordable test for detecting ciguatera toxins in fish does not exist. Even the enzyme immunoassay stick test[28] would be too expensive for a poor island economy, since its reagents cost approximately $5.00 per fish tested.

REFERENCES

1. **Gillespie, N. C., Lewis, R. J., Pearn, J. H., Bourke, A. T. C., Holmes, M. J., Bourke, J. B., and Shields, W. J.,** Ciguatera in Australia: occurrence, clinical features, pathophysiology and management., *Med. J. Aust.*, 145, 584, 1986.
2. **Bagnis, R. A., Kuberski, T., and Laugier, S.,** Clinical observations on 3,009 cases of ciguatera (fish poisoning) in the South Pacific, *Am. J. Trop. Med. Hyg.*, 28, 1067, 1979.
3. **Tatnall, F. M., Smith, H. G., Welsby, P. D., and Turnbull, P. C.,** Ciguatera poisoning, *Br. Med. J.*, 281, 948, 1980.
4. **Engleberg, N. C., Morris, J. G., Jr., Lewis, J. N., McMillan, J. P., Pollard, R. A., and Blake, P. A.,** Ciguatera fish poisoning: a major common-source outbreak in the U.S. Virgin Islands, *Ann. Intern. Med.*, 98, 336, 1983.
5. **Morris, J. G., Jr., Lewin, P., Hargrett, N. T., Smith, C. W., Blake, P. A., and Schneider, R.,** Clinical features of ciguatera fish poisoning: a study of the disease in the U.S. Virgin Islands, *Arch. Intern. Med.*, 142, 1090, 1982.
6. **Lawrence, D. N., Enriguez, M. B., Lumish, R. M., and Maceo, A.,** Ciguatera fish poisoning in Miami, *JAMA*, 244, 254, 1980.
7. **Russell, F. E.,** Ciguatera poisoning: a report of 35 cases, *Toxicon*, 13, 383, 1975.
8. **Withers, N. W.,** Ciguatera fish poisoning, *Ann. Rev. Med.*, 33, 97, 1982.
9. **Hanno, H. A.,** Ciguatera fish poisoning in the Virgin Islands (letter), *JAMA*, 245, 464, 1981.
10. **Gelb, A. M. and Mildran, D.,** Ciguatera fish poisoning, *N.Y. State Med. J.*, 79, 1080, 1979.
11. **Ho, A. M. H., Fraser, I. M., and Todd, E. C.,** Ciguatera poisoning: a report of three cases, *Ann. Emerg. Med.*, 15, 1225, 1986.
12. **Palafox, N. A., Jain, L. G., Pinano, A. Z., Gulick, T. M., Williams, R. K., and Schatz, I. J.,** Successful treatment of ciguatera fish poisoning with intravenous mannitol, *JAMA*, 259, 2740, 1988.
13. **Thomas, P. K.,** Clinical features and differential diagnosis, in *Peripheral Neuropathy*, Dyck, P. J., Thomas, P. K., Lambert, E. H., and Bunge, R., Eds., W. B. Saunders, Philadelphia, 1984, 1169.
14. **Pearce, R., Hines, C., Jr., Burns, T. W., and Clark, C. E.,** Ciguatera (fish poisoning), *South. Med. J.*, 76, 560, 1983.
15. **Yasumoto, T., Nakajima, I., Oshima, Y., and Bagnis, R. A.,** A new toxic dinoflagellate found in association with ciguatera, in *Toxic Dinoflagellate Blooms*, Taylor, D. L. and Seliger, H. H., Eds., Elsevier North-Holland, New York, 1979, 65.
16. **Allsop, J. L., Martin, L., Lebris, H., Pollard, J., Walsh, J., and Hodgkinson, S.,** Les manifestations neurologiques de la ciguatera, *Rev. Neurol.*, 142, 590, 1986.
17. **Bidard, J. N., Vijverberg, H. P. M., Frelin, C., Chungue, E., Legrand, A. M., Bagnis, R. A., and Lazdunski, M.,** Ciguatoxin is a novel type of sodium channel toxin, *J. Biol. Chem.*, 259, 8353, 1984.
18. **Capra, M. and Cameron, J.,** The effects of ciguatoxin on mammalian nerves, *Proc. Fifth Intl. Coral Reef Cong.*, 4, 457, 1985.
19. **Freedman, S. B., Miller, R. J., Miller, D. M., and Tindall, D. R.,** Interactions of maitotoxin with voltage-sensitive calcium channels in cultured neuronal cells, *Proc. Natl. Acad. Sci. USA*, 81, 4582, 1984.
20. **Miller, D. M. and Tindall, D. R.,** Physiological effects of HPLC-purified maitotoxin from a dinoflagellate, *Gambierdiscus toxicus*, in *Toxic Dinoflagellates*, Anderson, D., White, A. W., and Baden, D. G., Eds., Elsevier Science, New York, 1985, 375.
21. **Coombe, I. F., Capra, M. F., Flowers, A. E., and Cameron, J.,** Pathological changes in the mammalian gut following administration of ciguatoxin, in *Progress in Venom and Toxin Research*, Gopalakrishnakone, P. and Tan, C. K., Eds., First Asia-Pacific Congress on Animal, Plant and Microbial Toxins, Singapore, 1987, 19.
22. **Terao, K., Ito, E., Sakamaki, K., Igarashi, K., Yokoyama, A., and Yasumoto, T.,** Histopathological studies of experimental marine toxin poisoning. II. The acute effects of maitotoxin on the stomach, heart and lymphoid tissues in mice and rats, *Toxicon*, 26, 395, 1988.
23. **Jones, H. R., Jr.,** Acute ataxia associated with ciguatera-type (grouper) tropical fish poisoning, *Ann. Neurol.*, 7, 491, 1980.
24. **Banner, A. H., Sasaki, S., Helfrich, P., Alender, C. B., and Scheuer, P. J.,** Bioassay of ciguatera toxin, *Nature (London)*, 189, 229, 1961.

25. **Hokama, Y., Banner, A. H., and Boylan, D. B.,** A radioimmunoassay for the detection of ciguatoxin, *Toxicon*, 15, 317, 1977.
26. **Hokama, Y., Abad, M. A., and Kimura, L. H.,** A rapid enzyme immunoassay for the detection of ciguatoxin in contaminated fish tissues, *Toxicon*, 21, 817, 1983.
27. **Emerson, D. L., Galbraith, R. M., McMillan, J. P., and Higerd, T. B.,** Preliminary immunologic studies of ciguatera poisoning, *Arch. Intern. Med.*, 143, 1931, 1983.
28. **Hokama, Y.,** A rapid, simplified enzyme immunoassay stick test for the detection of ciguatoxin and related polyethers from fish tissues, *Toxicon*, 23, 939, 1985.
29. **Kimura, L. H., Hokama, Y., Abad, M. A., Oyama, M., and Miyahara, J. T.,** Comparison of three different assays for the assessment of ciguatoxin in fish tissues: radioimmunoassay, mouse bioassay and *in vitro* guinea pig atrium assay, *Toxicon*, 20, 907, 1982.
30. **Sakamoto, Y., Lockey, R. F., and Krzanowski, J. J.,** Shellfish and fish poisoning related to the toxic dinoflagellates, *South. Med. J.*, 80, 866, 1987.
31. **Hughes, J. M. and Merson, M. H.,** Fish and shellfish poisoning, *N. Engl. J. Med.*, 295, 1117, 1976.
32. **Asai, S., Krzanowski, J. J., Lockey, R. F., Anderson, W. H., Martin, D. F., Polson, J. B., Bukantz, S. C., and Szentivanyi, A.,** The site of action of *Ptychodiscus brevis* toxin within the parasympathetic axonal sodium channel h gate in airway smooth muscle, *J. Allergy Clin. Immunol.*, 73, 824, 1984.
33. **Sakamoto, Y., Krzanowski, J. J., Lockey, R., Martin, D. F., Duncan, R., Polson, J., and Szentivanyi, A.,** The mechanism of *Ptychodiscus brevis* toxin induced rat vas deferens contraction, *J. Allergy Clin. Immunol.*, 76 117, 1985.
34. **Reider, N. B., Goertz, N. I., Hall, J. D., Eidson, M., and Hull, H. F.,** Scromboid fish poisoning — New Mexico, 1987, *Morb. Mort. Weekly Rep.*, 37, 451, 1988.
35. **Taylor, S. L.,** Histamine food poisoning: toxicology and clinical aspects, *CRC Crit. Rev. Toxicol.*, 17, 91, 1986.
36. **Koenig, M. G., Spickard, A., Cardella, M. A., and Rogers, D. E.,** Clinical and laboratory observations on Type E botulism in man, *Medicine.*, 43, 517, 1964.
37. **Dolman, C. E.,** Type-E (fish-borne) botulism: a review, *Jpn. J. Med. Sci. Biol.*, 10, 383, 1957.
38. **Rosen, L., Loison, G., Laigret, J., and Wallace, G. D.,** Studies on eosinophilic meningitis. 3. Epidemiologic and clinical observations on Pacific Islands and the possible etiologic role of *Angiostrongylus cantonensis*, *Am. J. Epidemiol.*, 85, 17, 1967.
39. **Kuberski, T. and Wallace, G. D.,** Clinical manifestations of eosinophilic meningitis due to *Angiostrongylus cantonensis*, *Neurology*, 29, 1566, 1979.
40. **Morgan, D. P.,** Recognition and Management of Pesticide Poisoning, U.S. Environmental Protection Agency, Washington, D.C., 1989.
41. **Settipane, G. A.,** The restaurant syndromes, *N. Engl. Reg. Allergy Proc.*, 8, 39, 1987.
42. **Werner, S. B.,** Food Poisoning, in *Maxcy-Rosenau Public Health and Preventive Medicine, 12th Ed.*, Last, J. M., Ed., Appleton-Century-Crofts, Norwalk, CT, 1986, 311.
43. **Halstead, B. W.,** Fish poisonings — their pharmacology, diagnosis, and treatment, *Clin. Pharmacol. Therap.*, 5, 615, 1964.
44. **Goldfrank, L. R., Lewin, N. A., and Weisman, R. S.,** Fish, in *Goldfrank's Toxicologic Emergencies*, Goldfrank, L. R., Flomenbaum, A., Weisman, R. S., Howland, and Kulberg, A. G., Eds., Appleton-Century-Crofts, Norwalk, CT, 1986, 516.
45. **Sims, J. K.,** A theoretical discourse on the pharmacology of toxic marine ingestions, *Ann. Emerg. Med.*, 16, 1006, 1987.
46. **McNeal, E. T., Lewandowski, G. A., Daly, J. W., and Creveling, C. R.,** [^{3}H]Batrachotoxinin A 20 alpha-benzoate binding to voltage-sensitive sodium channels: a rapid and quantitative assay for local anesthetic activity in a variety of drugs, *J. Med. Chem.*, 28, 381, 1985.
47. **Lange, W. R., Kreider, S. D., Hattwick, M., and Hobbs, J.,** Potential benefit of tocainide in the treatment of ciguatera: report of three cases (letter), *Am. J. Med.*, 84, 1087, 1988.
48. **Henry, J. A. and Cassidy, S. L.,** Membrane stabilizing activity: a major cause of fatal poisoning, *Lancet*, 1, 1414, 1986.
49. **Bowman, P. B.,** Amitriptyline and ciguatera (letter), *Med. J. Aust.*, 140, 802, 1984.
50. **Davis, R. T. and Villar, L. A.,** Symptomatic improvement with amitriptyline in ciguatera fish poisoning (letter), *N. Engl. J. Med.*, 315, 65, 1986.
51. **Calvert, G. M., Hryhorczuk, D. O., and Leikin, J. B.,** Treatment of ciguatera fish poisoning with amitryptyline and nifedipine, *Clin. Toxicol.*, 25, 423, 1987.
52. **Dawson, J. M.,** Fish poisoning in American Samoa, *Hawaii Med. J.*, 36, 239, 1977.
53. **Rayner, M. D.,** Mode of action of ciguatoxin, *Fed. Proc.*, 31, 1139, 1972.
54. **Lewis, N. D.,** Disease and development: ciguatera fish poisoning, *Soc. Sci. Med.*, 23, 983, 1986.
55. **Winchester, J. F.,** Active methods for detoxification: oral sorbents, forced diuresis, hemoperfusion and hemodialysis, in *Clinical Management of Poisoning and Drug Overdose*, Haddad, C. M. and Winchester, J. F., Eds., W. B. Saunders, Philadelphia, 1983, 154.

56. **McLachlan, R. S.,** Ciguatera poisoning (letter), *J. Can. Med. Assoc.*, 121, 267, 1979.
57. **Halstead, B. W.,** *Poisonous and Venomous Marine Animals of the World,* U.S. Government Printing Office, Washington D.C., 1967.
58. **Lee, C.,** Fish poisoning with particular reference to ciguatera, *J. Trop. Med. Hyg.*, 83, 93, 1980.
59. **Heimbecker, R. O.,** Ciguatera poisoning — snowbirds beware (editorial), *Can. Med. Assoc. J.*, 120, 637, 1979.
60. **Vogt, R. L. and Liang, A. P.,** Ciguatera fish poisoning — Vermont, *JAMA*, 255, 2727, 1986.
61. **Helfrich, P., Piyakarnchana, T., and Miles, P. S.,** Ciguatera fish poisoning. I. The ecology of ciguateric reef fishes in the Line Islands, *Bernice P. Bishop Mus. Occas. Pap.*, 23, 305, 1968.

Chapter 2

LEGAL IMPLICATIONS OF CIGUATERA (A CASE HISTORY)

Joe Maran

TABLE OF CONTENTS

I. THE INJURY

On September 12, 1985 John O'Shea, age 56, arrived at The Hamilton Princess Hotel in Bermuda with his wife Virginia. They were there with a group of 80 to participate in a wholesale auto parts dealers convention. During the evening meal on September 13, 1985, John was served, along with every other member of the group, fillet of grouper fish. Some 5 or 6 h later 14 members of the group, including John, took ill, experiencing nausea, vomiting, dizziness, diarrhea, and cramps. Several of the group were seen by the hotel physician. In John's case, he became violently ill, with relentless vomiting throughout the night. Finally at 8:00 a.m. in the morning of September 14, 1985, the house physician recommended hospitalization. On the way to King Edward VII Memorial Hospital by ambulance, John suffered a cardiac episode, shock, and suffered significant interruption of blood and oxygen supply to his brain, with resultant hypoxic encephalopathy. Since the Bermuda Hospital did not have adequate facilities and equipment to care for John, he was flown to the Beth Israel Medical Center in Newark, New Jersey on September 18, 1985. After the patient stabilized, he was discharged on 10/21/85. John continued as an outpatient in physical therapy and was finally discharged on August 4, 1986. At present, John continues to suffer from slurred speech, memory loss, motor dysfunction, and a loss of intelligence measured by IQ tests to be 35 points.

II. INVESTIGATION

The author was retained as legal counsel on October 7, 1985. After some hasty intensive legal research, counsel reached out for Frank Verdiramo, a trusted, experienced investigator. In-depth briefings were held and Frank was persuaded to drop everything and travel to Bermuda. He arrived at The Hamilton Princess Hotel on October 12, 1985 and returned a week later.

Frank related all of his aborted attempts to interview employees, Board of Health Officers, town officials, hospital personnel, and the media. Bermuda, being dependent on tourism, had clammed up! Frank did bring back a one-page report signed by Dr. Cooke indicating a diagnosis of "some form of fish poisoning". Of course the hospital record did not contain any hint of fish poisoning and Dr. Cooke did not identify the fish poisoning as being ciguatera. However, this was the first big break in the case. The second jewel that Frank brought back was a copy of an article on ciguatera poisoning written by Professor Donald P. deSylva, Ph.D., a marine biologist out of the University of Miami, a potential expert witness.

III. HISTORY OF PERSONAL INJURY LAW

Now the research began in earnest. At common law, inherited from England by the founders of our country, everyone with the exception of government was responsible for their own negligence. The U.S. legal system of compensation for injury was based on fault. If someone was negligent and that negligence proximately caused an injury, then that person was liable to the injured party for compensation.

As the years went by legislation was passed that either added or subtracted from the common law. Most notable was the legislation that permitted suits against governmental entities. This was a departure from the common law, because at common law the King and subsequent governments were considered sovereign and could not be sued. However, negligence law and theory does not offer a person inflicted with ciguatera poisoning a remedy. Ciguatera cannot be detected in advance in any practical way. Therefore, there is no way to prove that the party selling or serving a reef fish was negligent in failing to discover the presence of ciguatera. Hence, if the hotel, restauranteur, or purveyor of fish is not negligent, they are not liable for serving fish contaminated with ciguatera. Since the liability of the seller of goods to the ultimate consumer on the basis of negligence is fraught with limitations, it was expected that some attempt would be made to carry his responsibility even further, and to find some ground of strict liability, which would make the seller, in effect, an insurer of the safety of the product. This was socially desirable, even though he had exercised all reasonable care and even where there was no privity of contract between the victim and the target defendant. Contract theories were tried out, but the ultimate consumer was rarely in contract with the manufacturer or seller of a product.

In the case history under discussion, the contract was between the Princess Hotel and the New Jersey Automotive Wholesalers Association, who booked the convention for its members. The first case, on the heels of a prolonged agitation over food and drink, which discarded the requirement of privity of contract was *Mazetti v. Armour* in 1913.[1] It was followed rapidly and then slowly, over almost half a century, by other courts, which found strict liability as to defective food and drink,[2] until by 1960 the majority of American courts had made it an established rule. The movement ran considerably ahead of any legal justification to support it. In 1960, less than three decades ago, a case was presented in New Jersey that is now regarded as the leading case in the country, *Henningsen v. Bloomfield Motors, Inc.*[3] It held both the manufacturer and distributor of an automobile liable for the ultimate injured party, without privity of contract on an implied warranty of safety carried over from the food cases.

What followed was the most rapid and altogether spectacular overturn of an established rule in the entire history of the law of torts (personal wrongs). A commission was established to clarify and modernize the law in these areas and to make uniform the law among the various jurisdictions, culminating in a proposed law entitled *Uniform Commercial Code*. The first state to adopt the Code was Massachusetts in 1958. New Jersey adopted it in 1963, and eventually every state in the union adopted the Uniform Commercial Code. The applicable provision relevant here reads as follows:[4]

12A:2-314. Implied Warranty: Merchantability; Usage of Trade.

1. Unless excluded or modified (12A:2-316), a warranty that the goods shall be merchantable is implied in a contract for their sale if the seller is a merchant with respect to goods of that kind. Under this section the serving for value of food or drink to be consumed either on the premises or elsewhere is a sale.
2. Goods to be merchantable must be at least such as (a) pass without objection in the trade under the contract description; (b) in the case of fungible goods, are of fair average quality within the description; (c) are fit for the ordinary purposes for which such goods are used; (d) run, within the variations permitted by the agreement, of even kind, quality and quantity which each unit and among all units involved; (e) are adequately contained, packaged, and labeled as the agreement may require; and (f) conform to the promises or affirmations of fact made on the container or label if any.
3. Unless excluded or modified other implied warranties may arise from course of dealing or usage of trade.[5]

The first state to apply a tort theory of strict liability, generally apart from the Uniform Commercial Code, was California.[6] That decision and the final acceptance of the proposal of the American Law Institute[7] in 1964 were immediately relied upon for the adoption of strict liability in tort throughout the country by way of judicial decision.

A. THREE ALTERNATIVE THEORIES

This now means that a claimant seeking damages against a merchant seller has three alternative theories available, all of which are often utilized in the same case. These are (1) negligence in tort; (2) strict liability for breach of warranty, express or implied; and (3) strict liability in tort.

IV. THE LITIGATION

Before a law suit could be filed there were two other issues to be addressed to wit: (1) a qualified expert who would be willing to testify; (2) venue and jurisdiction. Professor deSylva filled the bill and a commitment was obtained. As to venue, Bermuda was to be avoided because of Frank's investigation. New Jersey was the better venue if we could obtain jurisdiction. A defendant could always attack jurisdiction on constitutional grounds. The United States Supreme Court[8] has held that "due process" requires that a foreign corporation have certain minimum contacts with a jurisdiction to satisfy the traditional notions of fair play and substantial justice. A cursory check of state and telephone records indicated that the potential defendant, The Hamilton Princess Hotel, was not present within the states. Frank was dispatched to interview the president of New Jersey Automotive Wholesalers Association and to review their file to determine what contacts the defendant had with New Jersey, especially in the booking of the convention. It looked positive.

A complaint was filed in the Superior Court of New Jersey in the county where plaintiff resided on December 4, 1985.[9] Defendants filed an answer on February 12, 1986 of general denial and lack of jurisdiction. On May 8, 1986 defendants filed a motion to dismiss the complaint for lack of jurisdiction returnable June 6, 1986. Defendants maintained that Princess Hotels International did not own or operate The Hamilton Princess Hotel, but merely acted as an independent management consultant and that The Hamilton Princess was owned by a Bermuda corporation. Plaintiffs contended through affidavits of New Jersey Automotive Wholesalers Association personnel, copies of correspondence initiated by defendants, and advertising promotion in New Jersey that New Jersey had jurisdiction. Plaintiffs prevailed. Defendants next filed a motion on July 18, 1986 to add seven additional third-party defendants:

1. Quality Meat Packers of Toronto
2. Romanzini of France
3. Zwenenberg Company of Holland
4. Ilde de France Company
5. Bermuda Import and Export Company
6. Hamarus of New York
7. Tuner Fisheries of Boston
8. John Doe Companies

It was alleged that all the companies supplied contaminated food to defendants if, in fact, any food was contaminated.

Plaintiffs now had a dilemma: Should they file suit against all these additional defendants and become embroiled in a quagmire? Should they run the risk of limiting their cause of action against Princess only? After much discussion and analysis, it was decided. Focus on Princess only!

The dye was cast and the technical preliminaries were out of the way. Now the real work on the merits could begin. Extensive discovery of facts was important to both sides. Plaintiffs were seeking to develop facts that would support plaintiffs theories of liability and damages. The defense would seek to establish some basis to defend themselves. What would be their defense? We could only speculate at this point. Plaintiffs, of course, had the burden of proof to establish a *prima facie* case. Failure to do that results in a dismissal at the conclusion of plaintiffs case by the court, on the grounds that there is not enough evidence to submit the case to the jury. The most important issues to address were Was there ciguatera? Did the ciguatera cause a cardiac episode? Did the cardiac episode cause the shock and denial of oxygen and blood supply to the brain? Did these sets of facts cause brain damage and neurologic deficits? Legally the defense would argue that there was no proximate cause between the ciguatera and the resulting injuries.

In litigation there is a discovery period where both sides have a right to submit written questions called *interrogatories* to their adversary for answering. Additionally either party may take testimony under oath of other parties or witnesses. This takes place outside the courtroom before a court reporter informally in a private office in the presence of all the attorneys. The defense is entitled to medical examinations of the plaintiff by physicians of their choosing. All this occurs before trial. In present day litigation, each party is entitled to know in advance of the trial the positions of their adversaries, the identity of witnesses both lay and expert, and a synopsis of what they are going to testify to. There are very few surprises at trial, contrary to the television or film portrayals of trials.

Expert testimony was vital and legally required in this case.[4] A jury is never permitted to speculate as to cause and effect in medicine, science, or other areas of expertise. Therefore, even though the law imposes strict liability on the part of a seller or server of food for poisonous fish, proximate cause still has to be established between the ciguatera and the injury. This can only be done through the testimony of experts.

We had Dr. Cooke, who diagnosed some form of fish poisoning. Dr. deSylva opined that it was ciguatera, but he was not a physician. Counsel interviewed and retained plaintiff's treating physicians in the different specialities to piece the puzzle together. Dr. Michael Markowitz, a cardiologist who had also treated plaintiff prior to his ingesting the grouper, opined that plaintiff's cardiac arrest was brought on and caused by vomiting from the ciguatera. Of course Dr. Markowitz did, as he is legally entitled to, rely on the finding of Dr. deSylva, the marine biologist, as to the properties of ciguatera. Next Dr. Jeffrey Frankel, a neurologist, opined that the cardiac arrest caused plaintiff to go into shock, causing him to suffer an acute anoxic encephalopathy, resulting in brain damage.

It is also necessary for plaintiff to prove his damages. A. Wallace Deckel, Ph.D., a clinical neuropsychologist, measured John's neurologic cognitive deficits utilizing the Wechsler Adult intelligence test, Hooper Visual Organization test, Rey-Osterrith Complex figure test, auditory verbal learning test, Wechsler memory scale, Boston naming test, work fluency test, time perception test, various interlearned tests, and other miscellaneous tests. By comparing the results of these tests with preinjury intelligence tests, Dr. Deckel was able to opine that John lost 35 points of his intelligence quotient by reason of the ciguatera, relying on all the other expert findings. Dr. Harvey Goldberg, a physical medicine and rehabilitation physician, opined that John's neurologic impairments caused him to be permanently disabled, which was causally related to the ciguatera. Dr. Gary Clark, Director of the Brain Trauma Program of Kessler's Institute for Rehabilitation, supplied the technical expertise to fill in the gaps in the medical mechanics in explaining the chain of causation impacting on the brain.

How do you prove physical pain and mental suffering? How do you demonstrate these intangible hurts to a jury? Counsel retained Ernest Schuster, a video film specialist to create an "A Day in the Life of" film showing John's activities at Kessler's, his home, and his business. This may sound like Hollywood and gilding the lily, but it is of vital importance in demonstrating John's disabilities to the jury.

When it became apparent that the defense was going to take the position that, although the hotel menu indicated that grouper was being served, they ran out of grouper and actually served pollack, plaintiff countered by retaining a food scientist, Marvin Winston, President of Winston Laboratories. Pollack is not a reef fish and could not produce ciguatera. Mr. Winston analyzed the menu and opined that assuming pollack was served and ciguatera was not possible, then plaintiff suffered from a type of food poisoning contained in all the other food ingested by plaintiff. The defense's position on pollack being served was devastating to plaintiff's case and Winston Laboratories, not having any food to analyze, was skating on thin ice!

Finally, Paul Edmonds, C.P.A., provided his expertise to calculate *in futuro* the economic impact upon John in not being able to run his business.

Experts must submit their opinions in formal reports and must be ready to testify in court at trial, as reports are not admissible in evidence. They are only used to apprise all parties of their opinions before trial. Under case law, experts may express their opinions within the realm of reasonable medical probability or within the realm of reasonable scientific certainty.[10] They do not have to be 100% positive.[11] Opinions as to possibility are inadmissible.[12] Experts may rely on the opinions of other experts.[13] In this regard the law is merely recognizing that in all scientific inquiry it is common for one expert to premise an opinion on those of fellow technicians in related or cognate fields of science.[14] To safeguard the interests of justice to all parties, the trial court will permit vigorous and extensive cross-examination of expert witnesses to test the basis of their opinions. In fact, an expert's bare conclusions, unsupported by factual evidence, are inadmissible as a mere net opinion.[15] It therefore follows that the evidence, data, and the totality of the facts on the basis of which the expert arrived at his opinion must be made known to the court, so that it may evaluate the validity of the opinions and conclude what weight, if any, it should give to that opinion.[16]

In all, plaintiff's assembled a team of ten experts.[17] The defense, pursuant to court rules, elected to take the depositions of all plaintiff's experts, with the exception of the video expert and Dr. Cooke, who was out of the jurisdiction.

Finally, in the spring of 1987, all interrogatories had been answered on all sides and depositions had been completed. The case was ready for trial. But wait! The defense still had another thrust in their legal arsenal. They made a motion seeking to have the law of Bermuda, the place of occurrence, govern the case. Bermuda is under the dominion of the British Commonwealth and therefore, Bermuda applies English law. Only one case could be found under English law dealing with a hotel serving poisonous fish,[18] decided in 1938. In that case there was no finding of negligence and the court found for plaintiff on the sale theory at common law based on an implied warranty of fitness. The case made for interesting reading, being 50 years old, because the husband ordered for his wife and she became ill. The defense argued that there was no privity of contract between the wife and the hotel, because it was the husband's obligation to pay. The enlightened court held that it made no difference who did the ordering, but that since the wife consumed the fish she was obligated to pay for it and therefore there was privity and affirmed the award to the wife. However, it is important to note that English law was still concerned with privity of contract, which would complicate plaintiff's path through the legal maze. There was no English legislation that could be found abrogating privity. The New Jersey Court reserved decision pending a plenary hearing at trial set for September 8, 1987.

By this time all of the third-party defendants brought in by Princess had either been dismissed on summary judgment or Princess decided not to proceed against them. In either case it was felt that there was insufficient proof that any one of them supplied this particular fish that plaintiff actually ingested.

There were numerous settlement conferences held by the parties throughout the summer of 1987. After a full day of negotiations on September 3, 1987, the case was amicably settled. The terms included a cash payment of $900,000, plus $5000 per month, compounded at 3% annually, for the rest of John's life, which actuarially was expected to approximate 17 years, for a total payout of slightly over two million dollars. When last seen in May of 1988, John was in a good frame of mind, adjusting to his limitations, spending his time traveling with his wife Virginia.

V. CLOSING ARGUMENTS

Clearly no one would voluntarily trade an injury for money. Unfortunately we do not have the power to return a person to the state of health they once enjoyed. We can only compensate them monetarily. How has the Law of Torts impacted upon the problems of ciguatera? Pecuniary compensation is not in itself the ultimate object or a sufficient justification of legal liability. It is simply the instrument by which the law fulfills its purpose of penal coercion. The well-known Swedish Jurist Lundstedt pointed out that one requires a rare case of serious injury, but one forgets the infinitely greater number of cases where injury has not been done, owing to the fact that a social order, including the law of torts, is operative.

The prophylactic factor of preventing future harm has been quite important in the field of torts. The courts are concerned not only with the compensation of the victim, but with admonition of the wrongdoer. When the decisions of the courts become known, and the defendants realize that they may be held liable, there is a strong incentive to prevent the occurrence of the harm. Not infrequently one reason for imposing liability is the deliberate purpose of providing that incentive. A manufacturer or a server of food who is made liable to the consumer for defects in the product or contamination in the food will do what can be done to see that there are no such defects. This idea of prevention shades into that of punishment of the offender for what the offender has already done, since one admitted purpose of punishment itself is to prevent repetition of the offense. There are those who believe that punishment or retaliation is an important and proper aim of the law in assessing damages. To the extent that punitive damages are given, however, both prevention and retaliation become accepted objects of the administration of the law of torts. By way of analogy in the civil rights legislation, there is a provision for awarding treble damages if the defendants conduct is egregious. The legislative intent was surely to prevent one human being from violating the civil rights of another. Another example that is more on point is the Ralph Nader Institute. This organization is the consumer watchdog over the manufacturing industry. They investigate potential defects in products that render them unsafe and dangerous, and publish their findings. Ralph Nader was a tort lawyer who won a large class action award. From there he formed his organization to focus on preventing the distribution of defective products. After *Henningsen*,[3] which in 1960 held the manufacturer liable to the injured party for product defects without privity of contract, the automobile industry increased their efforts to put out a safer product. It was only after tort law imposed a duty on the manufacturer that we started to have safety features such as safety belts. Machine manufacturers, after a few adverse awards, started to put protective shields in front of danger points. All of the warning signs put on products to warn consumers of the potential dangers came into being because of the new tort law decisions.

A word should be said about motivation. Some pessimists might challenge the theory of tort law operating as a preventive force by citing that insurance companies actually pay the damage awards. Firstly, many manufacturers or hotel chains are self-insured. Secondly, if a company has too many claims, their premiums go up. Thirdly and most importantly, reputation is an extremely valuable asset. Most often there is a high correlation between reputation and profits.

Hopefully the fishing industry and the restaurant community will become aware of their liability for selling or serving reef fish contaminated with ciguatera, and they will unite for self-preservation and clean up their act. They can opt to not serve reef fish at all. They can also launch a campaign to raise money for ciguatera research, with a goal of either finding a cure for ciguatera in the fish or discovering an inexpensive practical method to detect ciguatera. Where there is a will (plus funding), there will be a way within the realm of reasonable scientific probability to detect ciguatera.

REFERENCES

1. *Mazetti v. Armour & Co.*, 135 P. 633 (1913).
2. Narrated in Regier, The Struggle for Federal Food and Drugs Legislation, 1933, I *Law & Con. Prob.* 3.
3. *Henningsen v. Bloomfield Motors,* 32 N.J. 358 (1960) the development is narrated in Prosser, *The Fall of the Citadel*, 1966, 50 Minn. L. Rev. 791.
4. N.J.S.A. 12A:1-314.
5. Louisiana is the only state that did not adopt this particular provision.

6. *Greenman v. Yuba Power Products, Inc.*, 377 p. 2d 897 (1962).
7. Section 402A, Restatement of Torts 2d.
8. *International Shoe Co. v. State of Washington,* 326 U.S. 310 (1945).
9. *O'Shea v. Princess Hotels International, Inc.*, et al. N.J. Superior Court; Law Division, Union County, Docket No. L-093613-85.
10. *Johnesee v. Stop & Shop Cos., Inc.,* 174 N.J. Super. 426 (App. Div. 1980).
11. *State v. Johnson,* 42 N.J. 146, 171 (1964).
12. *Schwartz v. Luancing,* 218 N.J. Super. 434 (Law Div. 1986).
13. Rule 56, Uniform Rules of Evidence.
14. Tyree, "The Opinion Rule", 10 Rutgers L. Rev. 601, 611 (1956).
15. *Buckelew v. Grossbard,* 87 N.J. 512, 524 (1981).
16. *Bowen v. Bowen,* 96 N.J. 36 50 (1984).
17. Gary S. Clark, M.D., Director, Brain Trauma Programs Kessler Institute for Rehabilitation, Inc., Saddle Brook, NJ; William R. Cooke, M.D., Woodbourne Hall 1 Gorham Road, Pembroke 5 32 Bermuda; A. Wallace Deckel, Ph.D., (Internal Medicine) 547 East Broad Street Westfield, NJ; Donald P. deSylva, Ph.D., Professor, Division of Biology and Living Resources University of Miami Rosenstiel School of Marine and Atmospheric Science Division of Biology and Living Resources 4600 Rickenbacker Causeway, Miami, FL; Paul Edmunds, C.P.A., 170 Kinnelon Road, Suite 23, Kinnelon, NJ; Jeffrey Frankel, M.D. (Psychiatrist), Essex Neurological Associates, P.A. 340 East Northfield Road, Livingston, NJ; Harvey Goldberg, M.D., Diplomate: American Board of Physical Medicine and Rehabilitation 522 Neptune Avenue, Suite 209, Brooklyn, NY; Michael D. Markowitz, M.D., F.C.C.P., P.A., 769 Northfield Avenue, West Orange, NJ; Ernie Schuster, President (Videos), VTH Associates Box 714, Millburn, NJ; and Marvin E. Winston, President, Winston Laboratories, Inc., 25 Mt. Vernon Street, Box 361, Ridgefield Park, NJ; sources of information.
18. *Lockett v. A.&M. Charles, Ltd.* 4 All. E.R. 170 (K.B. 1938).

Chapter 3

NEUROLOGICAL STUDIES ON THE EFFECTS OF CIGUATOXIN ON MAMMALIAN NERVE

John Cameron and Michael F. Capra

TABLE OF CONTENTS

I. CLINICAL REVIEW

Ciguatera is the most common form of fish food poisoning encountered in humans.[1,2] The clinical syndrome of ciguatera poisoning has been well described by many authors over the years.[3-8] A useful definition of ciguatera poisoning proposed by Lawrence et al.[4] requires that both gastrointestinal and paresthetic (dysesthetic) symptoms be experienced within 36 h after eating fish. In 129 cases studied by Lawrence et al.,[4] an incubation period ranging from 2 to 30 h, with a mean of 6 h, was found following ingestion of toxic fish flesh. The first symptoms to develop are usually gastrointestinal in nature, with intense watery diarrhea, nausea, vomiting, and abdominal pain being frequently described. These symptoms tend to settle within 12 to 24 h but are then followed by an acute neurologic disturbance, which can persist up to 2 to 3 weeks. The neurologic symptoms are quite intense and severe, usually manifesting as paresthesia and dysesthesia in the arms, legs, and perioral region; myalgia and cramps; weakness; arthralgia; and dental pain. A characteristic and perhaps pathognomic feature of ciguatera poisoning is the frequent occurrence of a paradoxical sensory disturbance in which the victims interpret cold as a tingling, burning, or "dry ice-like" sensation, and less commonly, hot objects as feeling cold.[3] Generalized motor incoordination, weakness, ataxia, diminished reflexes, and mildly impaired peripheral sensation are frequently found on examination.[9] The neurologic disturbance may persist for 1 to 2 weeks, but it is not uncommon for victims to experience ongoing, and at times recurring, symptoms for months and even years after the acute intoxication.[3,4,9,10]

The toxin also exerts an effect on the central nervous system, causing at times prominent headache, confusion, vertigo, visual and auditory hallucinations, memory disturbance, and infrequently convulsions and coma.

Cardiovascular anomalies have also been described, with prominent bradycardia, arrhythmias, and hypotension being frequently seen in the acute phase of the disturbance.[4,11]

Mortality associated with ciguatera poisoning is reported at less than 1% in the Pacific region[12] and is due to either respiratory paralysis[13] or severe dehydration, particularly in young children.[1] Diagnosis of ciguatera poisoning is made purely on a clinical assessment since, at present, there is no specific or reliable test for ciguatoxin detection, apart from bioassay of suspect fish.

Extraction techniques performed on toxic fish samples have revealed the presence of several closely related toxins, with the principal component causing the clinical disturbance being called *ciguatoxin*.[14-16] The action of these associated toxins probably explains the slight variations in the clinical manifestation of ciguatera poisoning observed at times in different localities and outbreaks. In particular, the poisoning associated with the parrotfish (*Scarus gibbus*) presents initially as a ciguatera-like disturbance, however, after 5 to 10 days a characteristic and prominent cerebellar disturbance associated with staggering gait, dysmetria, resting, and kinetic tremor develops and may persist for several weeks.[17] The cerebellar disturbance appears to be due to scaritoxin, a toxin that has similar properties to ciguatoxin and is found in close association with ciguatoxin in toxic parrotfish flesh.[17]

Despite the many reports detailing the clinical manifestation of ciguatera poisoning, very little has been documented as to the electrophysiologic disturbance that ciguatoxin causes in the peripheral nervous system in humans. Isolated case reports on small numbers of victims subjected to electric studies have revealed varying results, with little in the way of any consistant abnomality being demonstrated.

Over the last 5 years our research group has investigated the effect of ciguatoxin extract on the electric properties of the peripheral mammalian nervous system. This chapter summarizes some of the findings of this work performed over this period of time. It is necessary, however, to briefly review the neuropharmacology of ciguatoxin and the normal electrophysiologic events occurring in the peripheral mammalian nerve following the passage of an electric impulse, in order to interpret these experimental findings.

II. NEUROPHARMACOLOGY OF CIGUATOXIN

Ciguatoxin is believed to be the principal compound responsible for the symptomatology of ciguatera poisoning. Ciguatoxin is a heat-stable, lipid-soluble polycyclic ether compound with a molecular weight of 1111.7 Da. Murata et al.[57] have recently reported a proposed chemical structure for ciguatoxin extracted from moray eel (*G. javanicus*) with a molecular formula of $C_{60}H_{86}O_{19}$. Ciguatoxin occurs in minute quantities in toxic fish flesh (0.5 to 10.0 ppb) and can only be extracted through lengthy and expensive procedures.[19] Ciguatoxin is an extremely toxic substance causing death in mice at doses of 0.45 μg/kg.[18]

Initial studies performed on nerve-muscle preparations using crude extracts of ciguatoxin suggested that the toxin acted as an anticholinesterase agent.[20-23] Later studies, however, by Rayner et al.[24] and Ogura et al.[25] were unable to demonstrate any anticholinesterase-type activity after using a more purified toxin. It was concluded that the anticholinesterase activity demonstrated in the earlier studies was due to biologically active contaminants present in the crude toxin extract used. Rayner et al.[24] were first to demonstrate that ciguatoxin acted solely on excitable membranes. Boyarsky and Rayner[26] later reported that ciguatoxin produced depolarization in the pedal ganglion cells of *Aplysia*. Further studies by Setliff et al.,[27] Rayner and Kosaki,[28] and Rayner[29] have demonstrated an increased permeability of frog skin and muscle to Na^+ after exposure to ciguatoxin.

It is now generally agreed that ciguatoxin acts on all excitable cell membranes by opening voltage-dependent sodium channels.[29-33] This widespread effect accounts for the various sensory, motor, autonomic, and muscular disturbances observed in ciguatera poisoning.

Lombet et al.[58] have demonstrated that ciguatoxin competitively inhibits the binding of [H^3]-brevetoxin-3 to rat brain membranes with the affinity of ciguatoxin for the Na^+ channel being at least 20 to 50 times higher than that of brevetoxin. These results indicate that ciguatoxin and brevetoxins act at the same binding site (receptor site 5) on the sodium channel.

Perhaps the best insight into the action of ciguatoxin has been provided by Bidard et al.,[33] using cultured neuroblastoma cells. These studies have demonstrated that ciguatoxin creates a partial depolarization of the resting cell membrane potential, causing also spontaneous oscillations of membrane polarization and repeated action potential discharges. Ciguatoxin was also found to act synergistically with other sodium channel activators, such as veratridine, batrachotoxin, pyrethroid insecticides, and sea anemone and scorpion toxins, stimulating Na^+ isotope entry through voltage-dependent sodium channels. This influx was antagonized by tetrodotoxin and Ca^{2+}. This work also demonstrated that ciguatoxin had no action on slow Ca^{2+} channels. In the same group of experiments, ciguatoxin was found to form a stable but slowly reversible attachment to the Na^+ channel. This relatively stable attachment would account for the persistence of neurologic symptoms for up to 1 to 2 weeks after onset.

Further studies using voltage-clamp technique on frog myelinated nerve fibers have revealed that ciguatoxin opens voltage-dependent Na^+ channels at resting membrane potentials.[32]

Animal studies have demonstrated that ciguatoxin can produce death by blocking phrenic nerve conduction, resulting in respiratory failure. This was initially proposed to be a central effect of the toxin,[34] however, more recent work by Lewis[31] suggests the failure is due to a peripheral action of the toxin.

III. ELECTROPHYSIOLOGY OF MAMMALIAN NERVE

The membrane potential of large nerve fibers in the resting state is about −70 mV. This resting membrane potential is created by leakage of Na^+ and K^+ across the axonal membrane through potassium-sodium leak channels and also by the action of the Na^+-K^+ pump. The net effect is the accumulation of Na^+ on the outside of the nerve membrane and a buildup of K^+ on the inside of the membrane.[35]

Nerve signals are transported by action potentials, which are rapid changes in nerve membrane potential that pass along the nerve membrane. Following nerve fiber stimulation, the resting negative membrane potential is rapidly depolarized beyond 0 mV to approximately +20 to 30 mV. This rapid depolarization accounts for the rapid upstroke of the nerve action potential and is due to a sudden change in membrane permeability to Na^+ resulting in a large influx of Na^+ into the nerve fiber. This stage is followed by a period of repolarization, during which the nerve membrane suddenly becomes refractory to the passage of Na^+ and at which time there is a rapid diffusion of K^+ to the exterior to reestablish normal negative membrane polarity.[36] Associated with this is the propagation of the action potential along the nerve membrane.

Recent voltage clamp studies on isolated mammalian nerve by Horackova et al.,[37] Chungue et al.,[17] Brismar,[38] Chiu and Ritchie,[39] and Ritchie and Chiu[59] on rats and rabbits have demonstrated that a transient inward Na^+ current is responsible for the initial fast depolarization during the mammalian action potential. The outward current responsible for membrane repolarization is predominantly a voltage-insensitive passive leak of Na^+. The voltage-sensitive K^+ current is absent and therefore does not seem to play any role in the normal events during repolarization in the mammalian nerve. This observation is further supported by the virtual absence of potassium channels in the mammalian node region.[39]

This total dependence of the mammalian nerve on a normal Na^+ conductance probably accounts for the high susceptibility of the mammal to ciguatoxin. A sequence of events, namely, absolute refractory period (ARP), relative refractory period (RRP), supernormal period (SNP), and subnormal period has been observed in myelinated and unmyelinated nerve fiber in both the peripheral and central nervous systems in mammals, amphibians, and humans.[40-43]

After the passage of an impulse, an axon becomes totally inexcitable for a fraction of a millisecond to a further stimulus (test stimulus), and this period is referred to as the absolute refractory period. During this period the Na^+ channels are temporarily inactivated and no amount of stimulus will reactivate the channels to produce a further impulse.

This period is followed by the relative refractory period, during which there is a progressive return to normal Na^+ channel activation and normal membrane polarization.

A period of supernormality extends from the end of the RRP for approximately 15 ms. During this stage there is a slight shift of the membrane resting potential, due to transient Na^+ channel activation. This period is followed by one of subnormality, extending up to 100 ms, usually peaking around 60 ms. During this phase the membrane potential is slightly hyperpolarized.

This sequence of events is easily demonstrated in mammalian nerve *in vivo* and provides a convenient indirect method of assessment of Na^+ channel function.

IV. ELECTRIC STUDIES IN MAMMALS

A. RAT STUDIES

To investigate the electrophysiologic effects of ciguatoxin on the peripheral mammalian nervous system, we have conducted a series of studies *in vivo*, using the ventral coccygeal nerve in the rat tail as the experimental model. For these studies semipurified ciguatoxin was extracted from known toxic mackerel and barracuda fish samples and purified using a method similar to that reported by Nukina et al.[44] Crude extract was partially purified on silicic acid and alumina columns. Since biologically active but non-ciguatoxin-related substances may also be extracted in the purification method, a control extract for these experiments was also obtained using known nontoxic mackerel flesh.

The ciguatoxin extract from toxic fish produced hypersalivation, tachypnea, diarrhea, irritability, ataxia, and hind-leg weakness in rats following intraperitoneal injection. The LD_{50} was assessed at 52.2 mg/kg in mice. The nontoxic fish extract produced no clinical abnormalities. Mixed nerve velocity, absolute and relative refractory period studies, and supernormal

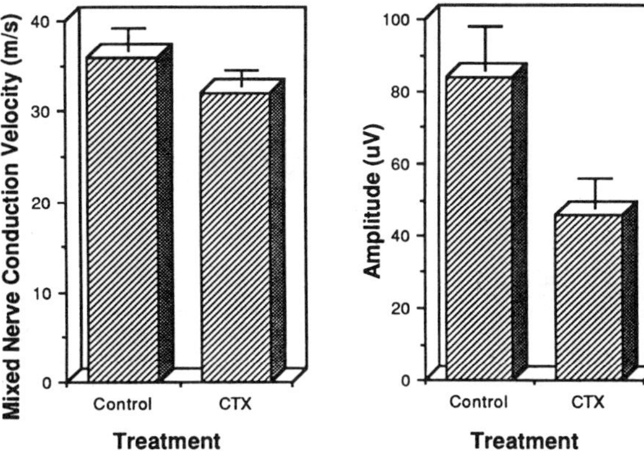

FIGURE 1. A comparison of the effect of ciguatoxin (CTX; 0.05 μl/g of 5×10^{-9} M) on the mixed nerve velocity and amplitude of the rat tail nerve (21 controls, 22 treated). Standard errors of the means are shown.

studies were performed in these experiments using the methodology documented by Capra and Cameron[10] and Parkin and LeQuesne.[45] For the absolute and refractory period studies, supermaximal conditioning and test stimuli were applied, whereas for the supernormal studies the test stimulus intensity was reduced to produce a mixed nerve action potential response that was one third of that obtained with supramaximal stimulation. Supernormality was determined as a percentage increase in the conditioned test response amplitude (CS) to that obtained from an unconditioned test stimulus (UCS). There was a particular interest in studying the action of ciguatoxin on peripheral nerve through ARP, RRP, and SNP studies since any Na^+ channel disturbance was more likely to be demonstrated through these techniques than with simple mixed-nerve conduction studies.

There was no significant difference between the refractory and supernormal periods assessed in the control animals and those animals subjected to intraperitoneal injection of the control nontoxic mackerel extract. One could conclude, therefore, that the extraction method was not inadvertently concentrating other biologically active neurotoxins with the potential to produce spurious results, a problem commonly encountered by earlier workers.

The ciguatoxin extract produced a significant slowing of mixed nerve conduction velocity and a significant reduction in the mixed nerve amplitude in the treated rats (Figure 1). The toxic extract also produced significant prolongation of the ARP (Figure 2), which in these experiments was defined as the interstimulus interval at which a nerve action response to the test stimulus was just perceptible. No significant prolongation, however, was demonstrated in the relative refractory studies (Figure 2). For the purpose of these experiments, the RRP was defined as the period of time following the end of the absolute refractory period to the time at which the latency of the test stimulus response equalled the latency of the conditioning stimulus response.

Perhaps the most significant finding to emerge from these particular studies was the exaggerated and prolonged response of the SNP in the treated rats. Both the magnitude and duration of this response were increased significantly over the interstimulus intervals recorded (Figure 3).

B. HUMAN STUDIES

In 1987 two outbreaks of ciguatera poisoning occurred on the east coast of Australia. The first outbreak occurred in Sydney and was traced to Spanish mackerel caught in Hervey Bay, a known endemic region off the coast of southern Queensland. A further outbreak of ciguatera poisoning

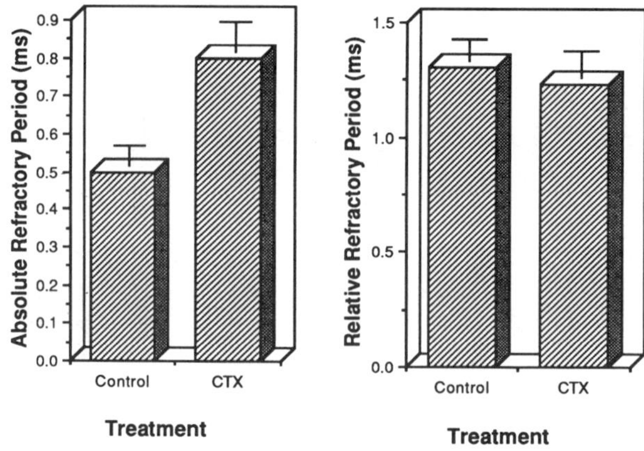

FIGURE 2. A comparison of the effect of ciguatoxin (CTX; 0.05 μl/g of 5×10^{-9} M) on the absolute and relative refractory periods of the rat tail nerve (21 controls, 22 treated). Standard errors of the means are shown.

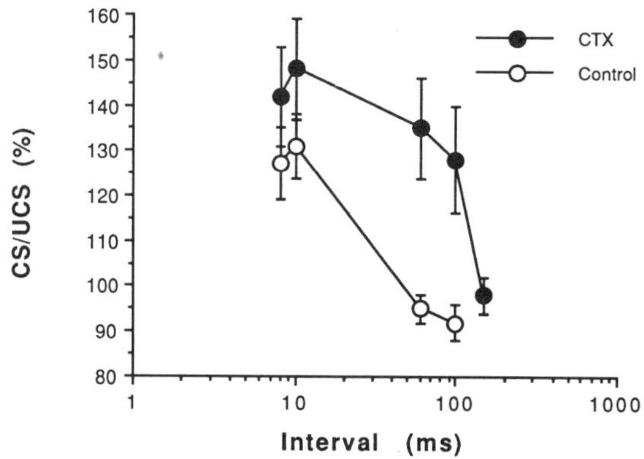

FIGURE 3. A comparison of the effect of ciguatoxin (CTX; 0.05 μl/g of 5×10^{-9} M) on the supernormal period of the rat tail nerve (21 controls, 22 treated). Standard errors of the means are shown.

occurred in Maryborough, a large provincial town servicing the Hervey Bay area. The fish responsible for this outbreak was never identified, but it was thought to have come from the Hervey Bay region.

Electric studies were performed on seven victims from the Sydney outbreak and eight victims from the Maryborough outbreak. These cases represented the more severely affected of those interviewed.

Sensory conduction velocity, absolute and relative refractory, and supernormal studies were performed on the sural nerve. Significant slowing of sensory conduction velocity was demonstrated, however, the sensory potential amplitude was not significantly affected (Figure 4). Both ARP and RRP, however, were quite significantly prolonged compared to the control values (Figure 5).

Perhaps the most significant finding, again, was the increased amplitude and duration of the SNP in these victims (Figure 6). The human findings were virtually identical to those demonstrated in the rat studies, except the RRP was not significantly prolonged in the rat, and the sural amplitude was not significantly affected in the human study.

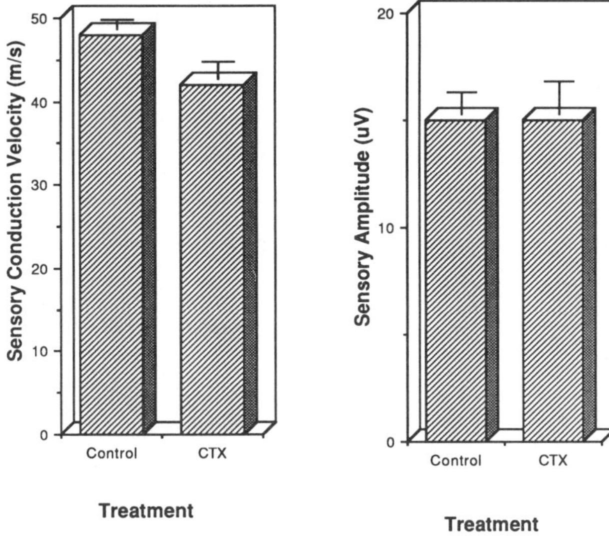

FIGURE 4. A comparison of sural nerve conduction velocity and amplitude between a group of 15 ciguatera victims (CTX) and 15 control patients. Standard errors of the means are shown.

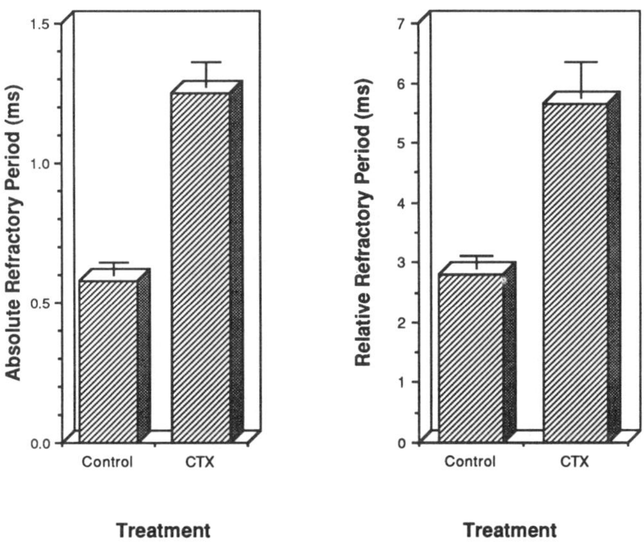

FIGURE 5. A comparison of the sural nerve absolute and relative refractory periods of 15 victims of ciguatera poisoning (CTX) and 15 control patients. Standard errors of the means are shown.

The electrophysiologic changes demonstrated in both the human and rat studies are suggestive of a disturbance causing prolonged sodium channel activation.[45]

Only isolated reports documenting electrophysiologic studies on cases of ciguatera poisoning have been described. The numbers of victims studied in these reports have been quite small and the results are generally conflicting. Ayyar[46] reported nine cases of ciguatera poisoning due to a large barracuda, and demonstrated only distal slowing in motor and sensory conduction studies, which he attributed to demyelination in the peripheral nerve. Nakano,[47] however, found

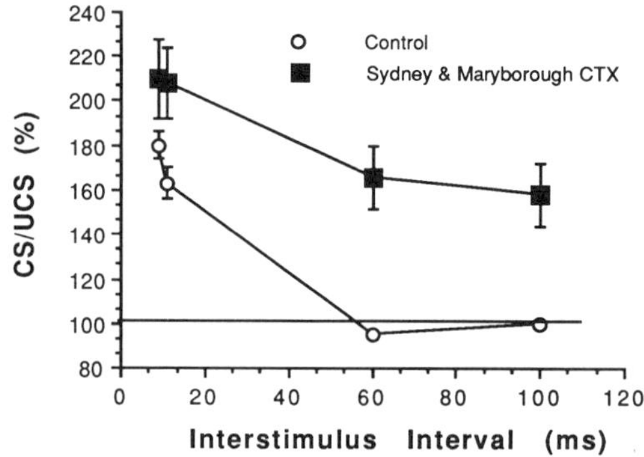

FIGURE 6. A comparison of the sural nerve supernormal period in 15 victims of ciguatera poisoning (CTX) and 15 control patients. Standard errors of the means are shown.

normal motor and sensory conduction in seven cases studied, although some neuromuscular fatigue was demonstrated in two cases. EMG studies revealed a myopathic disturbance, and muscle biopsies taken from three of these cases suggested some changes attributed to a toxic myopathy. Jones[48] reported normal nerve conduction studies on one case studied 7 d from the onset of symptoms.

Allsop et al.[49] described three cases of fish poisoning referred to as ciguatera poisoning. Significant slowing of motor conduction velocity was found in all three cases, while significant slowing of sensory conduction velocity, distal latencies, sensory amplitudes, and F-wave latencies were found in one case studied in detail over the course of the illness. Brain-stem auditory-evoked studies and somatosensory studies remained within normal limits, suggesting that no significant central electric disturbance was present. These electric abnormalities gradually resolved with recovery in this one patient. Sural nerve biopsy performed on this particular case demonstrated edema in the adaxonal layer of the Schwann cell cytoplasm, with axonal compression and vesicular degeneration of the myelin. Ataxia was a prominent feature that developed during the course of the illness in these three cases. Ataxia presenting at this particular stage of fish poisoning would suggest that these clinical and electric findings described were more likely due to scaritoxin than typical ciguatoxin poisoning.

As yet there is no specific treatment for the neurologic disturbance associated with ciguatera poisoning. Treatment is directed to symptomatic and supportive management.[50,51]

Ciguatoxin is a known Na^+ channel toxin that opens voltage-dependent channels, causing an increased permeability of the nerve membrane to Na^+. Local anesthetic agents are known to impair the flow of Na^+ into nerve fibers by binding to the inner aspect of the Na^+ channel when in the activated state.[52] Some preliminary studies by Lewis[31] on guinea-pig atria demonstrated that lidocaine, and to a lesser extent procaine, modified the effect of ciguatoxin. A further study by Legrand et al.[53] using anaesthetized cats to monitor respiratory and cardiovascular effects of ciguatoxin found that lidocaine appeared highly effective in counteracting the effects of ciguatoxin. In a recent report[54] tocainide, an orally effective lidocaine, appeared to control the acute and chronic neurologic symptoms of ciguatera poisoning in three cases.

The effect of lidocaine was studied in a series of experiments performed in our unit using the rat model. Intraperitoneal lidocaine (70 mg/kg) was found to significantly reduce the amplitude and duration of the supernormal period in treated rats towards the control values (Figure 7). Further studies are necessary, particularly controlled clinical trials, to ascertain whether intravenous perfusion of xylocaine or oral anaesthetic agents such as tocainide are useful in the relief of the neurologic manifestations of the disturbance.

An interesting aspect of ciguatera poisoning is the well-documented exacerbation or re-

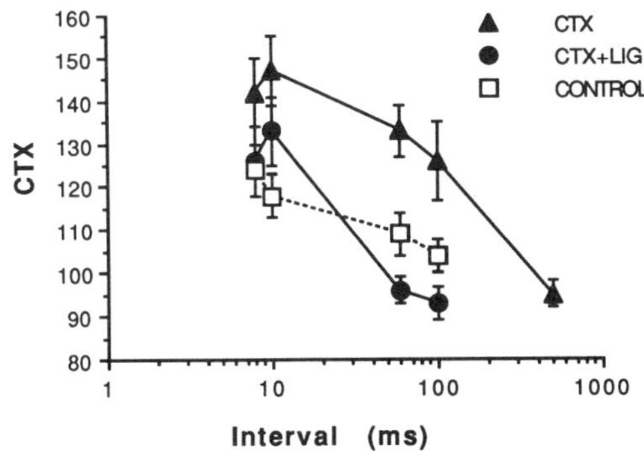

FIGURE 7. A comparison of the effects of ciguatoxin (CTX; 0.05 μl/g of 5×10^{-9}M) in the presence of lidocaine (CTX + LIG; 1 mg/kg) on the rat tail nerve. Each point represents data derived from ten animals. Standard errors of the means are shown.

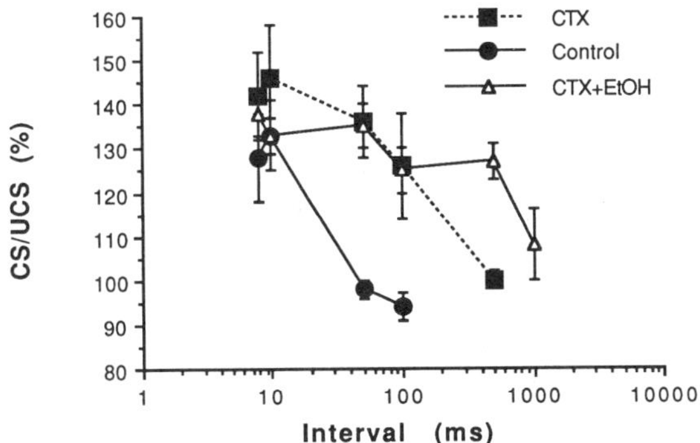

FIGURE 8. A comparison of the effect of alcohol (EtOH; blood concentration 0.05%) in the presence of ciguatoxin (CTX; 0.05 μl/g of 5×10^{-9}M) on the rat tail nerve. Each point represents data derived from ten animals. Standard errors of the means are shown.

emergence of neurologic symptoms following the ingestion of ethyl alcohol. This aspect was also studied in rats poisoned with ciguatoxin. Intraperitoneal ethyl alcohol (blood level 0.05%) was found to significantly prolong the abnormal supernormal response observed in ciguatoxin-treated rats (Figure 8). These findings support the clinical impression that alcohol may potentiate the neurologic disturbance in ciguatera poisoning. The basis of this action is still undefined, however, several mechanisms can be proposed. One possibility is that alcohol leaches toxin deposited in the body lipid stores, thereby increasing the availability of toxin to react with Na^+ channels. Ethanol has also been demonstrated to alter Na^+ conductance in excitable tissue and, in particular, to cause a depolarizing effect in mammalian nerve.[55,56] A synergistic effect between alcohol and ciguatoxin at the receptor site is therefore the more likely explanation for the exacerbation of the sensory symptoms.

V. SUMMARY

Ciguatoxin is a powerful neurotoxin that acts by opening voltage-dependent channels on excitable membranes. This effect can be indirectly studied, *in vivo*, using basic neurophysiologic techniques to assess refractory and supernormal periods following nerve excitation.

These studies in rats and humans have demonstrated an almost identical slowing of mixed nerve conduction velocity and prolongation of the ARP and SNP. These effects were antagonized by lidocaine and exacerbated by alcohol.

The rat model, therefore, provides a very useful *in vivo* model with which to study the neurologic action of ciguatoxin and antagonistic agents.

REFERENCES

1. **Withers, N. W.,** Ciguatera fish poisoning., in *Annual Reviews of Medicine*, Creger, Coggins, and Hancock, Eds., Annual Review, Palo Alto, CA, 1982, 97.
2. **Ragelis, E. P.,** Ciguatera seafood poisoning. Overview, in *Seafood Toxins*, Ragelis, E. Ed., American Chemical Society Symposium Series 262, Washington, D.C., 1984, 25.
3. **Bagnis, R. A., Kuberski, T., and Laugier, S.,** Clinical observations on 3,009 cases of ciguatera (fish poisoning) in the South Pacific, *Am. J. Trop. Med. Hyg.*, 28, 1067, 1979.
4. **Lawrence, D. N., Enriguez, M. B., Lumish, R. M., and Maceo, A.,** Ciguatera fish poisoning in Miami, *JAMA*, 244, 254, 1980.
5. **Morris, J. G., Jr., Lewin, P., Smith, C. W., Blake, P. A., and Schneider, R.,** Ciguatera fish poisoning epidemiology of the disease on St. Thomas, U.S. Virgin Islands, *Am. J. Trop. Med. Hyg.*, 31, 574, 1982.
6. **Capra, M. and Cameron, J.,** Epidemiological and social surveys on the incidence of and the attitudes towards ciguatera poisoning in two Australian communities, *Proc. Fifth Intl. Coral Reef Cong.*, 4, 489, 1985.
7. **Gillespie, N. C., Lewis, R. J., Pearn, J. H., Bourke, A. T. C., Holmes, M. J., Bourke, J. B., and Shields, W. J.,** Ciguatera in Australia: occurrence, clinical features, pathophysiology and management, *Med. J. Aust.*, 145, 584, 1986.
8. **Russell, F. E.,** Ciguatera poisoning: a report of 35 cases, *Toxicon*, 13, 383, 1975.
9. **Halstead, B. W.,** *Poisonous and Venomous Marine Animals of the World*, Darwin Press, Princeton, NJ, 1978.
10. **Capra, M. and Cameron, J.,** The effects of ciguatoxin on mammalian nerves, *Proc. Fifth Intl. Coral Reef Cong.*, 4, 457, 1985.
11. **Bagnis, R. A.,** La ciguatera aux iles Marquises: aspects cliniques et epidemiologiques, *Bull. World Health Org.*, 49, 67, 1973.
12. **Lewis, N. D.,** Ciguatera, Health and Human Adaptation in the Island Pacific, Doctoral Dissertation, Univ. California, Berkeley, 1981.
13. **Dawson, J. M.,** Fish poisoning in American Samoa, *Hawaii Med. J.*, 36, 239, 1977.
14. **Scheuer, P. J., Takahashi, W., Tsutsumi, J., and Yoshida, T.,** Ciguatoxin: isolation and chemical nature, *Science N.Y.*, 155, 1267, 1967.
15. **Miller, D. M.,** *Dinoflagellates Responsible for Ciguatera Food Poisoning*, Annual Summary Report to U.S. Army Medical Command, 1988.
16. **Yasumoto, T., Bagnis, R. A., and Vernoux, J. P.,** Toxicity of the surgeon fishes-II. Properties of the principal water-soluble toxin, *Bull. Jpn. Soc. Sci. Fish.*, 42, 359, 1976.
17. **Chungue, E., Bagnis, R. A., Fusetani, N., and Hashimoto, Y.,** Isolation of the two toxins from a parrotfish, *Scarus gibbus*, *Toxicon*, 15, 89, 1977.
18. **Tachibana, K.,** Structural Studies on Marine Toxins, Doctoral Dissertation, Univ. of Hawaii, 1980.
19. **Yasumoto, T., Raj, U., and Bagnis, R.,** Seafood poisoning in tropical regions, in *Symposium on Seafood Toxins in Tropical Regions*, Laboratory of Food Hygiene, Faculty of Agriculture, Tohoku University, Kagoshima, Japan, 1984, 1.
20. **Li, K.,** Ciguatera fish poison: a potent cholinesterase inhibitor, *Science*, 147, 1580, 1965.
21. **Banner, A. H.,** Marine toxins from the Pacific, I-Advances in the investigation of fish toxins, in *Animal Toxins*, Russell, F. E. and Saunders, P. R., Eds., Pergammon Press, Oxford, 1967, 157.
22. **Kosaki, T. I. and Anderson, H. H.,** Marine toxins from the Pacific, III comparative bioassay of ciguatoxin(s) in the mouse and chicken, *Proc. West. Pharmacol. Soc.*, 11, 126, 1968.
23. **Kosaki, T. I. and Stephens, J.,** Pupillary miosis to ciguatoxin(s) (from *Gymnothorax javanicus*), *Fed. Proc.*, 26, 322, 1967.
24. **Rayner, M. D., Kosaki, T. I., and Fellmeth, E. L.,** Ciguatoxin: more than an acetylcholinesterase, *Science*, 160, 70, 1968.
25. **Ogura, Y., Nara, J., and Yoshida, T.,** Comparative pharmacological actions of ciguatoxin and tetrodotoxin, a preliminary account, *Toxicon*, 6, 131, 1968.

26. **Boyarsky, L. L. and Rayner, M. D.,** The effect of ciguatera toxin on *Aplysia* neurons, *Proc. Soc. Exp. Biol. Med.*, 134, 332, 1970.
27. **Setliff, J. A., Rayner, M. D., and Hong, S. K.,** Effect of ciguatoxin on sodium transport across the frog skin, *Toxicol. Appl. Pharmacol.*, 18, 676, 1971.
28. **Rayner, M. D. and Kosaki, T. I.,** Ciguatoxin: effects on Na^+ fluxes in frog muscle, *Fed. Proc.*, 29, 548, 1970.
29. **Rayner, M. D.,** Mode of action of ciguatoxin, *Fed. Proc.*, 31, 1139, 1972.
30. **Ohizumi, Y., Shibata, S., and Tachibana, K.,** Mode of the excitatory and inhibitory actions of ciguatoxin in the guinea pig vas deferens, *J. Pharmacol. Exp. Therap.*, 217, 475, 1981.
31. **Lewis, R. J.,** Ciguatera and Ciguatera-Like Substances in Fishes, Especially *Scomberomorus commersoni* from Southern Queensland, Doctoral Dissertation, Univ. Queensland, Australia, 1985.
32. **Benoit, E., Legrand, M., and Dubois, J. M.,** Effects of ciguatoxin on current and voltage clamped frog myelinated nerve fibre, *Toxicon*, 24, 357, 1986.
33. **Bidard, J. N., Hank, P. M., Vijverberg, C., Chungue, E., Legrand, A. M., Bagnis, R. A., and Lazdunski, M.,** Ciguatoxin is a novel type of sodium channel toxin, *J. Biol. Chem.*, 259, 8353, 1984.
34. **Cheng, K. K., Li, K. M., and Quinctillis, Y. H. M.,** The mechanism of respiratory failure in ciguatera poisoning, *J. Pathol.*, 97, 89, 1969.
35. **Guyton, A. C.,** *Textbook of Medical Physiology*, W. B. Saunders, Philadelphia, 1986.
36. **Hodgkin, A. L. and Huxley, A. F.,** A quantitative description of membrane current and its application to conduction and excitation in nerve, *J. Physiol.*, 117, 500, 1952.
37. **Horackova, M., Nonner, W., and Stampfli, R.,** Action potentials and voltage-clamp currents of single rat Ranvier nodes, *Proc. Intl. Union Physiol.*, 7, 198, 1968.
38. **Brismar, T.,** Potential clamp analysis of membrane currents in rat myelinated nerve fibres, *J. Physiol.*, 298, 171, 1980.
39. **Chiu, S. Y. and Ritchie, J. M.,** Ionic and gating currents in mammalian myelinated nerve, in *Demyelinating Disease: Basic and Clinical Electrophysiology*, Waxman, S. G. and Ritchie, J. M., Eds., Raven Press, New York, 1981, 313.
40. **Gilliat, R. W. and Willison, R. G.,** The refractory and supernormal periods of the human median nerve, *J. Neurol. Neurosurg. Psychiat.*, 26, 136, 1963.
41. **Tackmann, W. and Lehmann, H. J.,** Refractory period in human sensory nerve fibres, *Eur. Neurol.*, 12, 277, 1974.
42. **Hopf, H. C., Lowitzsch, K., and Galland, J.,** Conduction velocity during the supernormal and late subnormal periods in human nerve fibres, *J. Neurol.*, 211, 293, 1976.
43. **Stohr, M.,** Activity-dependent variations in threshold and conduction velocity of human sensory fibres, *J. Neurol. Sci.*, 49, 47, 1981.
44. **Nukina, M., Koyanagi, L. M., and Scheuer, P. J.,** Two interchangeable forms of ciguatoxin, *Toxicon*, 22, 169, 1984.
45. **Parkin, P. J. and LeQuesne, P. M.,** Effect of a synthetic pyrethoid deltamethrin on excitability changes following a nerve impulse, *J. Neurol. Neurosurg. Psychiat.*, 45, 337, 1982.
46. **Ayyar, D. R. and Mullaly, W. J.,** Ciguatera: clinical and electrophysiologic observations, *Neurology*, 28, 345, 1978.
47. **Nakano, K. K.,** Ciguatera poisoning: an outbreak on Midway Island. Clinical, electrophysiological and muscle biopsy findings, *J. Neurol. Orthop. Surg.*, 4, 11, 1983.
48. **Jones, H. R., Jr.,** Acute ataxia associated with ciguatera-type (grouper) tropical fish poisoning, *Ann. Neurol.*, 7, 491, 1978.
49. **Allsop, J. L., Martin, L., Lebris, H., Pollard, J., Walsh, J., and Hodgkinson, S.,** Les manifestations neurologiques de la ciguatera, *Rev. Neurol. (Paris)*, 142, 590, 1986.
50. **Bagnis, R. A.,** Clinical aspects of ciguatera (fish poisoning) in French Polynesia, *Hawaii Med. J.*, 28, 25, 1968.
51. **Sorokin, M.,** Ciguatera poisoning in north-west Viti Levu, Fiji Islands, *Hawaii Med.*, 34, 207, 1975.
52. **Ritchie, J. M. and Greene, N. M.,** Local anaesthetics, in *Goodman and Gilman's. The Pharmacological Basis of Therapeutics.*, Gilman, A. G., Goodman, L. S., and Gilman, A., Eds., Macmillan, New York, 1980, 301.
53. **Legrand, A. M., Lotte, C., and Bagnis, R.,** Respiratory and cardiovascular effects of ciguatoxin in cats: antagonistic action of hexamethonium, atropine, propranolol, phentolamine, yohimbine, prazosin, verapamil, calcium and lidocaine, *Proc. Fifth Intl. Coral Reef Cong.*, Antenne Museum-EPHE, Moorea, French Polynesia, Tahiti, 1985, 463.
54. **Lange, R. W., Kreider, S. D., Hattwick, M., and Hobbs, J.,** Potential benefit of tocainide in the treatment of ciguatera: report of three cases, *Am. J. Med.*, 84, 1087, 1988.
55. **Wright, E. B.,** The effects of asphyxiation and narcosis on peripheral nerve polarisation and conduction, *Am. J. Physiol.*, 148, 174, 1947.
56. **Moore, J. W., Ulbright, W. and Takata, M.,** Effect of ethanol on the sodium and potassium conductances of the squid axon membrane, *J. Gen. Physiol.*, 48, 279, 1954.

57. **Murata, M., Legrand, A. M., Ishibashi, Y., and Yasumoto, T.,** Structures of ciguatoxin and its cogener, *J. Am. Chem. Soc.,* 1989, 111.
58. **Lombet, A., Bidard, J.-N., and Lazdunski, M.,** Ciguatoxin and brevetoxins share a common receptor site on the neuronal voltage-dependent Na^+ channel, *FEBS Lett.,* 219(2), 355—359, 1987.
59. **Ritchie, J. M. and Chiu, S. Y.,** Distribution of sodium and potassium channels in mammalian myelinated nerve, in *Demyelinating Disease: Basic and Clinical Electrophysiology,* Waxman S. G. and Ritchie, J. M., Eds., Raven Press, New York, 1981, 329—342.

Chapter 4

CIGUATERA IN AUSTRALIA

Michael F. Capra and John Cameron

TABLE OF CONTENTS

I. INTRODUCTION

The circumtropical distribution of ciguatera poisoning and its close association with coral reefs are well known. As the Australian Great Barrier Reef is the longest strip of coral reef in the world, extending 2000 km along the Queensland coast from Cape York in the north to the vicinity of Bundaberg in the south (Figures 1 and 2), it is not surprising that many cases of human ciguatera poisoning occur in Australia each year. Australians, especially those living along the east coast, have become increasingly aware of ciguatera over the past decade. This increased awareness is due primarily to the electronic and print media publicizing, and frequently sensationalizing, the sporadic, and sometimes large, outbreaks of ciguatera poisoning.

Headlines such as "Deadly poison discovered in Queensland mackerel", "Deadly mackerel toxin hits 42 victims", "Poisoned by fish — Sydney Warning", and "It's the nicest fish that kill you" have undoubtedly alerted the public to the consequences of consuming fish that carry ciguatoxin.

The earliest reference to ciguatera of historic connection to Australia is attributable to William Anderson, who was the surgeon's mate on Captain Cook's ship, "The Resolution", during Cook's second voyage of discovery to the South Seas. It was Cook's first voyage to the South Seas that led to the discovery of the east coast of Australia and the subsequent settlement of Sydney in 1788 by the British. Anderson, in a letter published in the *Philosophical Transactions of the Royal Society of London* in 1776,[1] gives a detailed description of an incident in which several of Cook's officers were poisoned in 1774 after eating fish from the Island of Malicolo in the Pacific nation of Vanuatu to the east of north Queensland. Anderson gives an account of the symptoms of the victims that closely match those in any modern review of ciguatera poisoning and he also makes the observation "... that in treating the disorder we could have no method founded on experience to pursue and therefore were obliged to palliate the symptoms from the analogy they bore to those that occur in other diseases". It is interesting to note that although our knowledge of ciguatera poisoning has increased greatly since Anderson's account of 213 years ago, the treatment of the disorder is still essentially symptomatic.

The first properly documented cases of ciguatera in Australia were reported by Paradice.[2] Paradice described a number of cases of ciguatera from the Cairns region of north Queensland (Figure 2), including an incident in which a whole family was poisoned. The species of fish responsible for all of the poisonings was the Chinaman fish, *Paradicichthys venenatus* (now *Symphorus nematophorus*).

The dangers of consuming Chinaman fish and the possible medical sequelae were reviewed by Whitley[3,4] and Cleland.[5] Whitley[6] recommended that a second fish from Queensland waters, the red bass, *Lutjanus coatesi* (now *L. bohar*), should be avoided as its flesh, like that of the Chinaman fish, could be poisonous at certain times. In 1943, Whitley[7] expanded his list of possible ciguateric fish to include sweetlips (*Lethrinus* and *Lethrinella*) and hinds (*Epinephelus*), and suggested that trevallies and mackerel may also be poisonous. No direct evidence was presented by Whitley to link these additions to actual ciguatera poisoning, and he suggested that reports of poisoning from these fish may be due to their contamination with pathogenic bacteria, rather than the presence of toxins within their flesh. Goat fish (family Mullidae) and sea pike or barracuda (*Sphyraena*) were also listed as possible ciguateric fish on the basis of information from Hawaii and the West Indies; however, there was no evidence, at that time, of any intoxication resulting from their consumption in Australia. No further published work on ciguatera poisoning in Australia could be found until Barnes[8] comments in the *Medical Journal of Australia* "... that the extreme paucity of published records gave the impression that ciguatera was no problem in Australian waters. This impression was false. In the Cairns district alone over one hundred cases had been recognized in a 3 year period and these represented only a token of the true incidence." These comments of Barnes' foreshadowed a brief revival in interest in ciguatera in the late 1960s[9,10] that carried into the 1970s.[11-14] However, most of the work on ciguatera in Australia has been done in the period 1980 to the present.

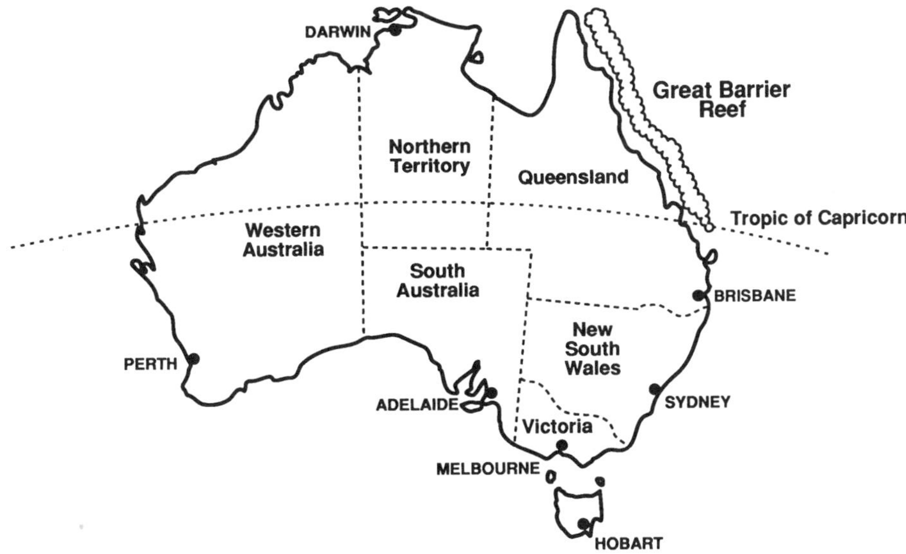

FIGURE 1. Map of Australia showing the states and state capitals. The extent of the Great Barrier Reef is shown. Ciguateric fish are caught in the waters of Queensland and the Northern Territory, however, there are no reports of toxic fish from the tropical waters of Western Australia.

The remainder of this chapter will review the current state of knowledge of ciguatera in Australia and the contribution made by Australian workers to the general understanding of ciguatera.

II. FISH RESPONSIBLE FOR CIGUATERA IN AUSTRALIA

Chinaman fish and red bass, as noted, were assessed as potential sources of ciguatera poisoning by Whitley.[3,4,6] These two species and a third species, the paddle-tail, *Lutjanus gibbus*, are now widely recognized as poisonous and cannot be sold legally in Queensland.[15] These species can, however, be eaten by the many amateur fishermen who fish the tropical waters of Australia, but fortunately they seem to avoid the consumption of Chinaman fish and paddle-tail. In certain parts of Queensland and the Northern Territory, some amateur fishermen consume the red bass, *L. bohar*, which is a species notorious throughout the Pacific as a potential source of ciguatera. Capra[16] bioassayed samples of Chinaman fish, red bass, and paddle-tail captured from reefs within a 60-km radius of Cairns and found a sufficiently high incidence of toxicity to preclude the human consumption of these species from this locality (Table 1).

Broadbent,[10] while confirming the toxicity of Chinaman fish and red bass, reported that over 50% of the cases of ciguatera poisoning in Queensland were caused by the coral trout, *Plectropomus maculatus*. Coral trout is a highly prized eating fish in Australia. It can be found on the menus of good seafood restaurants and commands a high price in retail outlets in Queensland and New South Wales. Broadbent also attributed 25% of the cases of ciguatera poisoning to the flowery cod, *Epinephelus fuscoguttatus*, and the spotted cod, *E. tauvini*.

Data from the 1960s indicated that 80 cases of ciguatera poisoning between Cairns in the north and Gladstone in the south of Queensland were due to the consumption of the narrow barred Spanish mackerel, *Scomberomorus commersoni*.[10] Spanish mackerel, also a highly valued eating fish, is the basis of an economically important industry in Queensland. In a single incident in 1966, 30 people were poisoned after eating Spanish mackerel and, in the following year, in another single incident, 33 people were poisoned. In each case the fish had been caught off Gladstone on the central Queensland coast.[9] In 1968, 12 people were poisoned after eating a Spanish mackerel that had been caught south of Gladstone above Fraser Island.[11]

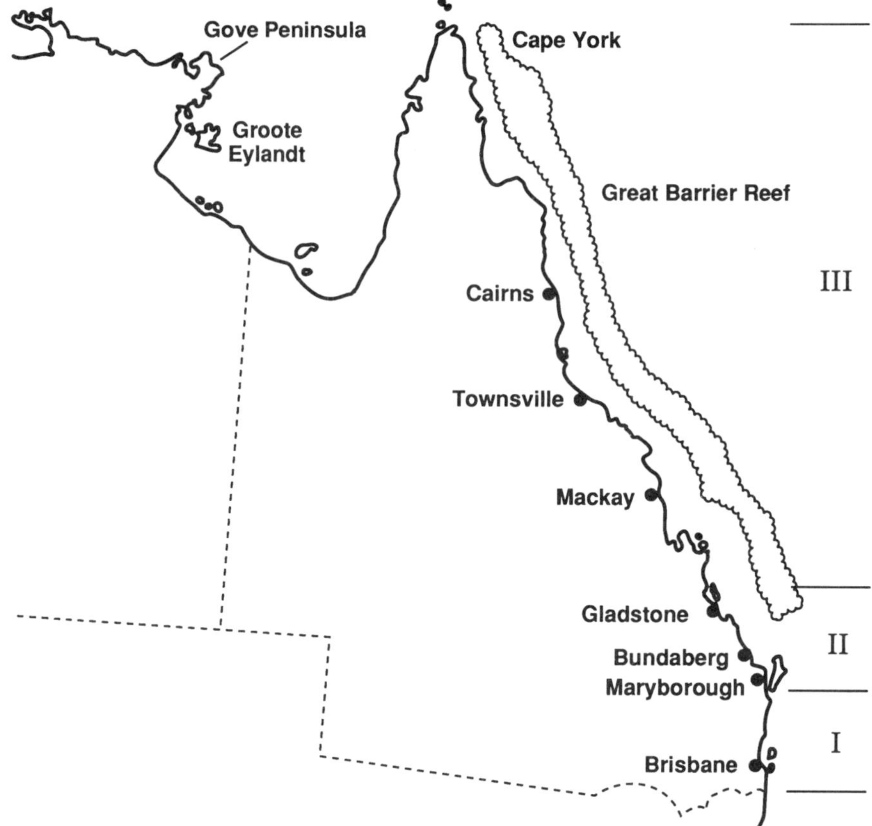

FIGURE 2. The coast of Queensland and part of the coast of the Northern Territory. The extent of the Great Barrier Reef is shown. The three zones of Lewis and Gillespie (1988) (I, II, and III) are marked on the map.

Published accounts of ciguatera and the fish responsible for human intoxication in the 1970s are few. Edmonds[12] described the Chinaman fish, red bass, and paddle-tail as particularly dangerous and listed the coral trout, Spanish mackerel, reef cod, barracuda, emperor, groper, surgeonfish, and Yankee whiting as causing occasional problems. Mitchell[14] reported an intoxication of a family of five after the consumption of a queenfish, *Scomberoides lyscon*.

A valuable data base on ciguatera and the fish responsible for human intoxication has been compiled by the Queensland Health Department and the Fisheries Section of the Queensland Department of Primary Industries from 1965 to the present time. Gillespie et al.,[17] Gillespie,[18] and Lewis and Gillespie[19] have published material from this data base on the species of fish responsible for ciguatera in Queensland. The top ten species responsible for human intoxication in Queensland over the period 1965 to 1984 are shown in Table 2.[17]

The top ten species of fish accounted for 473 cases of human intoxication between 1965 and 1984; a further 16 species of fish caused 40 cases of ciguatera, while 14 cases resulted from the consumption of nonspecified fish. It is worth noting that only those cases of ciguatera that were reported to the Health Department or Fisheries officers are included in the Queensland data base. Ciguatera in Australia is not a notifiable disease and many cases go unrecorded each year. The list of species published by Gillespie et al.[17] represents those most commonly responsible for ciguatera in Queensland. However, the list is not comprehensive and other species of fish do cause ciguatera from time to time.

TABLE 1
Estimated Incidence of Toxicity in Three Banned Fish Caught in North Queensland Waters

Common name, species	Incidence toxic fish/1000
Red bass, *Lutjanus bohar*	43
Chinaman fish, *Symphorus nematophorus*	68
Paddle-tail, *Lutjanus gibbus*	182

TABLE 2
Top Ten Species Responsible for Human Ciguatera Poisoning in Queensland (1965 to 1984)[17]

Fish species	Number of intoxications
Narrow barred Spanish mackerel (*Scomberomorus commersoni*)	226
Mackerel (unspecified) (*Scomberomorus* spp.)	134
Barracuda (*Sphyraena jello*)	29
Coral trout (*Plectropomus* spp.)	27
Flowery cod (*Epinephelus fuscoguttatus*)	14
Red emperor (*Lutjanus sebae*)	13
School mackerel (*Scomberomorus queenslandicus*)	9
Spotted mackerel (*Scomberomorus munroi*)	8
Giant dart (*Scomberoides commersonianus*)	8
Spotted cod (*Epinephelus tauvini*)	5

The other major part of Australia where ciguatera is endemic is the Northern Territory, where a data base similar to that of Queensland's is unavailable. The Northern Territory Health Authorities have published a list of approximately 20 species that should be avoided in ciguatera-prone waters.

The largest single outbreak of human ciguatera poisoning in Australia occurred in 1987, when 63 people were poisoned after the consumption of Spanish mackerel.[20] Mackerel, in particular the narrow barred Spanish mackerel, are responsible for the vast majority of outbreaks and the greatest number of people poisoned. Most of the toxic Spanish mackerel were caught in the waters of southern Queensland. Hervey Bay, between the mainland and Fraser Island (Figure 3) is notorious for the production of toxic mackerel. Platypus Bay, in particular, has produced so many toxic mackerel and barracuda over the past 10 years that its waters are now closed to the capture of these fish. A distinct pattern in the species of fish causing ciguatera has emerged in Queensland. In an analysis of the Queensland data base by Lewis et al.,[21] data on 617 individual cases of ciguatera poisoning have been collected from 225 outbreaks for the period 1965 to 1987 and have shown that ciguatera poisoning south of Gladstone is most likely to be caused by the ingestion of mackerel species, while north of Gladstone the majority of cases are

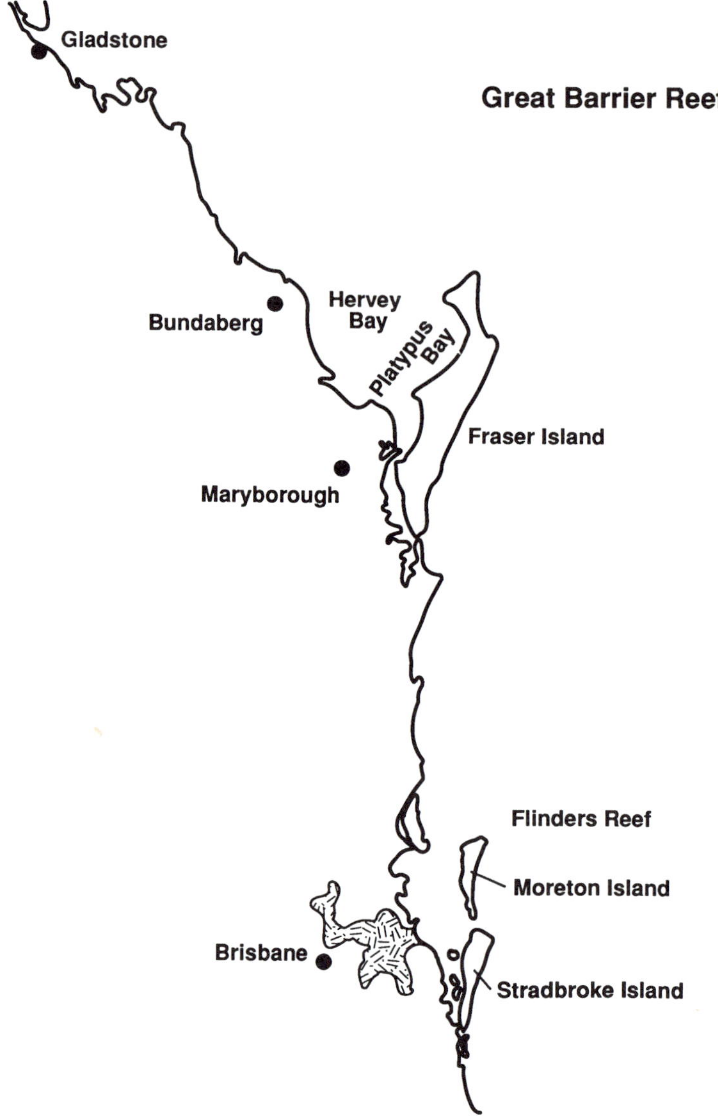

FIGURE 3. The south and central coast of Queensland. The waters of Hervey Bay, in particular the Platypus Bay Region on the western shore of Fraser Island, have produced many toxic fish over the past 10 years.

due to the consumption of non-mackerel species. Many demersal species have been implicated in causing ciguatera poisoning north of Gladstone, although cods (*Epinephelus* spp.) and coral trouts (*Plectropomus* spp.) are the principal groups involved.[17]

No data are available on the actual incidence of toxicity in commercially important species of fish from Australia. Two of the principal species involved, Spanish mackerel and coral trout, are the bases of economically important industries in which many tonnes of fish are captured each year for retail sale. The Australian catch of Spanish mackerel in 1979 to 1980 was just over 1000 tonnes and the Queensland catch represented a large proportion of this.[22] With such large tonnages of fish being consumed, there are relatively very few cases of human intoxication; nevertheless, there still exists a risk of poisoning.

III. DISTRIBUTION AND INCIDENCE OF CIGUATERA IN AUSTRALIA

Cases of ciguatera poisoning have in the main been confined to Queensland and the Northern Territory (see Figure 1). Much of Western Australia is in the tropics, yet no confirmed cases of ciguatera have been reported from that state. Although firm evidence is unavailable, the geographic and temporal incidence of ciguatera appears to vary. Barnes[8] reported a high incidence of ciguatera poisoning over a 3-year period in the early 1960s in Cairns. By the early 1980s the number of patients presenting with symptoms of ciguatera in Cairns had greatly declined.

A reef adjacent to Bremmer Island, a small island a few kilometers from Gove in the Northern Territory, was notorious for producing toxic fish in the early 1980s.[23] Much of the toxin used by the authors in their pharmacological studies was extracted from fish caught in the vicinity of Bremmer Island. Gove is a mining town with a large itinerant population. In the absence of local knowledge, many people fished the waters of Bremmer Island and became ill after eating their catch. Local Gove fishermen held many theories as to the origins of the toxicity of the Bremmer reef. One of the more plausible theories implicated an alumina processing plant discharge that was carried by currents towards Bremmer Island. However, sufficient data was never obtained to support any theory, and by 1986 the toxicity of the area had shown a marked decline.

Within Queensland over the past 25 years there has been an apparent southern shift in the incidence of ciguatera. Barnes[8] reported over 100 cases of ciguatera in Cairns. In 1966/67 outbreaks of ciguatera resulted from the consumption of fish from central Queensland.[9,11] Gillespie,[15] however, noted that almost all of the 200 plus recorded cases of ciguatera for the period 1976 to 1980 occurred in southeast Queensland. A total of 257 cases of human ciguatera intoxication, following consumption of Spanish mackerel captured in central and southern Queensland between 1976 and 1983, were reported by Lewis.[24,25] It is difficult to determine whether this perceived southern shift is due to a real increase in ciguatera in Queensland's south or an underrecording of cases in the north. It may also be attributable to more refined diagnoses and reporting of ciguatera in the south of the state.

Since the initial report of Paradice,[2] there have been many reports of single and multiple incidents of human ciguatera intoxications in Australia. There is even a report of intoxication in cats.[26] Published reports of human ciguatera poisoning in Australia are given in Table 3. The majority of reports have emanated from Queensland, and it should be noted that the same cases have been recorded several times as updates of the Queensland data base were published.[15,17,21]

Analysis of the Queensland data base[17-19,21] has shown a nonuniform distribution of ciguateric fish along the Queensland coast. There have been no recorded incidents of poisoning from relatively long sections of the coast, in particular from the north of Rockhampton to the north of Mackay, and the north of Cairns to the tip of Cape York (see Figure 2). Lewis and Gillespie[19] and Lewis et al.[21] divided the Queensland coast into three zones, two of which were south of Gladstone and a third that extended from Gladstone to Cape York (see Figure 2). The numbers and percentages of cases due to mackerel ingestion are presented in Table 4.

The figures in Table 4 illustrate the apparent southern distribution of ciguatera in Queensland. In any interpretation of the Queensland data base it should be borne in mind that a significant underrecording of ciguatera may have occurred in north Queensland. Gillespie et al.[17] believe that over 2000 cases of ciguatera poisoning may have occurred without notification to either the Health Department or Fisheries officers in the Cairns and Townsville districts between 1965 and 1984. If this is the case, the perception of a southward shift in ciguatera may not be correct, and the predominance of cases from Spanish mackerel may merely reflect the underreporting of cases from the north, where mackerel accounts for only 30% of reports.

TABLE 3
Human Ciguatera Poisoning in Australia

Year(s)	Locality	Species	No. of people poisoned	Author
1924	Cairns (Qld)	Chinaman fish (*Symphorus nematophorus*)	Several	Paradice[2]
1960s	Cairns (Qld)	Unspecified	> 100	Barnes[8]
1960s	Queensland	Coral trout (*Plectropomus maculatus*), flowery cod (*Epinephelus fuscoguttatus*), spotted cod (*Epinephelus tauvini*)	Unspecified	Broadbent[10]
1960s	Queensland	Spanish mackerel (*Scomberomorus commersoni*)	80	Broadbent[10]
1964—1974	Townsville (Qld)	Unspecified	750	Broadbent, personal communication cited in Gillespie et al.[17]
1965—1984	Queensland	Mainly Spanish mackerel (*Scomberomorus commersoni*)	527	Gillespie et al.[17]
1965—1987	Queensland	Several, mainly mackerel	617	Lewis et al.[21]
1966—1967	Gladstone (Qld)	Spanish mackerel (*Scomberomorus commersoni*)	63	Tonge et al.[9]
1968	North Fraser Island (Qld)	Spanish mackerel (*Scomberomorus commersoni*)	12	Hasset[11]
1976	Hervey Bay (Qld)	Queenfish (*Scomberoides lyscom*)	5	Mitchell[14]
1976	Hinchinbrook (650 km north of Brisbane)	Coral trout (*Plectropomus maculatus*)	2	Mitchell[27]
1976—1980	Qld, mainly Southeast	Several	> 200	Gillespie[15]
1976—1983	Central and South Qld	Spanish mackerel (*Scomberomorus commersoni*)	257	Lewis[24]
1982	Great Barrier Reef (Qld) (location not specified)	Coronation trout (*Variola louti*)	7	Pearn et al.[28]
1984	Whitsunday Islands (Qld)	Snapper, species unknown	1	Bowman[29]
1985	Gove (N.T.)	Mackerel, species unknown	5	Capra and Cameron[30]
1987	Sydney (NSW) Fish originated in Hervey Bay (Qld)	Spanish mackerel (*Scomberomorus commersoni*)	63	Capra and Cameron[20]

TABLE 4
Zonal Distribution of Ciguatera in Queensland and the Percentage of Cases Due to Mackerel Ingestion

Zone	Number of cases	% due to mackerel
I (NSW border to southern tip of Fraser Island)	151	82%
II (southern tip of Fraser Island to Gladstone)	290	87%
III (Gladstone to Cape York)	112	30%

The situation in the Northern Territory is even less clear than in Queensland. Capra and Cameron[30] report a single incident in which five people were poisoned by mackerel caught off Bremmer Island. Gillespie et al.[17] note the paucity of published information from the Northern Territory and state that the only ciguatera-prone areas are around the Gove peninsula and near Connection Island off Groot Eylandt. Several cases of ciguatera were treated at the Health Station on Groote Eylandt during the mid-1980s.[23] The ciguateric areas of the Northern Territory are shown in Figure 2.

The largest single outbreak of ciguatera recorded in Australia occurred in 1987 in Sydney, New South Wales, when 63 people were poisoned after consuming Spanish mackerel. Sydney is well below the ciguatera-prone waters of tropical Australia, and the ciguateric fish were traced by the New South Wales Health Department to Hervey Bay in Queensland.

Although many individual cases and outbreaks of ciguatera have been recorded in Australia (Table 4), there are only two estimates of the actual incidence of ciguatera poisoning available.[16,30,31] Broadbent[31] estimates the annual incidence of ciguatera in the Townsville region to be three cases per 10,000 population. The basis of this estimate is not given.

Epidemiological surveys of two Queensland communities — Maryborough-Hervey Bay (just below the southern limits of the Great Barrier Reef) and Cairns (adjacent to the northern region of the Great Barrier Reef) — were reported by Capra[16] and Capra and Cameron.[32] In each of these communities a telephone survey of 5% of the private listings was undertaken. The sample sizes were 386 in Maryborough-Hervey Bay and 564 in Cairns. The survey figures indicated that 1.8% and 2.5%, respectively, of the Maryborough-Hervey Bay and Cairns communities at some time in their lives had suffered an episode of ciguatera poisoning. When these figures were adjusted on the basis of average life expectancy (Australian Government actuarial tables 1980 to 1982), an estimate of the annual incidence of ciguatera poisoning was obtained for each community. The annual incidence in Maryborough-Hervey Bay was 2.4 cases per 10,000 population and in Cairns it was 3.4 cases per 10,000. The figures are similar to the 4.0 cases per 10,000 population reported as average for the South Pacific region.[33] The higher incidence of ciguatera in the north than in the south of the state conflicts with the pattern in the Queensland data base and supports the proposition that there has been an underreporting of ciguatera in the north.

IV. SYMPTOMATOLOGY OF CIGUATERA IN AUSTRALIA

The initial observations of the symptoms of ciguatera in Australia were made by Paradice,[2] who described diarrhea and vomiting, with abdominal and joint pain followed by several days of weakness. Since this initial description there have been many reports on the symptoms exhibited by the victims of ciguatera in Australia.[4,5,9,11-14,17-21,25,27,28,31,34,35]

A wide range of symptoms, including gastrointestinal and neurological dysfunction,[17,21,36] is now associated with the ciguatera syndrome. Cardiovascular symptoms appear to be rare in

TABLE 5
A Comparison of the Frequency of Symptoms Between Two Australian Groups of Ciguatera Victims and Victims from Other Pacific Countries

Sign or symptom	Percentage of victims with sign or symptom			
	Sydney	Queensland	Fiji	French Polynesia
Nausea	83	55	—	43
Vomiting	50	35	30	38
Diarrhea	78	64	51	71
Abdominal pain	68	52	59	47
Headache	85	62	—	59
Vertigo	65	45	38	42
Dental pain	48	37	—	25
Joint pain	83	79	69	86
Muscle pain	93	83	—	82
Burning of skin on contact with cold water	80	76	55	88
Paresthesia of hands	88	71	—	—
Paresthesia of lips	78	66	52	89
Loss of energy	83	90	—	60
Tremor	30	31	—	27
Dyspnea	38	28	9	16
Sweating	48	43	34	37
Salivation	15	10	10	19
Pruritus	88	76	35	45
Skin rash	25	26	2	21
Chills	65	49	42	59
Neck stiffness	50	27	—	24
Dysuria	23	22	—	10

Australian victims of ciguatera poisoning; however, hypotension, cardiac arrhythmias, bradycardia, or tachycardia with extrasystoles can at times occur during an episode of poisoning.[12]

The symptoms exhibited by victims of ciguatera in Australia are generally very similar to those observed in other parts of the world, in particular, the South Pacific Region.[17] A comparison of the frequency of signs and symptoms exhibited by two sets of Australian victims of ciguatera — victims from the Queensland data base 1965 to 1984,[17] and victims from the 1987 Sydney outbreak[20] — and victims from Fiji[37] and the French Pacific Territories[38] is given in Table 5.

Similar responses among each of the groups for most signs and symptoms are apparent in Table 5. The one significant exception is pruritis, which seems to be much more common among the Australian victims of ciguatera poisoning. Whether this reflects a variation in the genetic makeup of the victims or a structural difference in the responsible toxins is purely conjectural.

The sporadic nature of ciguatera outbreaks along the east coast of Australia has made it difficult to assess the time course of symptoms. An opportunity was afforded by the 1987 Sydney outbreak to follow the recovery of 40 of the 63 victims over a period of 6 months. The type and duration of various signs and symptoms for the Sydney outbreak are given in Table 6.

The duration of symptoms for some victims of the Sydney outbreak was quite long. Even 6 months after the ingestion of toxic fish, several victims suffered from one or more symptoms (Table 7). One woman who consumed 1 kg of toxic fish in two 500-g portions over a 3-day period had eight of the symptoms and was debilitated to the extent that she was unable to resume employment 6 months after her initial poisoning.

Although many people have fallen victim to ciguatera in Australia, the mortality rate is very

TABLE 6
Type and Duration of Symptoms in 40 of the 63 Victims of the 1987 Ciguatera Poisoning Outbreak in Sydney

Symptom	Percent with symptom	Duration of symptom (days mean ± SE)
Nausea	83	17 ± 7
Vomiting	50	11 ± 9
Abdominal pain	68	9 ± 2
Diarrhea	78	5 ± 1
Headache	85	32 ± 9
Vertigo	65	24 ± 9
Memory disturbance	43	121 ± 18
Anxiety	60	60 ± 13
Depression	63	54 ± 11
Dental pain	48	18 ± 4
Joint pain	83	59 ± 10
Paresthesia of hands	88	50 ± 8
Paresthesia of lips	78	35 ± 8
Temperature perception reversals	80	45 ± 7
Muscle pain	93	40 ± 8
Loss of energy	83	49 ± 8
Difficulty walking	65	24 ± 7
Tremor	30	20 ± 7
Shortness of breath	38	16 ± 6
Sweating	48	12 ± 4
Watery eyes	33	15 ± 3
Salivation	15	12 ± 4
Itchy skin	88	36 ± 7
Skin rash	25	17 ± 3
Chills	65	9 ± 2
Neck stiffness	50	44 ± 14
Dysuria	23	24 ± 9
Hallucinations	13	46 ± 34
Visual defects	18	84 ± 34

TABLE 7
Symptoms Persisting in the 1987 Sydney Victims of Ciguatera 6 Months After Ingestion of Toxic Fish

Number of persistent symptoms	Number of victims with symptoms
1	11
2	5
3	1
4	2
8	1

low. There is only one documented fatality which was probably due to the ingestion of toxic fish.[9] In 1965, a 25-year-old woman died in north Queensland after eating several fillets of mackerel. The woman consumed the fish at 7 p.m., and 4 hours later she complained of "coldness, numbness, and an inability to move her limbs". Sweating and profuse vomiting preceded a series of spasmodic convulsions and a semicomatose state with incontinence of feces. By 2:45 a.m. she was in a coma with periodic convulsions. Death occurred at 5:20 a.m., just over 10 h after the consumption of the fish. Her husband, who also consumed the fish, vomited violently at midnight and their dog, who ate the vomitus, was ill for 24 h. No significant pathological signs were apparent at autopsy and various tissues that were examined histologically showed no signs of abnormality.

This probable fatality occurred at a time when there was little attention paid to ciguatera in Australia. By the early 1980s not only were the medical and scientific communities taking an interest in ciguatera, but the media had begun to examine outbreaks and to report on the often severe symptoms and sequelae. The death under unusual circumstances of a healthy businessman during a company convention on one of Queensland's tropical island resorts led the national media to speculate on the possible involvement of ciguatera and to review the cause, symptomatology, and medical sequelae of ciguatera poisoning.[39]

The many cases of ciguatera reported in Australia have described a syndrome similar to that reported in other parts of the world. At least one less-than-usual case in which a human fetus was intoxicated was reported in Queensland by Pearn et al.[28] and later reviewed by Sutherland.[34] Pearn et al.[28] presented the case report of a primigravida who was poisoned, at term, by a portion of a coronation trout (*Variola louti*) caught on the Great Barrier Reef. The woman and six other people who ingested the fish complained of typical ciguatera symptoms within 4 h of their meal. Tumultuous fetal movement with intermittent and peculiar fetal "shivering" began simultaneously with the woman's own systemic symptoms. The bizarre fetal movement continued maximally for 18 h and decreased over the following 24-h period. A male infant delivered by Caesarean section 2 d later had left-sided facial palsy and on the morning after birth some possible myotonia of the small muscles of the hand was noted. The infant required intensive care without ventilation for respiratory distress syndrome. At 6 weeks the infant was normal. Excruciating hyperesthesia of the nipples during attempted breast feeding was reported by the mother. This case appears to be the only report of fetal involvement in ciguatera and suggests that the toxin responsible for the ciguatera syndrome is capable of crossing the placenta.

V. PHYSIOLOGICAL AND PHARMACOLOGICAL STUDIES ON CIGUATOXIN IN AUSTRALIA

In Australia, ciguatoxin has been extracted from the tissues of mackerel[24,30,40] and barracuda.[24,41,42] Extraction of wild and cultured populations of *Gambierdiscus toxicus* derived from Australian waters has produced maitotoxin but not ciguatoxin.[43,44] Extraction of the benthic dinoflagellate *Ostreopsis siamensis* from the ciguatera-endemic region of Hervey Bay, Queensland, produced neither ciguatoxin nor maitotoxin, but a water-soluble toxin distinguishable from maitotoxin.[44]

Toxin extracted from the flesh and viscera of toxic mackerel and barracuda has been used in several Australian physiological and pharmacological studies. Table 8 summarizes these studies.

VI. CLINICAL AND PATHOLOGICAL STUDIES IN AUSTRALIA

Although there are many reports of the signs and symptoms of the victims of ciguatera in Australia, there is a lack of information in the literature on clinical studies and clinical measurements from the victims of ciguatera. Allsop et al.[55] made a number of clinical measurements and assessments on three victims of ciguatera. Abnormalities in reflexes and nerve conduction parameters were observed. The EEG was normal, as was the composition of the CSF in these patients. Clinical laboratory investigation of one patient revealed a mild neutrophil leucocytosis, a rise in the erythrocyte sedimentation rate, and a moderate rise in the level of lactic dehydrogenase, while creatinine phosphokinease levels were normal. Cameron and Capra[36] reported on electrophysiological findings from the victims of the 1987 Sydney ciguatera outbreak.

Pathological studies of ciguatera in Australia have also been minimal. Tonge et al.,[9] describing a possible ciguatera death, reported no gross abnormalities at autopsy, nor any subsequent abnormalities in tissues examined histologically. Allsop et al.[55] examined the sural nerve fibers from a victim of ciguatera and found a striking edema of the adaxonal Schwann cell cytoplasm.

In the authors' laboratory, Coombe et al.[56] showed significant pathological changes in the structure of the small intestine of mice given lethal doses of ciguatoxin. When mice were given lethal doses of ciguatoxin, a characteristic expansion was noted in the lamina propria within the tips of the villi of the small intestine. This expansion appeared to occur concomitantly with vascular and lymphatic degeneration, and a general disruption of the lamina propria. The expansion of the lamina at the villi tips was greater in mice with a longer death time. As the expansion increased, the villi tips ruptured and the luminal contents were lost into the lumen of the intestine. The extent of damage caused to the small intestine can be seen in Figure 4. There have been no previous reports of pathological changes in intestinal tissues following ciguatoxin administration. It is possible that the gut symptomatology in human ciguatera victims may not only be due to the functional actions of ciguatoxin on membrane channels, but may also reflect gross pathological changes in the intestinal lining.

VII. STUDIES ON FISH

The authors have been intrigued for some time by the fact that a single fish can carry sufficient toxin within its tissues to poison many humans, yet there is no evidence to suggest that such a fish shows any overt pathology. It has been established that the nerves of fish respond to ciguatoxin in a manner similar to those of mammals.[42,50,51] Changes in nerve conduction parameters in southern species of fish that never carry ciguatoxin (noncarrier) and northern species that can at times carry ciguatoxin (carrier) are similar to changes observed in mammalian nerves.[42,50] When $^{22}Na^{+}$ efflux rates were measured from the ouabain-blocked olfactory nerves of both carrier and noncarrier species, a significantly increased efflux rate existed in nerves that had been treated with ciguatoxin.[42,51] Capra et al.[54] have postulated that when fish ingest ciguatoxin in sublethal doses the toxin is sequested or partitioned away from target sites. The method of sequestration is unknown, although any elucidation of the mechanism may produce insights into the therapy of human ciguatera intoxication.

Differences in the susceptibility of fish to ciguatoxin have been noted by Capra et al.[54] When two small tropical pomacentrids, *Chromis nitida* and *Pomacentrus wardi*, were given intraperitoneal injections of ciguatoxin, it was found that *C. nitida*, a planktivore, was significantly more susceptible to the toxin than *P. wardi*, a browser. Although ciguatoxin produced deaths in each species, greater doses were required than those that would be typically lethal in mammals. The difference in susceptibility between the planktivore and the browser may reflect the niche occupied by each species. A planktivore is less likely to encounter ciguatoxin from the benthic dinoflagellate, *Gambierdiscus toxicus*, in its mode of feeding than is the browser. Fish normally exposed to ingestion of ciguatoxin might be expected to have a higher tolerance to the toxin than fish not likely to encounter the toxin in their normal mode of feeding. The intraperitoneal route of administration of toxin by Capra et al.[54] differs from the normal mode of ingestion and may account for the lethality of the toxin.

In addition to the use of the fish preparation to give insight into the mode of action of the toxin in carrier species, these preparations can be useful in studying the pharmacology of ciguatoxin. Flowers,[42] using the lateral line branch of the vagus nerve from the whiting, *Silago cilliata*, has investigated the possible antagonistic agents of ciguatoxin. In a study of duration of the supernormal period[36] from whiting nerves (Figure 5), Flowers[42] has shown that the prolongation of supernormality that follows treatment with ciguatoxin can be diminished with tetrodotoxin, verapamil, and lignocaine.

TABLE 8
Physiological and Pharmacological Studies in Australia

Preparation	Results	Author(s)
Rat phrenic nerve-diaphragm	Ciguatoxin produced a rapid inhibition of the responses to indirect stimulation and a slower inhibition to direct stimulation	Lewis and Endean[45]
Guinea-pig ileum and vas deferens	Ciguatoxin produced dose-dependent contractions of the ileum. The response was blocked by atropine, tetrodotoxin and low $[Na^+]$, and potentiated by eserine. It was suggested that ciguatoxin acts on the ileum by releasing acetylcholine from cholinergic nerve terminals. Ciguatoxin produced large transient contractions in the vas deferens.	Lewis and Endean[46]
Rat ventral coccygeal nerve	Changes in nerve – conduction parameters consistent with ciguatoxin acting as an opener of Na^+ channels	Capra and Cameron[30]
Guinea-pig atria and papillary muscles	Positive inotropic responses in atria and papillary muscles consistent with direct actions on the myocardium via voltage-dependent Na^+ channels and indirect actions on myocardial nerves	Lewis and Endean;[47] Lewis[48]
Several mammalian preparations	Ciguatoxin had direct effects on nerves and direct and indirect effects on muscles	Lewis[24]
Guinea-pig atria	Local anesthetics, lidocaine, and procaine antagonized the effect of ciguatoxin on heart muscle	Lewis[49]
Fish nerves	Changes in nerve conduction parameters consistent with ciguatoxin acting as an opener of Na^+ channels	Flowers;[42] Flowers et al.[50]
Fish nerves	Ciguatoxin increased the efflux rate of $^{22}Na^+$ from olfactory nerves, indicating an action on Na^+ channels	Flowers;[42] Capra et al.[51]

Guinea-pig atria and papillary muscles	High doses of ciguatoxin produce negative inotropy and arrhythmias via direct action on myocardial Na^+ channels and indirect action on neural Na^+ channels	Lewis[52]
Guinea-pig atria	Preliminary experiment suggest that *in vitro* mannitol can cause long-lasting reversal of the actions of ciguatoxin in the atria	Lewis[53]
Rat ventral coccygeal nerve	Several compounds antagonize the actions of ciguatoxin on mammalian nerves	Cameron and Capra[36]
Fish nerves	Ciguatoxin produces changes in the nerves of fish that are similar to the changes induced in mammalian nerves. Several compounds antagonize the neural responses to ciguatoxin	Flowers[42]
Whole fish	Ciguatoxin is lethal to fish, but at higher than mammalian doses	Capra et al.[54]

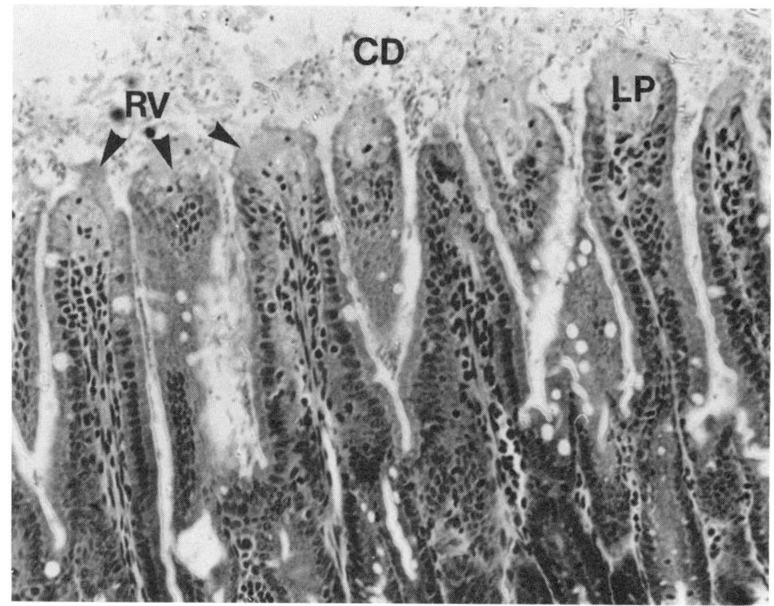

FIGURE 4. A hematoxylin and eosin stained section of the small intestine of a mouse exposed to a lethal dose of ciguatoxin. Note the expansion of the lamina propria (LP), the rupturing of villi tips (RV), and the presence of cellular debris (CD).

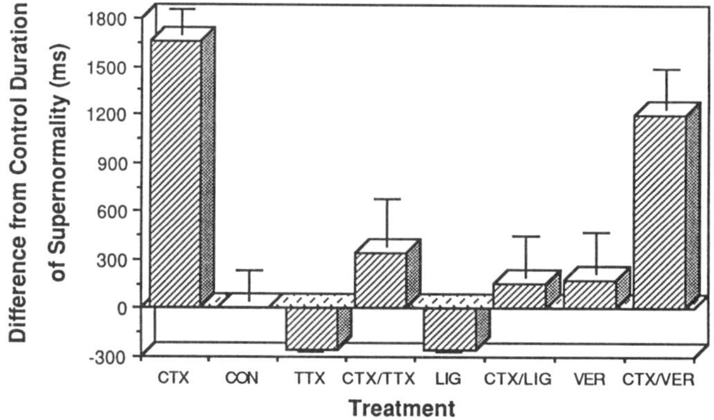

FIGURE 5. Supernormal studies from the isolated lateral line branch of the vagus nerve in the whiting, *Silago cilliata*. Differences from the control value (CON) are shown from various treatments. Ciguatoxin (CTX) greatly prolongs the duration of the supernormal period, while tetrodotoxin (TTX) and lignocaine (LIG) decrease the duration of supernormality. Verapamil (VER) also prolongs the duration of supernormality, but to a lesser extent than ciguatoxin. Tetrodotoxin, lignocaine, and verapamil all antagonize the prolongation of supernormality induced by ciguatoxin.

VIII. TREATMENT OF CIGUATERA IN AUSTRALIA

Since the observations of Anderson,[1] the treatment of ciguatera in Australia has remained essentially symptomatic,[17] not withstanding some interesting suggestions within the literature. Cleland[5] suggests the use of emetics in the initial phases of the disease and morphia to control the later pain and insomnia. Edmonds[12] also suggests the use of emetics, fluid and electrolyte replacement, calcium gluconate, mild sedation with diazepam, the use of opiates if needed, a steroid cover, and the possible use of atropine. In certain cases, Edmonds[12] felt that tensilon or neostigmine may prove useful, while vitamin B should be avoided. Bowman[32] successfully used amitriptyline to abolish the symptoms of ciguatera in a nonclinically depressed patient who had no neurotic traits. Gillespie et al.[17] noted that the long-term effects of ciguatera have been treated with varying degrees of efficacy using vitamin B_{12}, calcium gluconate, antihistamine agents, and amitriptyline. They also suggested that atropine may be useful in controlling persistent vomiting or diarrhea, as well as bradycardia and hypotension. Broadbent[31] suggests the use of antihistamines and mild antidepressants and the use of nonsteroidal anti-inflammatory drugs for the relief of prolonged arthralgia. He does, however, caution against "the cavalier administration of anticholinesterases and myriad cocktails of vitamins".

IX. INVOLVEMENT OF DINOFLAGELLATES IN CIGUATERA IN AUSTRALIA

The epiphytic dinoflagellate, *Gambierdiscus toxicus*, occurs in association with macroalgae in a variety of marine habitats along the Queensland coast.[18,57,58] Population densities are generally low (up to 25 cells/g of macroalgae), with the exception of Flinders Reef just north of Brisbane, where densities have at times been in excess of 1000 cells/g of macroalgae.[57] The population density of *G. toxicus* at Flinders Reef in 1985 was variable, with as few as 120 cells/g of macroalgae in May to June and as many as 2000 cells/g of macroalgae in September. The distribution of high cell numbers was patchy, although high densities were consistently found on the red algae *Digenia simplex*.[43] Bioassay of solvent extracts of biodetritus samples from Flinders Reef failed to confirm the presence of ciguatoxin, however, maitotoxin was characterized from the extracts. The lack of toxic fish from the Flinders Reef region, where high population densities of *G. toxicus* occur, led Gillespie et al.[43] to speculate on the existence of a possible "ciguatoxin inducing factor" that would need to be present before the population of *G. toxicus* could begin toxin production. Although ciguatoxin could not be found in *G. toxicus* from Flinders Reef, the possibility exists that some precursor compound from *G. toxicus* is bioconverted by fish to produce ciguatoxin.[21] This proposition was discounted after pooled liver samples from individual species of herbivorous and carnivorous fish had been bioassayed for ciguatoxin and proved to be negative.[21]

Bioassay data from Lewis et al.[58] indicates that where *G. toxicus* populations are high at Flinders Reef, there is an apparent absence of ciguatoxin in fish, while in the north of Queensland at John Brewer Reef, off Townsville, where there is a low population density of *G. toxicus*, the levels of ciguatoxin in *Ctenochaetus striatus* are high. It would seem that population densities of *G. toxicus* do not correlate with the ciguatoxin levels in Queensland fish. Holmes et al.[44] were unable to demonstrate the presence of ciguatoxin in cultured nonaxenic strains of *G. toxicus* from ciguatera endemic areas of Queensland and French Polynesia, and suggest that the involvement of *G. toxicus* in the biogenesis of ciguatera outbreaks may have to be reconsidered. Although *G. toxicus* has a widespread distribution in Queensland tropical waters, there is no direct evidence to link the presence of the dinoflagellate with the occurrence of ciguatoxin in fish.

X. CIGUATERA AND THE FISHING INDUSTRY IN AUSTRALIA

In Sydney in 1987, 63 people became ill after eating Spanish mackerel bought from various retail outlets. The outbreak was eventually traced to a single large wholesaler in Sydney. The initial information received by the New South Wales health authorities suggested that the offending fish had originated in northern New South Wales from an area well below the normal distribution of ciguatera. It was subsequently discovered that the toxic fish had, in fact, originated from a ciguatera-endemic area of Hervey Bay in Queensland and had passed through the Queensland fish markets en route to Sydney. Following the outbreak of poisoning and the confirmation of the involvement of ciguatera, the New South Wales Health Department initiated a criminal prosecution under the Pure Food Act of New South Wales against the wholesaler. This action went to court in late 1988 and was resolved in favor of the defendant in early 1989. The grounds upon which the case was resolved in the magistrates court were that the defendant "held an honest and reasonable belief in a state of fact which, if true, would make his actions innocent." The Health Department has contested this judgement and engaged a prominent Queens Counsel to appeal before the Supreme Court of New South Wales. The appeal has been lodged on the basis that a strict liability exists on the sellers of food and that the defense as accepted in the magistrates court is unavailable in the case of sellers of adulterated foods.

Fish tends to command a high retail price in Australia and so relatively expensive fish like Spanish mackerel is likely to be consumed by the more affluent members of the community. This, in general, was true of the 1987 ciguatera outbreak, where several professional people, including at least one lawyer, were poisoned. This type of person is more likely to engage in litigation, as has occurred in Sydney, where several people are now planning group and individual actions against the wholesale vendor. These actions are now likely to come before the courts in the near future. Irrespective of the outcome of the appeal proceedings of the Health Department before the Supreme Court, legal opinion suggests that any civil case brought by victims of the outbreak would have a good chance of success.

Success in any of the Sydney litigations will have a severe impact on Australia's northern fishing industry. If the Health Department prosecution of the wholesale vendor is successful, vendors may no longer risk buying fish that could carry ciguatoxin. Essentially this could mean that southern markets would no longer carry many of the species of fish that are currently caught in the northern waters of Australia. Successful civil litigations may involve considerable payment from the vendor's liability insurance, which in turn would make future liability cover for tropical fish difficult and expensive.

XI. CONCLUSION

Human intoxications resulting from the consumption of ciguateric fish occur in Australia. The fish responsible are captured from the waters of the Northern Territory and Queensland. Public awareness and scientific and medical interest in ciguatera have increased greatly during the past decade. Currently, in Australia, active research is being pursued into the involvement of dinoflagellates in ciguatera, the passage of ciguatoxin through the ecosystem, pharmacologic actions of ciguatoxin, the detection of ciguatoxin, and the treatment of ciguatera victims. Recent well-publicized outbreaks of ciguatera poisoning and a number of current and pending legal actions resulting from human intoxication will ensure that ciguatera and ciguatera research maintain a reasonably high profile.

ACKNOWLEDGMENTS

The authors wish to thank the Fishing Industry Research and Development Council and the Australian Research Council for their continuing support of ciguatera research.

REFERENCES

1. **Anderson, W.,** An account of some poisonous fish in the south seas, *Phil. Trans. R. Soc. London*, 66, 544, 1776.
2. **Paradice, W. E. J.,** Injuries and lesions caused by the bites of animals and insects, *Med. J. Aust.*, 2, 650, 1924.
3. **Whitley, G. P.,** Ichthylogical miscellanea, *Mem. Queensland Mus.*, 10, 8, 1930.
4. **Whitley, G. P.,** The Chinaman fish, *Aust. Mus. Mag.*, 4, 394, 1932.
5. **Cleland, J. B.,** Injuries and diseases in Australia attributable to animals (insects excepted), *Med. J. Aust.*, 2, 313, 1942.
6. **Whitley, G. P.,** A new fish reputed to be poisonous in Queensland, *Mem. Queensland Mus.*, 10, 175, 1934.
7. **Whitley, G. P.,** Poisonous and harmful fishes, *Coun. Sci. Indust. Res. Bull.*, 159, 1, 1943.
8. **Barnes, J.,** Ciguatera in Australia, *Med. J. Aust.*, 1, 1136, 1966.
9. **Tonge, J. I., Battey, Y., Forbes, J. J., and Grant, E. M.,** Ciguatera poisoning: a report of two outbreaks and a probable fatal case in Queensland, *Med. J. Aust.*, 2, 1088, 1967.
10. **Broadbent, G. D.,** Ciguatera in Queensland — report of a seminar on ichthysarcotoxism, 1968.
11. **Hassett, R.,** Ciguatera poisoning in fish and a 1968 outbreak in Bundaberg, *Proc. 34th Ann. Conf., Australian Institute of Health Surveyors* (Queensland Division), 58, 1973.
12. **Edmonds, C.,** *Dangerous Marine Animals of the Indo-Pacific Region*, Weddel Publishing, Newport, Victoria, Australia, 1974.
13. **Southcott, R. V.,** *Australian Venomous and Poisonous Fishes*, Southcott, Mitcham, South Australia, 1976, 16.
14. **Mitchell, K.,** Ciguatera, *Med. J. Aust.*, 2, 660, 1976.
15. **Gillespie, N. C.,** Fish poisoning causes concern in Australia, *Aust. Fish.*, 39, 28, 1980.
16. **Capra, M. F.,** Ciguatera poisoning: incidence and implications, A final report on Fishing Industry Research Trust Account Research Grant 82/33. Commonwealth Department of Primary Industries, Canberra, 1985.
17. **Gillespie, N. C., Lewis, R. J., Pearn, J. H., Bourke, A. T. C., Holmes, M. J., Burke, J. B., and Shields, W. J.,** Ciguatera in Australia: occurrence, clinical features, pathophysiology and management, *Med. J. Aust.*, 145, 584, 1986.
18. **Gillespie, N. C.,** Possible origins of ciguatera, in *Venoms and Victims*, Pearn, J. and Covacevich, J., Eds., Queensland Museum and Amphion Press, Brisbane, Australia, 1987, 31.
19. **Lewis, R. J. and Gillespie, N. C.,** Ciguatera, in *Venoms and Victims*, Pearn, J. H. and Covacevich, J., Eds., Queensland Museum and Amphion Press, Brisbane, Australia, 1988, 31-36.
20. **Capra, M. F. and Cameron, J.,** Ciguatera poisoning: pharmacology and pathology, A final report on Fishing Industry Research Trust Account Research Grant 83/41. Commonwealth Department of Primary Industries, Canberra, 1988.
21. **Lewis, R. J., Gillespie, N. C., Holmes, M. J., Burke, J. B., Keys, A. B., Fifoot, A. T., and Street, R.,** An analysis of the human responses to ciguatera in Australia, *Proc. Sixth Intl. Coral Reef Symp.*, 3, 61, 1988.
22. **Rohan, G. V.,** The market situation for tropical pelagic fish in Australia, in *Northern Pelagic Fish Seminar*, Grant, C. J. and Walter, D. G., Eds., Australian Government Publishing Service, Canberra, Australia, 1981, 144.
23. **Butler, G.,** Personal communication, Northern Territory Health Department, 1986.
24. **Lewis, R. J.,** Ciguatera and Ciguatoxin-Like Substances in Fishes, Especially *Scombermorus commersoni* from Southern Queensland, Doctoral Dissertation, University of Queensland, Brisbane, Australia, 1985.
25. **Lewis, R. J.,** Ciguatera in southeastern Queensland, in *Toxic Plants and Animals. A Guide for Australia*, Covacevich, J., Davie. P. and Pearn, J., Eds., 1987, 181.
26. **Clark, L. and Whitwell, G. B.,** Ciguatera poisoning in cats in Brisbane, *Aust. Vet. J.*, 44, 81, 1968.
27. **Mitchell, K.,** Ciguatera poisoning, in *Animal Toxins and Man*, Division of Health Education and Information, Queensland Health Department, Brisbane, Australia, 1981, 8.
28. **Pearn, J., Harvey, P., De Ambrosis, W., Lewis, R., and McKay, R.,** Ciguatera poisoning and pregnancy (letter), *Med. J. Aust.*, 1, 57, 1982.
29. **Bowman, P. B.,** Amitriptyline and ciguatera, *Med. J. Aust.*, 140, 802, 1984.
30. **Capra, M. and Cameron, J.,** The effects of ciguatoxin on mammalian nerves, *Proc. Fifth Intl. Coral Reef Cong.*, 4, 457, 1985.
31. **Broadbent, G. D.,** Ciguatera, *Aust. Family Pract.*, 16, 127, 1987.
32. **Capra, M. and Cameron, J.,** Epidemiological and social surveys on the incidence of and attitudes towards ciguatera poisoning in two Australian communities, *Proc. Fifth Intl. Coral Reef Cong.*, 4, 489, 1985.
33. **Yasumoto, T., Raj, U., and Bagnis, R.,** Seafood Poisoning in Tropical Regions, in *Symposium on Seafood Toxins in Tropical Regions*, Laboratory of Food Hygiene, Faculty of Agriculture, Tohoku University, Kagoshima, Japan, 1984, 1.
34. **Sutherland, S. K.,** *Australian Animal Toxins: The Creatures, their Toxins and Care of the Poisoned Patient*, Oxford University Press, Melbourne, Australia, 1985.
35. **Capra, M.,** Ciguatera poisoning, *Proc. Nutrit. Soc. Aust.*, 11, 63, 1986.

36. **Cameron, J. and Capra, M. F.,** Neurological studies on the effects of ciguatoxin on mammalian nerve, *Ciguatera Seafood Toxins*, CRC Press, Boca Raton, FL, 1990, chap. 2.
37. **Narayan, Y.,** Fish poisoning in Fiji, *Fiji Med. J.*, 8, 547, 1980.
38. **Bagnis, R. A., Kuberski, T., and Laugier, S.,** Clinical observations on 3,009 cases of ciguatera (fish poisoning) in the South Pacific, *Am. J. Trop. Med. Hyg.*, 28, 1067, 1979.
39. **Drewe, R.,** Death in paradise, *The Bulletin* (Australian Consolidated Press), p. 22, July 7, 1981.
40. **Lewis, R. J. and R. E.,** Occurrence of a ciguatoxin-like substance in the Spanish mackeral (*Scombermorus commersoni*), *Toxicon*, 21, 19, 1983.
41. **Lewis, R. J. and Endean, R.,** Ciguatera from the flesh and viscera of the barracuda, *Sphraena jello*, *Toxicon*, 22, 805, 1984.
42. **Flowers, A. E.,** The Effects of Ciguatera on Teleost Nerves, Master of Applied Science Thesis, Queensland University of Technology, Brisbane, 1989.
43. **Gillespie, N., Lewis, R., Burke, J., and Holmes, M.,** The significance of the absence of ciguatoxin in a wild population of *G. toxicus*, in *Proc. Fifth Intl. Coral Reef Cong.*, Antenne Museum-EPHE, Moorea, French Polynesia, 1985, 437.
44. **Holmes, M., Lewis, R., Gillespie, N., Fifoot, A., and Street, R.,** The absence of ciguatoxin on laboratory cultures of Australian and French Polynesian strains of *Gambierdiscus toxicus*, *Proc. Third Intl. Phycol. Cong.*, 18, 1988.
45. **Lewis, R. J. and Endean, R.,** Purification of ciguatoxin-like material from *Scombermorus commersoni* and its effects on the rat phrenic nerve diaphram, *Toxicon*, Supplement 3, 249, 1983.
46. **Lewis, R. J. and Endean, R.,** Mode of action of ciguatoxin from the Spanish mackerel, *Scombermorus commersoni* on the guinea-pig ileum and vas deferens, *J. Pharmacol. Exp. Therap.*, 228, 756, 1984.
47. **Lewis, R. J. and Endean, R.,** Direct and indirect effects of ciguatoxin on guinea-pig atria and papillary muscles, *Naunyn-Schmiedeberg's Arch. Pharmacol.*, 334, 313, 1986.
48. **Lewis, R. J.,** The cardiotoxic effects of ciguatoxin, in *Toxic Dinoflagellates*, Anderson, D. M., White, A., and Baden, D. G., Eds., Elsevier Science, Amsterdam, 1985, 379.
49. **Lewis, R. J.,** Interaction between ciguatoxin and local anaesthetics on the guinea-pig left atria, *Toxicon*, 23, 588, 1985.
50. **Flowers, A. E., Capra, M. F., and Cameron, J.,** The effects of ciguatoxin on nerve conduction parameters in teleost fish, in *Progress in Venom and Toxin Research*, Gopalakrishnakone, P. and Tan, C. K., Eds., First Asia-Pacific Congress on Animal, Plant and Microbial Toxins, Singapore, 1987, 411.
51. **Capra, M. F., Flowers, A. E., and Cameron, J.,** The effect of ciguatoxin on the rate of Na^+ efflux in unmyelinated olfactory nerves of teleosts, in *Progress in Venom and Toxin Research*, Gopalakrishnakone, P. and Tan, C. K., Eds., First Asia-Pacific Congress on Animal, Plant and Microbial Toxins, Singapore, 1987, 418.
52. **Lewis, R. J.,** Negative inotropic and arrhythmic effects of high doses of ciguatoxin on guinea-pig atria and papillary muscles, *Toxicon*, 26, 639, 1988.
53. **Lewis, R. J.,** Mannitol reverses the action of ciguatoxin *in vitro*, *Proc. Aust. Physiol. Pharmacol. Soc.*, 19, 237, 1988.
54. **Capra, M. F., Cameron, J., Flowers, A. E., Blanton, C. G., and Hahn, S. T.,** The effects of ciguatoxin on teleosts, *Proc., Sixth Intl. Coral Reef Symp.*, 3, 37, 1988.
55. **Allsop, J. L., Martinini, L., Lebris, H., Pollard, J., Walsh, J., and Hodgekinson, S.,** Les manifestations neurologiques de la ciguatera, *Rev. Neurol.* (Paris), 142, 590, 1986.
56. **Coombe, I. F., Capra, M. F., Flowers, A. E., and Cameron, J.,** Pathological changes in the mammalian gut following administration of ciguatoxin, in *Progress in Venom and Toxin Research*, Gopalakrishnakone, P. and Tan, C. K., Eds., First Asia-Pacific Congress on Animal, Plant and Microbial Toxins, Singapore, 1987, 405.
57. **Gillespie, N. C., Holmes, M. J., Burke, J. B., and Doley, J.,** Distribution and periodicity of *Gambierdiscus toxicus* in Queensland, Australia, in *Toxic Dinoflagellates*, Anderson, D. M., White, A., and Baden, D. G., Eds., Elsevier Science, New York, 1985, 183.
58. **Lewis, R. J., Gillespie, N. C., Burke, J. B., Holmes, M. J., Keys, A., and Fifoot, A.,** Ciguatoxin levels in fish in relation to population densities of *Gambierdiscus toxicus*, in *Aust. Mar. Sci. Assoc. Aust. Physical Oceanogr. Joint Conf.*, Marsh, H. and Heron, M. L., Eds., 1987, 36.

Chapter 5

EXTRACTION METHODS FOR MARINE TOXINS

Mark Jacyno and Donald M. Miller

TABLE OF CONTENTS

I. INTRODUCTION

A CDC (Center for Disease Control) report for 1972 to 1977 lists that marine-food-borne intoxications are responsible for 12.1% of all the reported food-borne disease outbreaks. However, one must keep in mind the fact that only 20% of the intoxications by dinoflagellate-tainted meat are reported, yet many people receive minute doses, resulting only in gastrointestinal disturbances, which are usually treated without the help of a physician. Diarrhetic (=diarrheic) shellfish poisoning (DSP), paralytic shellfish poisoning (PSP), neurotoxic shellfish poisoning (NSP), surf-borne respiratory inflammation, ciguatoxin (CTX), maitotoxin (MTX), scaritoxin, okadaic acid, hemolysins, icthyotoxins, and saxitoxin (STX) have all been traced back to dinoflagellate progenitors. Involved are 15 different genera, and of these 15 genera, 43 species of dinoflagellates have been found to be toxic, to date. Toxic dinoflagellates are benthic and epiphytic organisms that show no seasonal dependency for blooms. They inhabit coral reefs and lagoons associated with reefs due to the availability of preferred environmental conditions such as salinity, depth, light, temperature, and the continual presence of macroalgae.

The actual costs of a bout with dinoflagellate toxin intoxication have not been specifically published, however, the economic impact from one Canadian incident was documented. The average cost per case was $1860.[1] Hospitalization was determined as the greatest expense. It is assumed that up to 50,000 cases of ciguatera intoxication occur annually. There have been up to 3000 cases reported in the U.S., mainly in Hawaii and Florida. An additional $10,000,000 is lost annually to the Florida, Caribbean, and Hawaiian fishing industries due to fish bans and adverse publicity.[2] The annual cost of the PSP control program averages about one million dollars, and it is obvious that a good deal of money goes into monitoring and testing. From 1971 to 1977, 12 outbreaks and 68 cases of PSP were reported in the U.S. The source of intoxication were mainly clams. Also, in most of the cases the shellfish were caught and eaten at home; commercial distribution only accounted for two outbreaks. Illness usually occurs minutes to hours after ingestion and lasts hours to weeks. Symptoms include sensory abnormalities, cranial nerve dysfunction, gastrointestinal inflammation, and, at times, respiratory failure. Public health officials consider any detectable levels of *Gymnodinium breve* toxins per 100 g of shellfish meat as unfit for human consumption. As of now, Florida is the only state with a routine PSP surveillance. California, Washington, Alaska, Maine, Massachusetts, Hawaii, and Canada also have some experience in PSP surveillance.

All of this information points to one conclusion — the need for the development of assay systems that will prevent tainted food from reaching consumers. Purification/characterization of the "dinotoxins" will also lead to an understanding of the mode of action of these compounds and some viable modes of treatment for those who do become intoxicated.

In most cases the extraction of a particular toxin begins by trial and error, involving a lipid-water separation or some other variant. Later more sophisticated changes are made in the extraction scheme, and usually a bioassay is utilized to determine which fractions are toxic. Finally, enough of the toxin is separated for some structural determinations to be made. After this, the knowledge of the toxin and its biologic actions becomes logarithmic. For some of the toxins implicated in the ciguatera syndrome, the structures are known; for others, like ciguatera and maitotoxin, while conflicting first approximations have been proposed, we are still anticipating the structures. This chapter summarizes the available literature on the separation of ciguatera-type toxins.

II. DIARRHETIC SHELLFISH POISONING

DSP is one of the many forms of intoxications resulting from the ingestion of foods contaminated by dinoflagellate toxins. The symptoms of DSP are mainly gastrointestinal and include diarrhea, nausea, cramps, chills, and weakness. The symptoms occur within 4 h and can last up to 3 d, with no after effects or relapses.[3] No fatalities have been reported, but worldwide distribution of the dinoflagellates implicated in this syndrome make DSP a serious health and economic threat.

The dinoflagellates implicated as causative in the DSP syndrome are *Dinophysis fortii* and *D. accumulata*.[4] Other dinoflagellates that produce similar toxins are *Prorocentrum lima*, *P. concavum*, *Amphidinium carterii*, *A. klebsii*, and *Ostreopsis siamensis*.[5] The dinophysistoxins (DTXs), are polyether compounds that are all structurally related to okadaic acid, a C38 polyether fatty acid.[3]

DTX_1 was the first of the DSP toxins to be isolated, and was extracted from mussels. The structure of DTX_1 has been characterized and identified as 35-(S)-methyl okadaic acid. To date $DTX_{1\text{-}3}$, and the pectenotoxins$_{1\text{-}5}$ have been isolated from *D. fortii* and contaminated shellfish, namely, *Mytilus edulis*, *Patinopectin yessonusis*, *Tapes japonica*, and *Gomphina melanegis*.[3]

A. EXTRACTION FROM SHELLFISH

Shellfish suspected of being contaminated by DTX's can be extracted in the following manner. The digestive gland (hepatopancreas) is removed from the shellfish and extracted with acetone at room temperature. The acetone is evaporated off, and the residue is diluted up with water and extracted with diethyl ether.[3]

B. EXTRACTION FROM CELLS

Collected or cultured *D. fortii* or *D. accumulata* are extracted with methanol and acetone three times. The combined extracts are subjected to evaporation and resuspended in water. The aqueous solution is then extracted with diethyl ether.[3] The extract is then chromatographed in the same fashion as the mussel extracts.

C. CHROMATOGRAPHY

The ether-soluble residue is loaded on to a silicic acid column and eluted with benzene to benzene/methanol (9:1), then diethyl ether to diethyl ether/methanol (1:1). The toxic fraction is then further partitioned on a Sephadex LH-20 column using benzene/methanol (1:1). In this system, sample fractions are 10 ml in volume, with DTX_3 coming off the column in fractions 24 to 26, and fractions 28 to 31 contain $DTX_{1\text{-}2}$ and the pectenotoxins.

DTX_3 is further purified on a Lichroprep RP-8 column using methanol/water (20:1), and then on a μBondapak C_{18} column using methanol/water (93:7). DTX_3 is a colorless solid with a

TABLE 1
Rf Values of Diarrhetic Shellfish Toxins

Toxin	Rf value
DTX_1	0.42
DTX_2	—
DTX_3	0.57
PTX_1	0.43
PTX_2	0.71
PTX_3	0.49
PTX_4	0.53
PTX_5	0.41

minimum lethal dose in mice (ip) of 500 μg/kg. DTX_3 has been identified as 7-O-acyldinophysistoxin$_1$ and has no UV absorbance above 220 nm.

DTX_3 is subject to degradation by acid or alkali conditions, and by exposure to the air. To decrease toxin loss, the initial silicic acid column should be washed out with dilute NaOH and then with water prior to activation at 110°C.[3]

The pectenotoxins are separated from DTX_1 on a Lichroprep RP-8 column using methanol/water (17:3). DTX_1 fractions are then applied to an alumina column and eluted using methylene chloride/methanol (9:1). This separates all remaining pectenotoxins from the more acidic DTX's. The DTX fractions are eluted from the alumina column with the following solvents: chloroform, chloroform/methanol (9:1), chloroform/methanol (1:1), methanol, and methanol/1% ammonium hydroxide (1:1). DTX_1 is a white amphorous solid with a minimum lethal dose in mice (ip) of 160 μg/kg. DTX_1 has been identified as 35-S-methyl okadaic acid $C_{45}H_{88}O_{12}$, with a UV max at 220 nm.[3,4,6]

The pectenotoxins (PTXs), recovered from the Lichroprep RP-8 column are reapplied using the following solvent system: acetonitrile/methanol/water (2:2:3). The toxic fractions are then applied to a Develosil column to separate the five pectenotoxins using methylene dichloride/methanol (98:2). PTX_1 is a white crystalline solid with a minimum lethal dose in mice (ip) of 250 μg/kg. PTX_1 has been identified as $C_{47}H_{70}O_{15}$, with a UV max at 235 nm.[3] PTX_2 is also a white solid, with a minimum lethal dose in mice (ip) of 260 μg/kg. PTX_2 has also been identified as 43-deoxypectenotoxin$_1$.[3]

DTX_2 and $PTX_{3\text{-}5}$ are recovered in such small quantities that chemical analysis has yet to identify these toxic moieties, however, DTX_2 appears to be a related structurally to DTX_1 and DTX_3 but is a more polar molecule.[7]

D. THIN-LAYER CHROMATOGRAPHY

The toxic extracts have also been separated on TLC plates precoated with silica gel 60. The Rf values for the toxic moieties are obtained using benzene/acetone/methanol/6 N acetic acid (150:80:19:1). The toxins are visualized by spraying the plates with 50% sulfuric acid and then heating (Table 1).[3]

E. GAS CHROMATOGRAPHY

Gas chromatographic analysis of DTX_1 can also be carried out, as the values for the purified toxin have been obtained and standardized. The analysis is done on a Hitachi 163 unit equipped with a hydrogen flame ionization detector. DTX_1 is trimethylsilated with TRISIL "Z" by heating at 70°C for 10 min. A glass column containing 2% OV-101 on a 60/80 mesh uniport H.P. Column temperature is maintained at 315°C and the flow rate of the nitrogen gas is 30 ml/min.[3]

III. HEMOLYSINS AND OTHER MISCELLANEOUS TOXINS

The dinoflagellates associated with hemolysins and other toxic moieties are *Prorocentrum*, *Ostreopsis*, and *Amphidinium*. Other dinoflagellates suspected of producing diarrhetic-like poisonings are *P. minimum* and *P. micans*.[8,9]

A. EXTRACTION FROM *PROROCENTRUM*

Prorocentrum lima or *P. concavum* cells are extracted at room temperature, six times in acetone and then six times in methanol. The combined extracts are concentrated by evaporation and diluted up with water. The aqueous solution is then extracted with diethyl ether three times and then with 1-butanol three times.[6]

B. CHROMATOGRAPHY

PL_3 is separated from PL_1 and PL_2 on a silicic acid column with chloroform containing an increasing ratio of methanol (9:1), and then on silica gel 60 using chloroform/methanol (1:1). The toxic fraction is then applied to a Toyopearl H-W-40 column with methanol/water (1:1). The toxic eluent is reapplied to a silica gel 60 column with chloroform/methanol/water (25:10:1). The toxic fraction is then purified on a Develosil ODS-5 column using a linear gradient of acetonitrile/0.05 N acetic acid (1:9 to 3:7).[6] PL_3 is an amphorous solid with a minimum lethal dose in mice (ip) of 400 µg/kg. PL_3 has been identified as $C_{56}H_{85}NO_{12}$ with a UV max at 235 nm.

PL_2 is separated from PL_1 by using a basic alumina oxide column with the following solvent system: chloroform, chloroform/methanol (9:1) (PL_1 fraction elutes at this time), chloroform/methanol (1:1); methanol, and methanol/water (1:1). PL_2 is further purified by gel permeation on Sephadex LH-20 with chloroform/methanol (2:1). The final stage in the purification of PL_2 involves reverse-phase conditions and so is carried out on a Lichroprep RP-2 with methanol/water (3:1) at a rate of 1.0 ml/min. The toxic eluent is then chromatographed on a Develosil ODS column with methanol/water at 0.5 ml/min. PL_2 makes up the major toxic component in this extraction technique. PL_2 is a white crystalline solid with a minimum lethal dose in mice (ip) of 200 µg/kg. PL_1 is recovered in very small amounts and is believed to be a mixture of diol ester derivatives of okadaic acid.[6]

C. THIN-LAYER CHROMATOGRAPHY

The toxic moiety PL_2 from *Prorocentrum* can be separated on TLC plates using the following system. Crude extract or the purified PL_2 fraction is applied to plates precoated with silica gel 60 and one of two solvent systems may be employed: (1) chloroform/methanol/6 N acetic acid (80:20:1) or (2) chloroform/methanol/6 N acetic acid (90:9.5:0.5). Spots are visualized by spraying with 50% sulfuric acid in methanol and charring; the system 1 Rf of PL_2 is 0.48, and in system 2 the Rf is 0.53.[6]

D. GAS CHROMATOGRAPHY

Okadaic acids isolated from *Prorocentrum* (PL_2) are converted to trimethylsilyl derivatives by heating in TRISIL "Z" at 70°C for 10 min. These methyl derivatives can then be chromatographed on a Hitachi 163 G.C. unit equipped with a hydrogen flame ionization detector. The column is packed with 2% silicone OV-101 on a 60/80 mesh uniport H.P.[6]

E. EXTRACTION FROM *AMPHIDINIUM*

Cultured or collected cells of *Amphidinium carterii* or *A. klebsii*, are extracted with methanol at room temperature, concentrated by evaporation, resuspended in water, and then extracted with diethyl ether. The aqueous fraction is further extracted with 1-butanol, and both the ether fraction and the 1-butanol fraction are concentrated.[9]

F. CHROMATOGRAPHY

The dinoflagellate *Amphidinium* produces five hemolysins (HLs) of various potencies. $HL_{1\text{-}2}$ are separated from $HL_{3\text{-}5}$ on a silicic acid column using chloroform/methanol in a stepwise fashion. The toxic fractions are then applied to an ODS Q-3 column and $HL_{1\text{-}2}$ are eluted with methanol/water (9:1). $HL_{3\text{-}5}$ are further purified on a Toyopearl 40 column using methanol/water in a stepwise fashion.

$HL_{1\text{-}2}$ are the most abundant toxic components produced by *Amphidinium*. These compounds have been characterized as the following molecules: HL_1 is 0-β-D-galactopyranosyl(1-1)-3-0-octadecatetraenoyl-D-glycerol and HL_2 is 0-α-D-galactosyl-(1-6)-0-β-D-galactopyranosyl(1-1)-3-0-octadecatetraenoyl-D-glycerol. These compounds have been identified as intermediate metabolites of photosynthetic metabolism. HL_1 possesses 80% of the hemolytic activity of commercial saponin, while the structurally similar HL_2 only possesses 25% of the hemolytic activity of commercial saponin.

$HL_{3\text{-}5}$ appear to be structurally different from the galacto-sugar structures of $HL_{1\text{-}2}$. As the recovered quantities of these hemolytic fractions are so minute, only partial characterization has been accomplished. These fractions possess the following hemolytic activity as compared with commercial saponin: HL_3 — 100%, HL_4 — 9%, HL_5 — 2%.[9]

G. EXTRACTION FROM *OSTREOPSIS*

Little work has been done on the characterization of the toxins present in the dinoflagellate genus *Ostreopsis*. Extracts from *Osteropsis lenticularis*, *O. ovata*, and *O. siamensis* have all demonstrated toxic activity.[5,9-11]

Cultured *Ostreopsis* cells are dried, and then crushed and sonicated in methanol. The methanol extract is evaporated and partitioned with diethyl ether and water. This results in two toxic fractions, one water soluble and one ether soluble.[11]

The ether-soluble extract is evaporated to dryness and partitioned between hexane and aqueous methanol. The toxic methanolic fraction is dried and resuspended in acetone. The insoluble precipitate is collected, dried, and resuspended in methanol. Mouse bioassays of the crude ether-soluble fraction yielded an LD_{50} of 0.33 mg/kg mouse.[11]

The water-soluble extract is extracted with N-butanol and the water is discarded. The N-butanol fraction is then evaporated to dryness and extracted with acetone. The acetone- insoluble precipitate is collected, dried, and resuspended in methanol. Mouse bioassays of the crude water-soluble fraction yielded an LD_{50} of 0.10 mg/kg mouse.[11]

A study by Yasumoto[9] on the toxicity of dinoflagellates cultured from endemic South Pacific regions included cultured *Ostreopsis* cells, which were extracted in the following manner. Cells are extracted in boiling methanol, the methanol is evaporated off, and the residue is resuspended in water and extracted with diethyl ether two times and then with 1-butanol three times.[5] This extraction procedure produces three toxic fractions, water soluble, 1-butanol soluble, and diethyl ether soluble. At this point Yasumoto's work concentrated on preliminary toxicity studies and did not include further purification.

H. CHROMATOGRAPHY

The water-soluble toxic fraction can be further purified by evaporating the fraction to dryness and then redissolving it in methanol. This induces the formation of crystals, and the crystals are removed (crystals toxic to mice at 5.2 μg/mouse). The soluble portion of the water-soluble fraction is then applied to a C18 column with acetone as the mobile phase. This results in three fractions, and a fourth is collected off the column using methanol as the mobile phase. The second fraction possessed the most activity, 0.032 mg/kg mouse; this fraction has been designated ostreotoxin 1 (OTX_1).[11] The toxic activity falls off significantly in fraction 1 and fraction 3, indicating that the activity there may be carry over from the area of toxic activity in the second fraction. OTX_1 also exhibited an irreversible effect on isolated guinea-pig ileum preparations, but appears to affect the ileum in a manner that is different from maitotoxin. Toxic effects in mice also significantly differed from that of maitotoxin, especially in the observation period that followed survival of the LD_{50}. Survivors of OTX_1 LD_{50} exhibited adverse signs throughout and after the 48-h observation period. Survivors of MTX LD_{50} typically did not exhibit adverse reactions or signs after the initial 24 h.[11]

IV. BREVETOXINS

The dinoflagellate *Ptychodiscus brevis* is the progenitor of the red tide toxins, or brevetoxins. The *breve* toxins were named after *Gymnodinium breve*, the first of the dinoflagellates of this genus to be cultured successfully. These extracts from large-scale cultures of this organism led to the first purification scheme for this novel toxin. Brevetoxins are linear polyether compounds that are responsible for massive fish kills and human intoxications. Extracts were purified by HPLC and flash chromatography. Initially a series of toxins were isolated from cultures of the organisms: ichthyotoxic, neurotoxic, and hemolytic moieties, and a phosphorus-containing toxin of unrelated structure. Upon obtaining a crystalline toxin, Lin[12] in 1981 was able to establish the structure of the major component of the brevetoxins, brevetoxin B. These studies were followed by comparisons with NMR data that helped confirm the structure.[13] The brevetoxins are oxygenated polyether compounds, an unprecedented structure derived from a partially methylated carbon chain with an enal and a conjugated lactone terminal. This compound (BTX-B) has a molecular formula of $C_{50}H_{70}O_{14}$ (molecular weight of 894).[14] There have been six brevetoxins identified to date; these are BTX-A, BTX-B, BTX-C, GB-4, GB-5, and GB-6. BTX-A, BTX-B, BTX-C, GB-5, and GB-6 are the polyether compounds, and GB-4 is a novel phosphorus-containing toxin. GB-5 has only been collected in minute quantities and is a derivative of BTX-B.

The brevetoxins appear to cause many toxic effects. Hemolytic activity appears to be the most frequently associated action. An LD_{50} of 250 μg/kg has been reported in mice. Sasner[15] reported that the toxin produced neuromuscular blockade, and Padilla[16] reported induction of repetitive firing in the squid giant axon after applications of very small doses (0.005 μg/ml). From these reports and others, Risk[17] proposed that the brevetoxins undergo multivalent binding on excitable membranes near Na^+ channels and that the toxic effect is activation of Na^+ channels at resting potentials. Baden[18] also reported that the brevetoxins were highly cytotoxic. The brevetoxins are much more lipophilic than the saxitoxins, but poisonings in humans appear to be milder than exposure to saxitoxin. Neurotoxic symptoms include sensory abnormalities, diarrhea, and at higher doses, cardiac arrhythmias and acute apnea.[19]

Brevetoxin symptoms in humans occur about 30 to 60 min after ingestion. Symptoms include dizziness, tingling sensations in the extremities, dilated pupils, hot-cold reversals, cranial nerve dysfunction, and gastrointestinal disturbances, namely, vomiting and diarrhea. These symptoms usually last for 3 to 4 d, depending on the dose ingested. There have not been any human fatalities associated with the brevetoxins; a dose of 10,000 MU/kg can cause illness in humans.[14] Brevetoxins can accumulate in shellfish and in fish by direct or indirect means.[20] One interesting difference, though, is that the shellfish seem equally susceptible to the brevetoxins but tolerant of the saxitoxins.

A. EXTRACTION

Cultured *P. brevis* (*Gymnodinium*) cells are extracted with chloroform.[20] Extractions of cultured *Ptychodiscus* have also been successful using water acidified to pH 5.5 and diethyl ether.[12] However, in a more recent study, cells were extracted with methylene chloride, and the extract was then partitioned between petroleum ether and 90% methanol.[21]

B. CHROMATOGRAPHY

The methanolic extract of Shimuzu's method is loaded onto a silica oxide column and eluted with the following solvent system: methylene chloride/benzene/methanol (40:5:1) and then with methylene chloride/ethyl acetate/methanol (50:3:0.1). Brevetoxin-B (BTX-B) is removed at this point by crystallization in acetonitrile. Evaporation of the methanol or of acetonitrile allows BTX-B to come out of solution and form stout crystals. BTX-A is further purified by HPLC on silica oxide using isooctane/99% isopropyl alcohol (4:1). BTX-A forms needlelike crystals. BTX-B is also further purified by HPLC on a silica oxide column using isooctane/99% isopropyl alcohol (4:1). BTX-A and BTX-B are both icthyotoxic and neurotoxic. BTX-A is the most potent of these toxins and has been found to bind and interact with Na^+ channels on excitable membranes, causing a sustained depolarization.

Lin's method[12] involves repeated flash chromatography, and produces three fractions BTX-A, BTX-B, and BTX-C. BTX-B is then crystallized out of solution, as in Shimuzu's method.[21]

BTX-A is the most potent of the toxins recovered from *P. brevis*, with an LD_{50} in guppies of 4 μg/ml.[21] BTX-A forms crystals that are prism shaped with an mp of 197°C and has the molecular formula $C_{49}H_{70}O_{13}$.

BTX-B is the most prevalent toxin obtained yieldwise and has an LD_{50} in guppies of 16 μg/ml. BTX-B forms stout acicula crystals that have an mp of 295°C. BTX-B has the molecular formula $C_{50}H_{70}O_{14}$, with a weak UV max at 208 nm.

BTX-C is an unstable compound that tends to decompose with time once it has been isolated from the other compounds present in the crude extract. This toxic moiety has an LD_{50} in guppies of 30 μg/ml. BTX-C forms crystals with a mp of 291°C and has a UV max at 280 nm. BTX-C has the molecular formula $C_{49}H_{69}ClO_{14}$.

GB-4 is a phosphorous-containing compound with icthyotoxic activity. GB-4 has been isolated by extraction of cells in chloroform, then hexane, next benzene, and finally in chloroform again. This extract is applied to a 5-μm silica column and eluted with benzene/ethyl acetate (1:1) as the mobile phase and monitored at 280 nm.[22] GB-4 has an LD_{50} of 90 μg/ml in guppies. GB-4 has an mp of 82°C, and when the chloroform-soluble is recrystallized with benzene, GB-4 forms colorless needles. This compound has the formula $C_{10}H_{22}N_3O_3PS$ and has a UV max of 280 nm.

GB-5 makes up a minor component of the total toxin yield and elutes slightly ahead of BTX-B component in normal-phase chromatography on a silica oxide column using benzene/ethyl acetate (1:3) as the mobile phase. Any remaining BTX-B can be removed by a crystallization step, as noted above. The GB-5 can then be further purified by preparative TLC. GB-5 is an amphorous solid identified as 37-O-acetate of BTX-B.

GB-6 is another minor component that can also be isolated by preparative TLC. GB-6 is a crystalline solid that forms fine needles. This component has an LD_{50} in guppies of 75 μg/ml. GB-6 has an mp of 295°C and the molecular formula $C_{50}H_{70}O_{15}$.

C. THIN-LAYER CHROMATOGRAPHY

TLC of the BTXs is performed on silica oxide plates. BTX-B uses the solvent system benzene/ethyl acetate (1:3), resulting in an Rf value of 0.42. GB-5 uses the solvent system hexane/acetone (5:1). GB-6 also uses benzene/ethyl acetate, but in a (1:1) ratio. The Rf value for GB-6 in this system is 0.37.[23] BTX-A is developed using acetone/petroleum ether (30:70) on a plate with an inorganic fluorescence indicator and then visualized at 254 nm with a UV detector, producing an Rf value of 0.26.[24]

References have been made of TLC separations of BTX-C, however, the solvent system and Rf values have not been provided in the two papers concerning its structure (Chou[25] and Golik[26]). There is no information concerning the TLC solvent system or Rf factors for GB-4.

V. SAXITOXINS

Saxitoxins or PSP toxins were the first dinoflagellate toxins to be characterized. The dinoflagellates linked to the PSP syndrome are as follows: *Gonyaulax tamerensis*, *G. catenella*, *G. excavata*, (*Protogonyaulax*), *Pyrodinium bahamense*, *Gynmodinium catenatum*, and *Alexandrium affine*. To date 13 toxic moieties have been identified and characterized from these organisms.[7] There are also a large number of shellfish, xanthid crabs, marine gastropods, and finfish that regularly become tainted with some, if not all, of these toxic compounds during blooms of these dinoflagellates.[27]

The occurrence of this form of intoxication is widespread in tropical and temperate marine waters. Studies on cultured strains of *Gonyaulax* collected from different regions indicated that some strains varied widely in toxicity, with some being virtually nontoxic.[28] Although toxic and nontoxic species can coexist,[29] the generality has been noted that strains in temperate regions are much more virulent than tropical strains. Salinity has also been found to influence toxicity. The toxins produced by *Gonyaulax* are (1) saxitoxin, (2) neosaxitoxin, and (3) smaller amounts of the gonyautoxins 1-5 and the carbamoyl and sulfamate toxins.[8] Saxitoxin was first isolated from Alaskan butter clams in 1960 by Schantz.[30] Cultures of *Gonyaulax*, however, only produced small amounts of saxitoxin and instead produced more neosaxitoxin, and also small amounts of the gonyautoxins. Shimizu[31] worked out a purification scheme for isolation of the different toxins from mass cultures of the organism. Separation of the toxins was accomplished with Sephadex G-15 columns, as they are strongly basic and would elute in an increasing acetic-acid gradient. An interesting finding by Hall[32] was that the gonyautoxins could be converted to saxitoxin by treatment with acid. The gonyautoxins are also very unstable and undergo solvolysis and subsequent degradation after being separated.

Neosaxitoxin acts like saxitoxin and is structurally related to saxitoxin, as it only carries one guanidium-charged group. Also, reduction of neosaxitoxin with various agents leads to the formation of saxitoxin. There is growing evidence that a similar reaction may take place inside organisms; this could explain the larger amount of saxitoxin present compared to the gonyautoxins and neosaxitoxin.[8] The most stable of the purified toxins is saxitoxin. Saxitoxin is a very hydrophilic substituted tetrahydropurine base molecular formula $C_{10}H_{17}N_7O_4$ (molecular weight of 299). A hydrated ketone group at position 12 of the five-membered ring is essential for toxic activity; the molecule also contains two highly charged guanidium groups.[33]

Saxitoxin is a unique compound in that it is a very specific neurotoxin. This molecule binds with very high affinity to sodium channels in excitable tissues, blocking them, and thus blocking the production of action potentials. As this toxin is so specific in its action, it has become a neurophysiologic tool.[34]

Ingestion of saxitoxin-tainted shellfish results in neuromuscular paralysis, with death occurring from paralysis of respiratory muscles. The toxin produces its effects quickly, and as of yet there is no antidote. Strangely, the neurons of many shellfish appear to be very resistant to this toxin. Toxicity of this compound is measured in mouse units (MU), or the amount of toxin needed to kill a 20-g mouse in 15 min. Purified STX has a toxicity of 5500 MU/mg.[33]

PSP symptoms in humans occur about 30 min after ingestion. Symptoms include paresthesia or a burning/tingling sensation on the tongue, lips, and face, which gradually progresses to the neck, arms, legs, fingers, and toes. This later changes to numbness, and voluntary movements become difficult. Paralysis occurs, resulting in ataxia, loss of coordination, a constrictive sensation in the throat, and incoherent speech. Other symptoms include lightheadedness, weakness, dizziness, headache, salivation, intense thirst, and temporary blindness; gastrointestinal disturbances are not common. Following a toxic dose (estimated at 5000 to 20,000 MU), paralysis of the respiratory muscles can occur, resulting in respiratory arrest. There is no antidote, but treatment of symptoms has been successful in some cases. The mortality rate is about 15%.

TABLE 2
Nomenclature for Saxitoxin Group of Toxins

Carbamate toxins	Sulfamate toxins	Decarbamate toxins
STX	B_1	$dcGTX_3$
NeoSTX	B_2	$dcGTX_2$
GTX_1	C_3	
GTX_2	C_1	
GTX_3	C_2	
GTX_4	C_4	

A. EXTRACTION FROM DINOFLAGELLATES

Cells are centrifuged 1700 **xg** for 3 min at room temperature and then extracted with 0.05 M acetic acid. The cells are then frozen and thawed three times to lyse the cells and again centifuged at 1700 × *g* for 3 min. The supernant is filtered through a 0.45-μm filter and is ready for analysis.

B. EXTRACTION FROM SHELLFISH

The hepatopancreas (or in the case of *Saxidomus giganteus*, the siphon) is removed from the shellfish and blended in a Waring blender for 2 min in 0.1 N HCL. The extract is lypholized and resuspended in water. The sample is then centrifuged at 1000 × *g* and the supernatant is passed through an ultrafiltration membrane with a 10,000-D cutoff.

A portion of the extract can then be adjusted to 0.2 N HCL and heated to 100°C for 5 h to hydrolyze the sulfocarbamoyl toxins to their carbamate forms.

C. CHROMATOGRAPHY

Chromatography of the PSP toxins involves the use of an ion interaction column and detection of the resolved toxins by fluorescence derived from postcolumn oxidation with periodate.

Samples are loaded on a Hamilton PRP-1 10-μm column, which is equilibrated and heated to 35°C. The mobile phase consists of two solvent systems:

1. Water with 1.5 mM hexane and heptane sulfonate and 1.5 mM ammonium phosphate (PO_4), at pH 6.7
2. 25% acetonitrile with 1.5 mM hexane and heptane sulfonate, and 6.5 mM ammonium phosphate (PO_4), at pH 7.0

Gradient conditions are as follows, 0 to 11 min 100%A, 11 to 17 min 70%A and 30%B, 17 to 17.5 min 10%A and 90%B, 17.5 to 19 min 100%B, and 19 min+ 100%A.

The postcolumn reaction system consists of two pumps. The pump A reservoir contains 5 mM periodate in 0.1 M sodium phosphate at pH 7.8. The reaction is carried out in 1.0-ml coil held at 90°C at a flow rate of 0.5 ml/min. The pump B reservoir contains 0.75 M nitric acid at a flow rate of 0.3 ml/min.[28,35]

PSP toxins resolved in this manner are listed in Table 2.

D. THIN-LAYER CHROMATOGRAPHY

STX and decarbamoyl-STX comigrated during attempts to resolve these compounds on both silica gel G, plates of silica gel 60, and carboxymethyl cellulose plates. Seven different solvent systems were employed, but all failed to resolve the two moieties.[36] However, Oshima[37] reported the following Rf values for other PSP toxins on silica gel 60 plates developed in pyridine/ethyl acetate/acetic acid/water (75:25:30:15), as indicated in Table 3.

TABLE 3
Rf Values for Saxitoxins

Toxin	Rf value
STX	0.64
NeoSTX	0.72
GTX_1	0.92
GTX_2	0.82
GTX_3	0.74
GTX_4	0.84
GTX_5	0.58

TABLE 4
Characteristics of Saxitoxins

Toxin	Rf value	Color
STX (decarbomyl)	1.0	Blue
STX	0.89	Blue
GTX_2	0.58	Blue
NeoSTX (decarbomyl)	0.5	Yellow/green
NeoSTX	0.5	Yellow/green
GTX_3	0.39	Blue
GTX_5	0.32	Blue
GTX_1	0.26	Yellow/green
GTX_4	0.15	Yellow/green

E. ELECTROPHORESIS OF PSP TOXINS

Electrophoretic analysis of crude extracts from PSP dinoflagellates is performed on cellulose acetate strips, 2.56 × 30.72 cm, on a Thomas model 20 electrophoresis cabinet with a model 21 power supply. Samples are run for 3 h at 200 V (constant) and a 0.5 mA/strip. Electrolyte buffer consisted of 0.08 Tris acidified to pH 8.7 with HCL.

All of the toxic moieties migrate toward the cathode. NeoSTX and its acid hydrolysis product comigrate. GTX_2 also travels very close to NeoSTX. GTX_4 migrates very slowly from the origin, and GTX_5 travels very close to GTX_3 and GTX_1. The plates must be run for 3 h or GTX_5, GTX_4, and the acid hydrolysis products of STX and NeoSTX will not be resolved.[38]

Compounds and their relative mobilities are listed in Table 4.

VI. CIGUATERA-TYPE TOXINS: INTRODUCTION

Ciguatera-type toxins, exemplified by ciguatoxin and maitotoxin, have long plagued tropical and subtropical oceanic regions. This syndrome has generally been attributed to certain costal marine fishes. However, within the past decade a group of benthic dinoflagellates have been implicated as the causative agents of ciguatera.[9] Yasumoto found high levels of toxicity in samples of detritus collected from the surface of dead coral in the Gambier islands, as well as toxic samples recovered from the stomach contents of suspected ciguatoxic fish. Associated with the toxic samples were large numbers of dinoflagellates. The dinoflagellate was assigned the name *Diplopsalis adachi*.[39] However, it was later found that this dinoflagellate was in fact a new genus and was renamed *Gambierdiscus toxicus*.[40] This dinoflagellate is widely distributed in the Pacific, and to a lesser extent in the Atlantic.

In studies on the toxicity content of dinoflagellates, homogeneous samples of *G. toxicus* were obtained from detritus by seiving and decanting. This dinoflagellate attaches itself to algae in high numbers (as many as 500,000 cells per gram of algae). *G. toxicus* is presumed to be the dinoflagellate that produces ciguatoxin and maitotoxin. Toxin production varies during the different growth phases, and there is no evidence of toxin secretion/excretion into the culture medium.[10] Purified samples of these toxins given intraperitoneally to mice have resulted in death within 48 h at doses as low as 5 μg/kg.

The only definite producer of these compounds is *Gambierdiscus toxicus,*[10] however, *Prorocentrum concavum, Prorocentrum lima, Ostreopsis siamensis, Ostreopsis ovata*, and *Ostreopsis lenticularis* have also been implicated as possible sources.[5,10,11]

Intoxication by consumption of ciguatera-tainted fish leads to as many as 10,000 to 50,000 reported cases annually, and thus is responsible for the preponderance of seafood-related poisonings.[2] Although fatalities are rare, intoxicated individuals can become severely incapacitated and the neurologic symptoms have a tendency to reoccur sporadically years later. The symptomatology has been described in great detail in numerous publications.[2,41,42] The symptoms of intoxication are as follows: gastrointestinal inflammation/irritation, leading to diarrhea and causing dehydration to the point of cardiovascular and neurologic distress; severe pruritis; hot/cold reversal; tingling and numbness in extremities and mouth; and, in extreme cases, muscular paralysis and respiratory failure.[41] Neurologic symptoms can persist for months and can reoccur after recovery. The degree of toxicity can be appreciated from the minute quantities necessary for intoxication, 20 ng/kg being sufficient to induce severe intoxication in humans. One distinct feature of intoxication is the fact that effects vary from region to region; this phenomenon is partially due to different fish and different dinoflagellates endemic to each specific area. As of now, no specific treatment exists for ciguatera poisoning, however, some compounds, such as nifedipine and amitryptyline, may help to alleviate some of the symptoms,[43] and in a recent finding mannitol was found to also alleviate symptoms of intoxication.[44]

Despite many efforts over the past 20 years, the chemical composition of the ciguatera toxins have remained a mystery. The main factors behind this elusiveness are the difficulties in obtaining large samples of crude toxin, relative toxin instability during extraction and purification procedures, and the need for sensitive assays for each specific toxin.

As better extraction and purification techniques that increase toxin yield and purity become available, much of the conflicting data may be resolved. Quantities of isolated, pure samples can lead to thorough ^{1}H NMR investigation and highly specific bioassays that may help uncover each toxic fraction's mode of action. As of now, several extraction procedures exist; some investigators rely on viscera/flesh samples,[7,9,44-48] while some rely on cell culture extracts.[49-51] Of course, different investigators use different solvent/solvent partitioning methods as well. The purification step of choice is high-pressure liquid chromatography (HPLC), however, different investigators utilize different separation schemes.[7,46,51-54] This of course, only adds to the existing confusion, as similarities of purified toxins from different groups is at best questionable, due to a range of different sources, different solvent/solvent interactions, and different separation and collection techniques. Another disturbing feature of ciguatera-type toxins is that there is no assay for toxin purity, i.e., a sample may contain one or more forms of maitotoxin, ciguatoxin, and okadaic acid, and all in differing amounts, despite attempts to purify and isolate each toxic fraction.

VII. MAITOTOXIN

Initially isolated from surgeonfish by Yasumoto, maitotoxin is found only in fish viscera and cell culture extracts, but in large amounts, especially in *Gambierdiscus toxicus* cultures.[10] Maitotoxin has also been found to be associated with the benthic dinoflagellate *Prorocentrum lima*.[9,55] No chemical characterization for maitotoxin has been successful as of yet, however, an estimated molecular weight of 3300 amu has been proposed by Yasumoto.[9] Chemical analysis has revealed that the molecule contains no amino acid and no fatty acid moieties, as found in ciguatoxin. Maitotoxin is a hydrophylic compound that is soluble in methanol, ethanol, and water, and is highly polar.

It has been reported that maitotoxin acts as a Ca^{2+}-channel activator acting on voltage sensitive Ca^{2+} channels by increasing Ca^{2+} permeability across the cell membrane.[56-58] Maitotoxin is perhaps the most potent marine toxin (LD_{50} = 0.17 μg/kg in mice[45]) that acts in an irreversible manner on isolated ileum assays.[49,59]

A. EXTRACTION FROM DINOFLAGELLATES

The most thorough investigation into the chemical properties of maitotoxin was done by Yokoyama,[60] who obtained a colorless solid that was assumed to be pure by TLC. Yokoyama's method employs the following steps. Cultured *G. toxicus* is collected by filtration and extracted twice with methanol and twice with methanol/water (1:1) under reflux. The filtrates are combined and evaporated, with the residue being resuspended in methylene chloride. This is then extracted three times with an equal volume of methanol/water (4:1). The toxin extract is then concentrated under a vacuum to form an aqueous suspension that is extracted with butanol. The butanol is then evaporated off and the residue resuspended in chloroform/methanol (7:3); this makes up the crude extract.

B. CHROMATOGRAPHY

The crude extract is loaded onto a silica gel column (Mallinckrodt) that has been equilibrated with the chloroform/methanol (7:3) mixture. The column is washed with the same solvent mixture and then the toxin is eluted with chloroform/methanol (1:1). The toxic eluent is evaporated, redissolved in methanol/water (1:1), and loaded onto a C18 column (Fuji gel Q3). The column is washed successively with methanol/water 1:1, methanol/water 7:3, and finally with pure methanol. The toxic fraction elutes in the second solvent system (7:3) and is redissolved in acetonitrile/water (1:4), loaded on a Develosil C8 column, and eluted stepwise in the following fashion: acetonitrile/water 1:3, 3:7, 4:6, and 1:1. The toxic fraction elutes in the third solvent system (4:6) and is rechromatographed on Develosil C8 using acetonitrile/water (1:2). The toxic fraction (as revealed by bioassay) is further chromatographed on a Develosil TMS-5 column with methanol/acetonitrile (35:65). Eluents from the columns are monitored by a UV detector set at 225 nm. The bioassay used to determine the toxicity of column eluents is the mouse lethality test (ip). The resultant product is a colorless solid with a UV max of 230 nm and a LD_{50} in mice (ip) of 0.13 μg/kg.

C. EXTRACTION FROM FISH

Maitotoxin has been extracted from tainted fish.[61] Yasumoto found that specimens of *Ctenochaetus striatus* (surgeon fish) contained water and lipid-soluble toxins. Extraction of the water-soluble toxin (maitotoxin) was accomplished by mixing the viscera and gut contents of captured surgeon fishes with 70% and 96% ethanol. The ethanol is then concentrated, extracted with ether, and put into a cellophane dialysis bag. The material retained in the bag is then extracted with 1-butanol. An equal amount of ether is added to the 1-butanol fraction and extracted with water. The aqueous layer is then concentrated and acetone is added. The resulting precipitate is dissolved in a small amount of water, loaded onto a Sephadex G-100 column, and eluted with water. The crude toxic fraction elutes in a fast-moving band near the void volume.

D. CHROMATOGRAPHY

The fish extract is loaded onto a silicic acid column and eluted with chloroform/methanol (6:4). The toxic fraction collected is then subjected to gel filtration on a Sephadex G-25 column. The toxic fraction occurs just after the void volume and is then reapplied to a silicic acid column and eluted with 1-propanol/water (8:2). The toxic fraction is applied to a cellulose column and eluted with chloroform/methanol/water (5:15:1). The final product is a yellowish amphorous powder with an LD_{50} in mice (ip) of 15 mg/kg.

E. THIN-LAYER CHROMATOGRAPHY

Purified MTX (as per Yokoyama[60]) was developed on precoated plates of silica gel-60 with pentanol/pyridine/water (4:4:1) and visualized by charring the plates after spraying with sulfuric acid/methanol (1:1). In this solvent system MTX possesses an Rf of 0.43.

VIII. CIGUATOXIN

Initially isolated from red snapper and moray eel liver by Scheuer, ciguatoxin is found in fish viscera and musculature or in cell culture extracts of *Gambierdiscus toxicus,* but only in very minute quantities. Although no molecular structure for ciguatoxin has been established, ^1H NMR data suggest a molecular weight of 1111.7 amu.[46] The most probable conformation is an oxygenated long chain fatty acid with cyclic oxoether linkages. Ciguatoxin is soluble in methanol, ethanol, acetone, and 2-propanol, but not in benzene or water. Ciguatoxin also appears to be able to reversibly interconvert to a less polar form, referred to as *scaritoxin* by some, due to its long shape under appropriate conditions of basicity.[46] This interconversion may be facilitated within fish upon consumption (differing from species to species) or may be induced by purification techniques on certain basic chromatography columns.[48]

It has been reported that ciguatoxin acts as an Na^+ channel activator,[62] acting on voltage-sensitive Na^+ channels to increase Na^+ permeability across the cell membrane.[46,58] Ciguatoxin is also involved indirectly in norepinephrine release from adrenergic nerve terminals.[63] Ciguatoxin is a highly toxic hydrophobic compound (LD_{50} = 0.45 μg/kg in mice[46]) that acts in a reversible manner on isolated ileum assays.[64]

A. EXTRACTION FROM DINOFLAGELLATES

Extraction of ciguatoxin from cultured and/or wild *Gambierdiscus toxicus* has proven to be extremely difficult due to the minute amount of ciguatoxin produced by these organisms and the relative large amount of maitotoxin.[65] It appears that wild specimens accumulate more ciguatoxin than cultured specimens. Thus, most of the chemical work that has been done on ciguatoxin is on samples obtained from moray eel liver and viscera, and tainted reef fish. Past work by Tindall[10] and Miller,[53] and more recently by Legrand,[66] concentrated on purification of ciguatoxin from cultured dinoflagellates.

Extraction of cultured *G. toxicus* is accomplished by crushing the collected cells and then sonication in methanol at room temperature. The crude methanol extract is concentrated and extracted with ether/water (2:1) three times. This results in two toxic fractions, one ether soluble and one water soluble. The ether-soluble fraction is dried and extracted with hexane/aqueous methanol (1:2) three times. The methanol fraction is dried and is resuspended in warm acetone. The acetone is cooled to –20°C overnight, cold filtered, and the precipitate is collected and dried. The water-soluble fraction extracted with butanol/water (2:1) three times. The butanol fraction is dried and resuspended in warm acetone. This is cooled to –20°C overnight, cold filtered, and the precipitate is collected and dried.[53] Legrand's extraction method[66] involves the following procedures. Extract *G. toxicus* cells with acetone at room temperature and evaporate off the solvent. Resuspend residue in water and extract first with diethyl ether and then with 1-butanol, and evaporate off the solvent. Resuspend the residue in acetone and cool; this allows the maitotoxin to percipitate out of solution while the ciguatoxin remains soluble. The CTX fraction is applied to a Florisil column and eluted using the following gradient: hexane/acetone 4:1, acetone/methanol 9:1, and methanol. The toxic fraction (eluting in the 9:1 acetone/methanol) is subjected to reverse-phase chromatography on a Develosil ODS Lop column using an increasing aqueous methanol to methanol gradient. The toxic fraction (appearing in the 90% methanol range) is then purified by gel permeation chromatography on either a Sephadex LH-20 column or a Toyopearl HW-40 column using methanol and then methanol/water (85:15).

B. CHROMATOGRAPHY

Chromatography of crude extracts obtained by the method of Miller et al.[53] involves the following steps. The dried acetone percipitate is resuspended in methanol and applied to a silicic acid column and eluted with chloroform/methanol (1:1). The toxic fraction obtained is applied to an aluminum oxide column and eluted with methanol/water (1:1). The toxic fraction obtained is then chromatographed on Sephadex G-15 using water. The LD_{50} is 4.96 mg/kg in mice ip.[53]

Chromatography of crude extracts obtained by Legrand's extraction method are further purified on a Develosil ODS-7 column (8 × 250 mm) using a linear gradient starting with acetonitrile/water (85:15) to acetonitrile at a flow rate of 0.5 ml/min for 100 min. The toxic fractions come off the column at approximately 40, 75, and 80 min. Column eluents are monitored by a UV flow monitor set at 215 nm. Toxicity was assesed by mouse bioassay.

C. EXTRACTION FROM EELS

Ciguatoxin has been extracted from moray eel viscera *(Gymnothorax javanicus)*. The crude extract when chromatographically purified yields crystals that have an LD_{50} of 0.45 μg/kg (ip) in mice.[46] Eels are extracted in the method developed by Tachibana.[45] The viscera is extracted from captured eels, minced, and soaked in acetone. The acetone soluble material is then filtered and cooled to –20°C overnight. The solution is filtered and evaporated. The aqueous mixture is extracted with hexane and then backwashed with aqueous methanol. The methanol fraction is concentrated and saturated with NaCl, and then extracted with ethyl acetate. The ethyl acetate fraction is then dried with Na_2SO_4, filtered, and evaporated, yielding a brownish oil.

D. CHROMATOGRAPHY

Chromatography of eel extract is accomplished in the following fashion. The crude extract is loaded onto a BioSil-A column and eluted using a chloroform/methanol gradient. The toxic fraction recovered is loaded onto basic alumina and eluted with a chloroform/methanol/aqueous methanol gradient. This results in two toxic fractions, one polar and one less polar. The more polar fraction is recovered in much larger quantities than the less polar toxin; this may be an artifact created by the alumina column.[48] The more polar fraction is then applied to a Sephadex LH column and eluted with methylene chloride/methanol, and the toxic fraction is collected and rechromatographed. The toxic fraction is then applied to a C18 Hi-Flosil column and eluted with aqueous methanol. The toxic fraction recovered is then loaded into an HPLC Lichrosorb RP-18 column and eluted with aqueous methanol; this is repeated three times, yielding the purified ciguatoxin. The final HPLC trace on a C18 reverse-phase silica column produces a symmetrical peak, and when evaporated yields a colorless solid that is readily soluble in methanol, ethanol, and acetone. The CTX obtained by this procedure displays a UV absorbance at 215 nm. Proposed structures for CTX obtained by plasma desorption mass spectrometry and ^{1}H NMR are $C_{53}H_{77}NO_{24}$ or $C_{54}H_{78}O_{24}$, with a molecular weight of 1111.2 Da.[66]

E. EXTRACTION FROM FISH

Ciguatoxin has been extracted from the flesh of the fish, *Scomberomorus commersoni*.[47] The flesh of tainted fish is extracted with acetone in a Waring blender. The acetone-soluble material is stored at –18°C overnight. The acetone-soluble material is then evaporated, the pH is adjusted to 8, and the material is extracted with diethyl ether. The ether fraction is extracted with aqueous methanol. The methanol fraction is extracted with hexane. This procedure yields a crude methanol fraction that consists of a brownish oil.

F. CHROMATOGRAPHY

Chromatography of the crude fish extract is then applied to silicic acid 100-mesh column. The toxin is eluted with chloroform/methanol (9:1). The toxic fraction recovered is then chromatographed on DEAE-cellulose (acetate) column with chloroform/methanol (1:1). The toxic fraction is applied to a Sephadex LH-20 column and eluted with chloroform/methanol (2:1). The toxic fraction is rechromatographed on a Sephadex LH-20 column two times using 96% ethanol. The purified CTX is a clear oily material with an LD_{50} in mice (ip) of 0.72 mg/kg.

G. THIN-LAYER CHROMATOGRAPHY

Indelicato's method for TLC pigment analysis involves the following steps. Cultured *Gambierdiscus toxicus* cells are dried and then sonicated in acetone. The acetone extract is dried and resuspended in carbon disulfide. This extract is then spotted onto activated silica gel G plates. The plates are developed in hexane/acetone (6:4) in a sealed chamber.

TLC analysis of the crude ether-soluble material (CTX) by Dickey's method[49,54] involves the following procedure. Crude ether-soluble extract is applied to an activated silica gel G plate at a concentration of 0.4 mg. The plate is developed to 14 cm with chloroform/methanol/water (60:35:8), resulting in a good separation of the crude components. Upon acid-char treatment 16 components are resolved. The plate was then divided into eight zones, scraped, eluted, and assayed on mice at a concentration of 0.4 mg equivalents. Components appearing between Rfs 0.33 and 0.47, and 0.47 and 0.61 were found to be toxic by mouse bioassay. Both fractions exhibiting toxic activity co-chromatographed with green pigments.

H. DERIVATIZATION OF CIGUATOXINS FOR HPLC ANALYSIS

Some researchers have attempted to devise a fluorometric method for the detection of ciguateric toxins,[67] as the ciguatoxins appear to have poor UV and IR absorbances.[45] The method of Sick involves the following procedures. The crude methanolic extract from *Gambierdiscus toxicus* cells is semipurified by HPLC and oxidized to form derivatives. Periodic acid (0.065 M) and ammonium hydroxide (2.0 M) can be used to form mixtures of alkaline-oxidized derivatives. Samples and reagents are mixed for 1 min and maintained at a pH of 9.8. For HPLC analysis, the sample pH was adjusted to 5.0 with acetic acid to maximize the detection of the fluorescent derivatives. Elution off a cyano column is achieved using methanol/water (80:20) in a linear gradient run at a ramp rate of 4% per minute. Postcolumn derivatization is accomplished by using a system similar to that used in the analysis of the PSP toxins. Three reservoirs containing (1) periodic acid (0.065 M), (2) ammonium hydroxide (2.0 M), and (3) acetic acid (4.0 M) are connected to the postcolumn effluent line. A pump runs each reservoir, allowing reagents A and B and the column eluents to mix in a reaction coil (0.56 mm i.d. with an internal volume of 1.5 ml). The reaction coil is maintained at 50°C by using a water bath to ensure optimum derivatization of the column eluents. Pump C then mixes the acetic acid with the derivatives that come out of the reaction coil to lower the pH to 5.5 before the mobile phase enters the fluorometer, which is set at excitation and emission wavelengths of 340 and 410 nm, respectively. Derivatized toxin eluted from the detector at 18 to 20 min (flow rate of 1.8 ml/min). Comparisons of the detection limits, mouse bioassay vs. HPLC, show that the HPLC method is much more sensitive (0.81 MU for HPLC analysis vs. 9.70 MU for mouse time to death analysis).[67] Unfortunately, neither the parent toxic moieties nor the oxidation products formed in the derivatized *G. toxicus* extract have been identified.

IX. CONCLUSIONS

Many different toxins have been linked to dinoflagellate progenitors. These toxins show differing degrees of activity and affect different target "receptors". *Gambierdiscus toxicus*,[49,53,54,59] *Prorocentrum concavum*, *P. lima*, *Ostreopsis siamensis*, *O. ovata*,[9] *O. lenticularis*,[11] *Amphid-*

inium carteri, A. klebsii,[5,9] *Dinophysis fortii, D. accumulata,*[3] *Gonyaulax tamerensis, G. catenalla, G. excavata,*[27,32,37,68] *Gymnodinium catenatum,*[28] *Pyrodinium bahamense*, and *Ptychodiscus brevis*[20] all produce toxins that can kill mice. *Gambierdiscus toxicus, Amphidinium carteri, A. klebsii, Coolia monotis, Prorocentrum mexicanum,*[5,9] and *Ptychodiscus brevis*[16] all produce toxins with strong hemolytic activity.[5,9] *Prorocentrum concavum, Amphidinium carteri, A. klebsii,*[9] and *Ptychodiscus brevis*[69] also produce potent ichthyotoxins.

The literature surrounding extraction of dinoflagellate toxins and toxicity studies is confusing at best. Organisms, through reinvestigation, have been named and renamed so that now they can appear in the literature under two or three different names. *Gonyaulax* sp. changed to *Protogonyaulax* sp. and *Gymnodinium* sp. changed to *Ptychodiscus* sp.[70,71] Other problems involved with the isolation of dinoflagellate toxins are differences in the toxicity of flagellates from different regions, and even amongst differing strains from the same region.[29,72] Toxin production in dinoflagellates appears to be linked to some unkown factor, as toxin quality can be affected by culture techniques, resulting in a loss of production or even one or more of the toxic moieties.[10,73] This strangely enough can also occur in wild dinoflagellates, as some field studies indicate significant variation of toxin production amongst strains collected from the same area.[10,73] Another disturbing factor in the attempts to isolate dinoflagellate toxins is their tendency to undergo chemical transformations induced by the metabolic mechanisms of the ingesting animal[32] or by degradations/modifications that can occur during the extraction process.[48]

The toxins produced by dinoflagellates are in themselves very unique compounds. They are extremely potent, nonproteinacious compounds that serve an unkown function for the dinoflagellates. Some have proposed that the toxins are merely waste products, while others have suggested that the toxins are linked to the photosynthetic machinery of the dinoflagellate. This suggestion seems plausible in light of recent publications linking toxin production to pigment content.[74] This could also explain reports that toxins tend to comigrate with pigments in HPLC and TLC analysis of crude extracts.[49] The *Gonyaulax* sp. toxins (PSP tetrahyropurine), *Amphidinium* sp. toxins (hemolytic monoacylgalactolipids), and GB-4 (a phosphorous-containing compound) from *Pthychodiscus brevis* are all "atypical" in structure when compared with the oxygenated polyether structures of the dinoflagellates *Gambierdiscus* sp., *Ostreopsis* sp., *Ptychodiscus* sp., *Dinophysis* sp., and *Prorocentrum* sp. The toxins of the polyether type have been associated with the "ciguatera syndrome".[75] When comparing the extraction procedures, some similarities and some differences become evident. The PSP toxins are extracted under acidic conditions (0.05 M acetic acid or 0.1 HCL); this allows hydrolysis to occur so that the carbamate forms become more evident. PSP toxins are chromatographed on ion-exchange columns and must undergo postcolumn oxidation to produce products that are detectable by UV absorbance. The brevetoxins are also extracted under acidic conditions (diethyl ether and acidified water), however, methylene chloride was also used successfully. The brevetoxins are purified by flash chromatography and HPLC on silica oxide columns. Extraction of the polyetherlike toxins is dependent on the toxin source. Extractions from wild or cultured dinoflagellates involves methanol or methanol/acetone; extraction from fish or shellfish invariably employs acetone. This suggests that although CTX and okadaic acid may be similar in certain aspects, they may not be as closely related to the brevetoxins (namely, BTX-A, BTX-B, and BTX-C), as was previously thought.

Differences in the extraction procedures for ciguateric toxins (fish/eel vs. cells) tends to suggest that the toxic moieties are different, most likely involving the addition or loss of active or charged groups, such as the highly reactive hydroxyl groups. This is evident in extractions of ciguatoxin, as cells are extracted with methanol, a polar solvent, whereas extraction from fish/eels employs acetone, a less-polar solvent. Column purification of the polyetherlike toxins involves alumina oxide and reverse-phase (C18 and C8) columns.

ACKNOWLEDGMENTS

This study was supported by U.S. Army Medical Research and Development Command, contract DAMD17-87-C-7002. The views, findings, and opinions expressed herein are those of the authors and should not be construed as those of the Department of the Army.

REFERENCES

1. **Todd, E. C. D.,** Ciguatoxin in Canada, in *Toxic Dinoflagellates*, Anderson, D. M., White, A. W., and Baden, D. G., Eds., Elsevier Science, New York, 1985, 505.
2. **Regalis, E. P.,** Ciguatera sea food poisoning: an overview, in *Sea Food Toxins*, Regalis, E. P., Ed., American Chemical Society, Symposium Series 262, Washington, D.C., 1984, 25.
3. **Yasumoto, T., Murata, M., Oshima, Y., Matsumoto, G. K., and Clardy, J.,** Diarrhetic shellfish poisoning, in *Seafood Toxins*, Ragelis, E. P., Ed., American Chemical Society, Washington, D.C., 1984, 207.
4. **Yasumoto, T., Oshima, Y., Murakami, Y., Nakajima, I., Bagnis, R., and Fukuyo, Y.,** Toxicity of benthic dinoflagellates found in coral reef, *Bull. Jpn. Soc. Sci. Fish.*, 46, 327, 1980.
5. **Nakajima, I., Oshima, Y., and Yasumoto, T.,** Toxicity of benthic dinoflagellates in Okinawa, *Bull. Jpn. Soc. Sci. Fish.*, 47, 1029, 1981.
6. **Murakami, Y., Oshima, Y., and Yasumoto, T.,** Identification of okadiac acid as a toxic component of a marine dinoflagellate *Prorocentrum lima*, *Bull. Jpn Soc. Sci. Fish.*, 48, 69, 1982.
7. **Yasumoto, T.,** Recent progress in the chemistry of the dinoflagellate toxins, in *Toxic Dinoflagellates*, Anderson, D. W., White, A. G., and Baden, D. G., Eds., Elsevier Press, 1985, 259.
8. **Shimizu, Y.,** Dinoflagellate toxins, in *The Biology of the Dinoflagellates*, Taylor, F. J. R., Ed., Blackwell Scientific Publications, Oxford, 1987, chap 8.
9. **Yasumoto, T., Seino, N., Murakami, Y., and Murata, M.,** Toxins produced by benthic dinoflagellates, *Biol. Bull.*, 172, 128, 1987.
10. **Tindall, D. R., Dickey, R. W., Carlson, R. D., and Morey-Gaines, G.,** Ciguatoxigenic dinoflagellates from the Caribbean Sea, in *Seafood Toxins*, Ragelis, E. P., Ed., American Chemical Society, Washington, D.C., 1984, 225.
11. **Tindall, D. R. and Miller, D. M.,** Toxicity of *Ostreopsis lenticularis* from the British and United States Virgin Islands, in *Toxic Marine Phytoplankton Blooms*, Graneli, E., Sundstrom, B., Edler, L., and Anderson, D. M., Eds., Elsevier Press, New York, 1989,
12. **Lin, Y. Y., Risk, M., Ray, S. M., Van Engen, D., Clardy, J., Golik, J., James, J. C., and Nakanishi, K.,** Isolation and structure of brevetoxin B from the "red tide" dinoflagellate *Ptychodiscus brevis* (*Gymnodinum breve*), *J. Am. Chem. Soc.*, 103, 6773, 1981.
13. **Shimizu, Y., Shimizu, H., Scheuer, P. J., Hokama, Y., Oyama, M., and Miyahara, J. T.,** *Gambierdiscus toxicus*, a ciguatera-causing dinoflagellate from Hawaii, *Bull. Jpn. Soc. Sci. Fish.*, 48, 811, 1982.
14. **Carmichael, W.,** Algal toxins, in *Advances in Botanical Research*, Academic Press, London, 1986, 47.
15. **Sasner, J., Ikawa, M., Thurberg, F., and Alam, M.,** Physiological and chemical studies on *Gymnodinium breve* Davis toxin, *Toxicon*, 10, 163, 1972.
16. **Padilla, G. M., Kim, Y. S., Rauchman, E. J., and Rosen, G. M.,** Physiological activities of toxins from *Gymnodinium breve* isolated by high performance liquid chromatography, in *Toxic Dinoflagellate Blooms*, Taylor, D. and Seliger, H., Eds., Elsevier Science, New York, 1979, 351.
17. **Risk, M., Werbach-Perez, K., Perez-Polo, J. R., Bunce, H., Ray, S. M., and Parmentier, L. J.,** Mechanism of action of the major toxin from *Gymnodinium breve*, in *Toxic Dinoflagellate Blooms*, Taylor, D. and Seliger, H., Eds., Elsevier Science, New York, 1979, 367.
18. **Baden, D. G., Mende, T. J., and Block, R. E.,** Two similar toxins isolated from *Gymnodinium breve*, in *Toxic Dinoflagellate Blooms*, Taylor, D. and Seliger, H., Eds., Elsevier, New York, 1979, 327.
19. **Steidinger, K.,** A re-evaluation of toxic dinoflagellate biology and ecology, in *Progress in Phycological Research*, Round, F. E. and Chapman, V. J., Eds., Elsevier Press, New York, 1983, 147.
20. **Baden, D. G., Mende, T. J., Poll, M. A., and Block, R. E.,** Toxins from Florida's red tide dinoflagellate *Ptychodiscus brevis*, in *Seafood Toxins*, Ragelis, E. P., Ed., American Chemical Society, Washington, D.C., 1984, 359.
21. **Shimizu, Y., Chou, H. N., Bando, H., Van Duyne, G., and Clardy, J. C.,** Structure of brevetoxin A (GB-1 toxin), the most potent toxin in the Florida red tide organism *Gymnodinium breve (Ptychodiscus brevis)*, *J. Am. Chem. Soc.*, 108, 514, 1986.

22. **Alam, M., Sanduja, R., Hossain, M. G., and Van Der Helm, D.,** Isolation and X-ray structure of O,O-dipropyl(E)-2-(1-methyl-2-oxopropyllidene) phosphorohydrazidothioate (E)-oxime from the red tide dinoflagellate, *Gymnodinium breve*, *J. Am. Chem. Soc.*, 104, 5232, 1982.
23. **Chou, H. N., Shimizu, Y., Van Duyne, G., and Clardy, J.,** Isolation and structures of two new polycyclic ethers from *Gymnodinium breve* Davis (*Ptychodiscus brevis*), *Tetrahedron Lett.*, 26, 2865, 1985.
24. **Pierce, R. H., Brown, C., and Kucklick, J. R.,** Analysis of *Ptychodiscus brevis* toxins by reverse phase HPLC, in *Toxic Dinoflagellates*, Anderson, D. M., White, A. W., and Baden, D. G., Eds., Elsevier Science, New York, 1985, 309.
25. **Chou, J. and Shimizu, Y.,** A new polyether toxin from *Gymnodinium breve* Davis, *Tetrahedron Lett.*, 23, 5521, 1982.
26. **Golik, J., James, J. C., Nakanishi, K., and Lin, Y.,** The structure of brevetoxin C, *Tetrahedron Lett.*, 23, 2535, 1982.
27. **Oshima, Y., Kotaki, Y., Harada, T., and Yasumoto, T.,** Paralytic shellfish toxins in tropical waters, in *Seafood Toxins*, Ragelis, E. P., Ed., American Chemical Society, Washington, D.C., 1984, 161.
28. **Anderson, D. M., Sullivan, J. J., and Reguera, B.,** Paralytic shellfish poisoning in northwest Spain: the toxicity of the dinoflagellate, *Gymnodinium catenatum*, *Toxicon*, 27, 665, 1989.
29. **Yentsch, C. M., Dale, B., and Hurst, J. W.,** Coexistance of toxic and nontoxic dinoflagellates resembling *Gonyaulax tamarensis* in New England costal water (NW Atlantic), *J. Phycol.*, 14, 330, 1978.
30. **Schantz, E. J. and Magnusson, H. W.,** Observations on the origin of the paralytic poison in Alaska butter clams, *J. Protozool.*, 11, 238, 1964.
31. **Shimuzu, Y., Alam, M., Oshima, Y., and Fallon, W. E.,** Presence of four toxins in red tide infested clams and cultured *Gonyaulax tamarensis* cells, *Biochem. Biophys. Res. Commun.*, 66, 731, 1975.
32. **Hall, S. and Reichardt, P. B.,** Cryptic paralytic shellfish toxins, in *Seafood Toxins*, Ragelis, E. P., Ed., American Chemical Society, Washington, D.C., 1984, 114.
33. **Halstead, B. and Schantz, E.,** Paralytic shellfish poisoning, in *Paralytic Shellfish Poisoning*, World Health Organization, Geneva, Switzerland, 1984, 5.
34. **Lombet, A., Bidard, J.-N., and Lazdunski, M.,** Ciguatoxin and brevetoxin share a common receptor site on the neuronal voltage-dependent Na^+ channel, *FEBS Lett.*, 2, 1987.
35. **Sullivan, J. J., Jonas-Davis, J., and Kentala, L. L.,** The determination of PSP toxins by HPLC and autoanalyzer, in *Toxic Dinoflagellates*, Anderson, D. M., White, A. W., and Baden, D. G., Eds., Elsevier, New York, 1985, 275.
36. **Ghazarossian, V. J., Schantz, E. J., Schnoes, H. K., and Strong, F. M.,** A biologically active and hydrolysis product of saxitoxin, *Biochem. Biophys. Res. Commun.*, 68, 776, 1976.
37. **Oshima, Y., Buckley, L. J., Alam, M., and Shimizu, Y.,** Hetereogeneity of paralytic shellfish poisons. Three new toxins from cultured *Gonyaulax tamerensis* cell, *Mya arenia* and *Saxidomus giganteus*, *Comp. Biochem. Physiol.*, 57C, 31, 1977.
38. **Fallon, W. E. and Shimizu, Y.,** Electrophoretic analysis of paralytic shellfish toxins, *J. Environ. Sci. Health*, A19, 455, 1977.
39. **Yasumoto, T., Nakajima, I., Bagnis, R. A., and Adachi, R.,** Finding of a dinoflagellate as a likely culprit of ciguatera, *Bull. Jpn. Soc. Sci. Fish.*, 43, 1021, 1977.
40. **Adachi, R. and Fukuyo, Y.,** The thecal structure of a marine toxic dinoflagellate *Gambierdiscus toxicus* gen. et sp. nov collected in a ciguatera endemic area, *Bull. Jpn. Soc. Sci. Fish.*, 45, 67, 1979.
41. **Bagnis, R. A.,** Clinical aspects of ciguatera (fish poisoning) in French Polynesia, *Hawaii Med. J.*, 28, 25, 1968.
42. **Ogura, Y., Nara, J., and Yoshida, T.,** Comparative pharmacological actions of ciguatoxin and tetrodotoxin, a preliminary account, *Toxicon*, 6, 131, 1968.
43. **Calvert, G. M., Hryhorczuk, D. O., and Leikin, J. B.,** Treatment of ciguatera fish poisoning with amitryptyline and nifedipine, *Clin. Toxicol.*, 25, 423, 1987.
44. **Palafox, N. A., Jain, L. G., Pinano, A. Z., Gulick, T. M., Williams, R. K., and Schatz, I. J.,** Successful treatment of ciguatera fish poisoning with intravenous mannitol, *JAMA*, 259, 2740, 1988.
45. **Tachibana, K.,** Structural Studies on Marine Toxins, Ph.D. dissertation, University of Hawaii, 1980.
46. **Tachibana, K., Nukina, M., Joh, Y.-G., and Scheuer, P. J.,** Recent developments in the molecular structure of ciguatoxin, *Biol. Bull.*, 172, 122, 1987.
47. **Lewis, R. J. and R. E.,** Occurrence of a ciguatoxin-like substance in the Spanish mackerel (*Scombermorus commersoni*), *Toxicon*, 21, 19, 1983.
48. **Nukina, M., Koyanagi, L. M., and Scheuer, P. J.,** Two interchangable forms of ciguatoxin, *Toxicon*, 22, 169, 1984.
49. **Dickey, R. W.,** The Extraction, Purification and Characterization of Toxins from the Marine Dinoflagellates *Gambierdiscus toxicus* and *Prorocentrum concavum*, Ph.D. dissertation, Southern Illinois University, Carbondale, IL, 1984.
50. **Tindall, D. R. and Miller, D. M.,** Purification of maitotoxin from the dinoflagellate, *Gambierdiscus toxicus*, using high pressure liquid chromatography, in *Toxic Dinoflagellates*, Anderson, D. M., White, A. W., and Baden, D. G., Eds., Elsevier Science, New York, 1985, 321.

51. **Miller, D. M. and Tindall, D. R.,** Preparative HPLC separation of maitotoxin from crude extracts of *Gambierdiscus toxicus*, in *9th World Congress on Animal, Plant, and Microbial Toxins (IST)*, 1988.
52. **Lewis, R. J. and Endean, R.,** Ciguatoxin from the flesh and viscera of the barracuda, *Spyraena jello*, *Toxicon*, 22, 805, 1984.
53. **Miller, D. M., Dickey, R. W., and Tindall, D. R.,** Lipid soluble toxins from a dinoflagellate, *Gambierdiscus toxicus*, in *Seafood Toxins*, Ragelis, E. P., Ed., American Chemical Society Symposium Series 262, Washington, D.C., 1984, 241.
54. **Dickey, R. W., Miller, D. M., and Tindall, D. R.,** Extraction of a water-soluble toxin from a dinoflagellate, *Gambierdiscus toxicus*, in *Seafood Toxins*, Ragelis, E. P., Ed., American Chemical Society Symposium Series 262, Washington, D.C., 1984, 257.
55. **Tindall, D. R. and Miller, D. M.,** Purification and assay of two ciguatera toxins from the dinoflagellate, *Prorocentrum concavum*, *Toxicon*, 25, 155, 1986.
56. **Freedman, S. B., Miller, R. J., Miller, D. M., and Tindall, D. R.,** Interactions of maitotoxin with voltage-sensitive calcium channels in cultured neuronal cells, *Proc. Natl. Acad. Sci. USA*, 81, 4582, 1984.
57. **Takahashi, M., Ohizumi, Y., and Yasumoto, T.,** Maitotoxin, a Ca^{2+} channel activator candidate, *J. Biol. Chem.*, 257, 7287, 1982.
58. **Ohizumi, Y.,** Pharmacological actions of the marine toxins ciguatoxin and maitotoxin isolated from poisonous fish, *Biol. Bull.*, 172, 132, 1987.
59. **Miller, D. M. and Tindall, D. R.,** Physiological effects of HPLC-purified maitotoxin from a dinoflagellate, *Gambierdiscus toxicus*, in *Toxic Dinoflagellates*, Anderson, D. M., White, A. W., and Baden, D. G., Eds., Elsevier Science, New York, 1985, 375.
60. **Yokoyama, A., Murata, M., Oshima, Y., Iwashita, T., and Yasumoto, T.,** Some chemical properties of maitotoxin, a putative calcium channel agonist isolated from a marine dinoflagellate, *J. Biochem.*, 104, 184, 1988.
61. **Yasumoto, T., Bagnis, R. A., and Vernoux, J.-P.,** Toxicity of the surgeon fishes-II. Properties of the principal water-soluble toxin, *Bull. Jpn. Soc. Sci. Fish.*, 42, 359, 1976.
62. **Bidard, J.-N., Vijverberg, H. P. M., Frelin, C., Chungue, E., Legrand, A.-M., Bagnis, R. A., and Lazdunski, M.,** Ciguatoxin is a novel type of sodium channel toxin, *J. Biol. Chem.*, 259, 8353, 1984.
63. **Miyahara, J. T., Oyama, M. M., and Hokama, Y.,** Mechanism of norepinephrine release by ciguatoxin, in *Proc. Fifth Intl. Coral Reef Cong.*, Antenne Museum-EPHE, Moorea, French Polynesia, Tahiti, 1985, 467.
64. **Miller, D. M., Dickey, R. W., and Tindall, D. R.,** The effects of a lipid extracted toxin from the dinoflagellate *Gambierdiscus toxicus* upon nerve-muscle and intestinal preparations, *Fed. Proc.*, 41, 1561, 1982.
65. **Yasumoto, T.,** Toxins involved in ciguatera and the origins of the toxins, in *American Chemical Society, Hawaii Meeting, ABST 336*, Elsevier, New York, 1979, 71.
66. **Legrand, A.-M., Litaudon, M., Genthon, J. N., Bagnis, R. A., and Yasumoto, T.,** Isolation and some properties of ciguatoxin, *J. Appl. Phycol.*, 1, 183, 1989.
67. **Sick, L. V., Hansen, D.C., Babinchak, J. A., and Higerd, T. B.,** An HPLC fluorescence method for identifying a toxic fraction extracted from the dinoflagellate, *Gambierdiscus toxicus*, *Mar. Fish. Rev.*, 48, 29, 1987.
68. **Sullivan, J. J. and Wekell, M. M.,** Determination of paralytic shellfish poisoning toxins by high pressure liquid chromatography, in *Seafood Toxins*, Ragelis, E. P., Ed., American Chemical Society, Washington, D.C., 1984, 197.
69. **Kim, Y. S. and Padilla, G. M.,** Purification of the ichthyotoxic component of *Gymnodinium breve* (red tide dinoflagellate) toxin by high pressure chromatography, *Toxicon*, 14, 379, 1976.
70. **Taylor, F. J. R.,** Human and domestic animal fatalities as well as skin reactions associated with the rough trigger fish: *Canthidermis maculatus* (Bloch) in Dominica West Indies following hurricane David, *Rev. Int. Oceanogr. Med.*, 35, 1984.
71. **Taylor, F. J. R.,** The distribution of the dinoflagellate *Gambierdiscus toxicus* in the Eastern Caribbean, in *Proc. Fifth Intl. Coral Reef Cong.*, Antenne Museum EPHE, Moorea, French Polynesia, Tahiti, 1985, 423.
72. **Ballentine, D. L., Tosteson, T. R., and Bardales, A. T.,** Population dynamics and toxicity of natural populations of benthic dinoflagellates in southwestern Puerto Rico, *J. Exp. Mar. Biol. Ecol.*, 4, 201, 1988.
73. **Tosteson, T. R., Ballantine, D. L., Tosteson, C. G., Hensley, V., and Bardales, A. T.,** Associated bacterial flora, growth, and toxicity of cultured benthic dinoflagellates *Ostreopsis lenticularis* and *Gambierdiscus toxicus*, *Appl. Environ. Microbiol.*, 55, 137, 1989.
74. **Bomber, J., Tindall, D. R., Venable, C. W., and Miller, D. M.,** Resolution of the pigment compositon and low light response of fourteen clones of *Gambierdiscus toxicus*, in *Toxic Marine Phytoplankton Blooms*, Graneli, E., Sundstrom, B., Edler, L., and Anderson, D. M., Eds., Elsevier Press, New York, 1990, 305.
75. **Anderson, D. M. and Lobel, P. S.,** The continuing enigma of ciguatera, *Biol. Bull.*, 172, 89, 1987.
76. **Genenah, A. A. and Shimizu, Y.,** Specific toxicity of paralytic shellfish poisons, *J. Agric. Food. Chem.*, 29, 1289, 1981.

Chapter 6

ASSAYS FOR CIGUATERA-TYPE TOXINS

Claude A. Rakotoniaina and Donald M. Miller

TABLE OF CONTENTS

I. INTRODUCTION

The complexity of ciguatera fish poisoning or ciguatera intoxication cannot be overemphasized,[1,2] and there has been a continued search for assays that would either allow identification of toxic fish, identification of toxin, quantification of toxin, or identification of the mode of action. Ciguatera intoxications result from the ingestion of any of a large variety of tropical reef and in-shore fishes that contain toxins accumulated by way of the marine food web.[1-3] The marine food chain involves at least a benthic dinoflagellate, *Gambierdiscus toxicus* (and possibly *Prorocentrum* sp., *Ostreopsis* sp., *Ptychodiscus [Gonyaulax] sp*., and others)[4-6] and varied reef fishes, microphagous herbivores, detritivores, and larger piscivorous carnivores and omnivores, which accumulate the toxins.[1,2]

Ciguatera intoxications have been associated with a complex of syndromes including gastrointestinal, neurologic, and cardiovascular symptoms.[2,7-9] It is now generally accepted that several toxins may contribute to the complex of ciguatera syndromes observed.[10] They are ciguatoxin,[11-13] maitotoxin,[9,14,15] scaritoxin,[16-19] brevetoxin,[20] palytoxin,[21] and okadaic acid.[22,23] It has also been suggested that there may be relationships between the clinical and pathophysiologic features and the nature of the toxin(s) involved in ciguatera intoxications.[1,2,12,24]

A variety of *in vitro* and *in vivo* assay methods has been developed for the study of the complex pharmacologic, clinical, pathophysiologic, and immunologic aspects of ciguatera intoxications.[1-3] None of these methods has proven to be completely satisfactory for laboratory routine testing, field experience, or specific investigations, since they all have their limitations and undesirable pitfalls.[1,3,10,12,25,26] Among criteria to be considered in the development and choice of assay methods are practicality, sensitivity, and specificity.[26] In the case of ciguatera studies, concern has been expressed as to the use of techniques that would give results comparable to clinical records of human ciguatera intoxications.[1,12,25] Examples of *in vitro* techniques for ciguatera toxicity studies are immunoassay[26-29] and varied isolated organ or tissue assays.[26-29] *In vivo* studies for ciguatera toxicity include bioassays on intact fish, shrimp, crayfish, frog,[1,2,12,25] mosquito,[30-32] dog, pig, hamster, guinea pig,[1] and turtle.[25] At present, the most widely used bioassays have been in intact animals such as mouse,[25,31,33-38] rat,[35,38] cat,[33,39-42] mongoose,[25,33,43] rabbit,[38,44,45] and chick.[42,46,47]

The primary objective of this review is to summarize the published data on animal assays for ciguatera-type toxins. The previous literature does not contain a complete summarization of the many and different attempts to establish an adequate bioassay for these toxins. Special reference is given to the animal assays involving ciguateric fishes and fish extracts, as well as the two major ciguatera-type toxins, ciguatoxin and maitotoxin, in the forms of both extracts from fish and dinoflagellate cultures.

II. ANIMAL MODELS FOR CIGUATERA TOXICITY STUDIES

Animal assay methods for ciguatera toxicity studies may be divided into two broad categories: testing by quantitative feeding and injection of an extract of ciguateric materials. Because the reactions in humans result from the ingestion of fish, the first tests used in the investigation of ciguatera-type toxins was based on the responses of animals fed toxic fish. Initially, feeding assays for ciguatera toxicity were carried on with mice, cats, and puppies.[48,49] Technical, economic, and legal constraints have rendered the use of these species as test animals difficult, which may have led to the extension of feeding assays to other animals such as the mongoose and chick.[1,12,25,50]

Although feeding tests were necessary at first for screening fish for ciguatera toxicity, they were not satisfactory for further studies of the toxins. The first injection tests of ciguatoxic fish were initiated by Hiyama,[48] Halstead,[49] and Hashimoto,[51] and consisted of an intraperitoneal injection of an extract into mice. The extraction media for fish flesh or viscera varied from alcohol or water[48] to acidified or distilled water,[49] and acidulated methanol.[51]

At present, the ciguatera research community is faced with a wide range of choice regarding animal species, extraction media, routes of administration, and types of ciguateric materials to be used for different purpose and interests. Finding suitable test models that meet specific needs has been a continual concern and problem, to which much effort has been directed in the past.[1,50] One approach that might arrive at an acceptable choice might be to proceed to a careful analysis of animal models that have been used for ciguatera toxicity studies. For practical purpose and on the basis of scientific and economic considerations in relation to ciguatera toxicity studies to date, it may be appropriate to view previous whole-animal test models into two broad categories: animal species of minor interest (dog, rabbit, guinea pig, hamster, and turtle) and animal species of major interest (fish, rat, mouse, cat, mongoose, and chick).

A. VERTEBRATES OF MINOR INTEREST

1. Dog (*Canis familiaris*)

Dogs have been used as a bioassay and are more susceptible to ichthyosarcotoxins than either the cat or pig (Kawakubo and Kikuchi, 1942, cited by Halstead[1]), but presently are eliminated because of their excessive cost, legal problems associated with their procurement and maintenance,[1] and perhaps the amounts of toxin that would be required. Indeed, those investigators who have used dogs, used puppies to reduce the amounts of toxin.

2. Rabbit (*Oryctalagus cuniculus*)

Rabbits are sensitive to ciguatera toxins and are a useful model using the eye test[52] and immunologic assays, nevertheless, there is a dearth of literature available on rabbits as a test model. Kosaki and Anderson[52] found the ciguatoxin-induced pupillary miosis correlated well with the effects of the same toxin in the mouse and rat.

3. Hamster (*Cricetulus griseus, Mesocricetus auratus*)

Hamsters might be a satisfactory test animal, but are more expensive than mice and do not appear to be any more sensitive to ciguatera toxins.[1]

4. Turtle (*Pseudemys scripta*)

Turtles may develop recognizable symptoms, particularly to ciguatoxin,[25] when test fed, although they never eat enough to cause death. They have been rejected as a test animal because of the difficulties encountered in determining the amount of test meal ingested or in evaluating the symptoms they exhibit, inasmuch as their only reaction is to withdraw within their shell.[25]

B. VERTEBRATES OF MAJOR INTEREST

1. Mouse (*Mus mus*)

Mice are not difficult to procure and to maintain,[1,12] and have been the animal of choice (using intraperitoneal injection) to test for ciguatera toxicity. However, their use in ciguatera toxicity study is not without controversy concerning their sensitivity to ciguatera toxins, their reactions, and the form of ciguateric material to be administered.

a. Mouse Feeding Test

Mice feeding tests have proven to be of little value for the following reasons. One, because of the variation in physiologic response of individual mice to a given test sample, some test animals would react to toxic samples, whereas others would not.[1] Two, mice would avoid eating raw fish or fish-contaminated food,[25] thus rendering them unsuitable for quantitative assay. Three, when fed toxic fish, mice are less sensitive to ciguatoxin.[12,33]

b. Mouse Injection Test

Halstead[1] found mice to be the next most satisfactory test animal after cats and intraperitoneal injection to be the most effective route of administration. Other authors concluded that mice can be used for a toxicity test during purification,[12] provided highly purified aqueous extracts are used,[25] although some authors cited by Banner,[25] including Hashimoto, have indicated that the injection of aqueous extracts into mice could not be relied upon. Banner[25] found that satisfactory results for a quantitative test could be obtained by using a method based on intraperitoneal injection into standard mice or an alcoholic extract of fish flesh, which is subsequently purified by washing with petroleum ether and re-extracted with diethyl ether. Banner and Boroughs[33] found mouse intraperitoneal tests to be inefficient, because the mice are insensitive to small quantities of ciguatoxin injected intraperitoneally in aqueous extracts. With mouse assays, using intraperitoneal injections of aqueous extracts, there is the danger of false reactions, negative or positive, and failure to critically observe the reactions of the test animals.[1]

In determining the effects of size of mice on the reactions to a standard dosage, Banner[25] established that both the smallest and the largest injected mice are less sensitive and more variable in their reaction to ciguatera toxins than are those in 20 to 25 g range. Subsequent to Banner, Kimura et al.[34] conducted mouse bioassays on ciguatera toxins using extracts in Tween. Male and female Swiss mice weighing 15 to 20 g were each injected intraperitoneally with a ciguatoxic dose of 1000 or 2000 mg extract/kg body weight in 0.5 ml of 0.2% Tween 60 in 0.15 M NaCl.

Halstead et al.[53] advocated a procedure using aqueous extracts. Mice weighing 20 to 25 g were injected intraperitoneally with 1 ml of the supernatant fluid (a milky suspension) obtained from homogenization of fish portions (muscles, viscera, etc.) in water and centrifugation of the slurry for 25 min at 2000 rpm. He recognized three types of mouse reactions to poisonous fish.

Banner et al.[25] suggested a modification of Halstead and Bunker,[53] using crude homogenates of fish tissues. In this procedure, four mice weighing 15 to 25 g were used to test for toxicity of the aqueous extract. The reactions of the four mice were observed for 26 h and placed into four groups.[25] Each mouse was injected intraperitoneally with 1 ml of the clear supernatant fluid obtained from homogenization of fish flesh and centrifugation of the slurry at 2000 rpm (900 g) for 25 min.

Tachibana[54] introduced utilizing the time to death as an index for ciguatoxin. He stated, "When a reliable relationship between dose and death time is established, the experimental error of the LD_{50} should depend solely on the variation in sensitivity of an individual mouse to the toxin."

Tindall and others[55] have reported using mouse bioassay for routine determination of LD_{50} values for extracts of *G. toxicus, P. concavum, P. mexicanum*, and *Ostreopsis lenticularis.*[15] In this case, LD_{50} determinations are completed using female white mice weighing 19 to 21 g. Doses of toxic extract are suspended in 0.5 ml of 0.1% Tween 60 in 0.15 M NaCl and administered by intraperitoneal injection. All mice are observed for a period of 48 h. Following the method of Weil,[56] four dose levels are used with three repetitions at each level. The LD_{50}s are calculated from moving-average interpolation tables.

2. Rat (*Rattus rattus, R. norvegicus, R. exulans*)

Rats are satisfactory test animals but might also be more expensive than mice and are not any more sensitive to ciguatera toxins.[1] They are less sensitive to ciguatera toxins, even when fed toxic meal for weeks.[25]

3. Cat (*Felis catus*)

Cats have proven to be a satisfactory[33] and useful[1] test animal for ciguatera toxicity. They are quite sensitive to ciguatera toxins.[1,12,50] Cats do possess some potential disadvantages. First, they easily develop a vomiting reflex,[1,12,25,50] due to a rather narrow tolerance between the minimum toxic dose and a dose that induces a vomiting response. As a result, they often regurgitate part of the test meal, thereby making it difficult to estimate the amount of toxic fish retained[25,50] and causing an unparalleled response to the toxicity of ciguateric materials.[12] Second, cats are difficult to procure and to maintain.[1,12,33] They are subject to legal constraints in some countries.[1,12] Also, they are large test animals and therefore require large amounts of toxic sample.[50] Finally, cats are difficult to keep healthy.[12,50] They are highly susceptible to various viral infections that not only are difficult to control and may cause morbidity symptoms superposed on toxicity reactions, making it difficult to interpret the results, but also may cause a high mortality rate.[50]

a. Cat Feeding Test

Halstead[1] found oral cat feeding tests, particularly in kittens, to be the most reliable and sensitive bioassay for ciguatera toxins. In a study conducted on 26 cats in Tahiti, Bagnis and Fevai[40] obtained fairly homogenous clinical reactions from animals fed fish flesh. The same feeding test allowed the authors to further investigate the neuropathologic, hematologic, histopathologic, and pharmacologic effects of ciguatera toxins. Twenty-six cats weighing 300 to 1000 g and of age 4 to 8 weeks were starved 48 h. Each of the cats was fed 10% of body weight of ground ciguateric fish flesh. The base toxicity scale was established by Bagnis et al.,[7] based on symptomatology at the 48th h following ingestion.

4. Mongoose (*Herpestes mongo, H. auropunctatus*)

Mongooses have great advantages. They are highly sensitive to ciguatera toxins and exhibit symptoms characteristic of human and feline intoxications.[12,25] They do not regurgitate and thus give a quantifiable response that is related to the toxin ingested.[10,12,25] However, mongooses are not completely satisfactory as test animals, both biologically and economically.[1,12,25] First, those that have been used came from a wild population and therefore have shown great individual variation to ciguatera toxicity. Second, because of their viciousness, they are hard to catch and to handle. Third, they require too much test meal to permit the replicate testing necessary to establish an LD_{50}. Finally, they may be unavailable and prohibited by law in many regions.[1,12,25]

a. Mongoose Feeding Test

Mongoose feeding has been used as a standardized screening test to establish the degree of toxicity of a ciguateric meal. A roughly quantitative assay was designed and used extensively in Hawaii using trapped wild animals.[3,25] Mongoose feeding tests have permitted observations such as ciguatera toxin was not destroyed by drying at 102 to 108°C for 24 h, or by freezing for a period up to 6 months,[33] and ethanol could be used to efficiently extract the toxin from fish.[33]

Mongoose can be fed up to 15% of their body weight of raw fish, dried fish, or extracts that are mixed with raw eggs.[25] In determining the lethal dose in the mongoose, Banner and Boroughs[33] concluded that no ciguatoxic fish was found to be lethal under 5% of body weight, and no fish was used that did not cause death at 15% of body weight of the mongoose. The authors[25] classified the responses of the mongoose in five stages, based on the maximal response in the animals within 48 h after a single test feeding.

5. Chick (*Gallus gallus* sp., *G. domesticus*)

Chicks have been advocated to be a very satisfactory animal model for both the feeding and injection tests. They are readily available, easy to manage, of relatively small size, and unlikely to regurgitate. They are highly sensitive to ciguatera toxins and the effects of intoxication are cumulative.[33]

There have been some negative reservations attached to the use of chicks as a ciguatera toxicity bioassay in the past,[25,42] which may be explained in many ways. For example, negative results would be to be expected in the following cases:[46] (1) if the ciguateric meal, such as ground-dried flesh, were administered by voluntary feeding;[25] (2) if the ingested quantity of toxic homogenate per unit of the chick body weight were well below that necessary to induce ciguatera intoxication symptoms in cats;[42] and (3) if the test chickens were older than 30 d, inasmuch as the blood brain-barrier develops in 30 d, and central nervous effects could not be determined after this time.[41]

a. Chick Feeding Test

The chick feeding test for ciguatera toxicity is a very simple test system that could be advisable to local populations in economically depressed and ciguatera-endemic areas without scientific equipment. The test lasts 48 h at the most and therefore allows the suspected fish to be kept until completion of the investigation.[46]

A procedure for the chicken feeding test might include the following:[46] chicks weighing 70 to 100 g and 8 to 10 d old are force fed with 10% of their body weight in a ciguateric meal, generally minced and homogenized cooked tissue (e.g., fish liver). The response to liver feeding is observed after a 48-h period. Vernoux[46] has suggested the use of a chick feeding test as a valid preventive screening test for fish until immunologic methods are perfected and made available.

b. Chick Injection Test

For ciguatera toxicity study purposes, chicken injection tests have given satisfactory results for intravenous, intraperitoneal, and intramuscular bioassay.[52,57] Li[57] induced ciguatera by intramuscular injection in hen and reported pathomorphologic changes of the nervous system.

6. Fish

Studies on the effects of toxin on fish were started by Banner and others in 1960. In this study they tested the retention and accumulation of crude toxic extracts from fish when fed to the red snapper, *Lutjanus bohar*. Davin found that fish fed ciguatoxin- and maitotoxin-containing feed suffered behavioral changes. More recent studies by Capra and others[58] using fish extracts and dinoflagellate extracts have shown that fish are sensitive to intraperitoneal injections of toxin and that the fish are less sensitive to the toxin than the mouse.

C. INVERTEBRATES

Dose-response assays of toxin by injection into invertebrates such as insects has a long history. Miller and others[59] discovered that curare affects insects in the same manner. The small invertebrates require very little toxin (orders of magnitude less) for an assay. It comes as no surprise that ciguatera investigators later turned their attention to brine shrimp,[60] crayfish,[1-3,12,25] flies,[61] and mosquitos.[30-32] Nevertheless, technique is all important in the success of using these organisms.

III. CLINICAL AND PATHOPHYSIOLOGIC FEATURES OF CIGUATOXICATION IN EXPERIMENTAL ANIMALS

Banner[25] observed 58 mongooses fed ciguateric meal and reported no significant pathologic changes in both the acute and subacute cases. In the acute case of animals fed in a single feeding of 10% of body weight, there was no apparent relationship between the predominantly neurologic symptoms and the postmortem lesions. The only postmortem lesions noticed was a tendency to develop gastric ulcers, which probably resulted from the adaptation stress of wild mongoose. In the subacute case of mongoose fed intermittently with 1% of body weight, there was no pathologic change in the central nervous system, and there was at most evidence of hepatotoxic change. No immunization, sensitization, or toxin accumulation was observed by Hessel et al.[50] in two test cats fed ciguateric fish flesh in two different ways. Both a single-feeding test and a multiple-feeding test over a 6-week period did lead to dose-dependent symptoms, but neither of them generated immunization, sensitization, or toxin accumulation.

According to Banner,[3] the basic test for ciguatera intoxication through ingestion must be a feeding test on a sensitive animal and must be based on measured test meals given at a percentage of body weight. The animals to be tested are starved for 24 h and then either fed with a unique dose of ciguateric meal or extracts, or injected with ciguatoxic extracts. The test animals are observed for 48 h with their responses generally rated from 0 (no response) to 5 (death within 48 h).

IV. SIGNIFICANCE OF WHOLE ANIMAL ASSAYS IN CIGUATERA STUDY

Not all animals show sensitivity to ciguatera-type toxins,[33] and even if they do they may not respond quite the same way.[25] Banner et al.[25] reported the case of rats that did not show symptoms when fed (a week to several months) meal that was lethally toxic to mongoose.

Mongooses and cats[1] are both sensitive to ciguatoxin and exhibit similar symptoms. However, mongooses are superior to cats in that they are not likely to regurgitate, and therefore they respond quantitatively to toxic meal.[12,25]

Cats appear to be much more sensitive than mice.[31] Alternately, comparison of the reactions of mongoose test fed to those of injected mice shows varied situations. Banner et al.[25] observed a difference in symptoms in mongooses and mice that was further demonstrated to be a difference in reaction of the two species to the same type of ciguatera toxin. Banner and Boroughs[33] found that mice showed no symptoms when fed toxic fish, even at twice the dose in percentage of body weight that was lethal to the mongoose. Yasumoto and Scheuer[13] were unable to detect a marginally toxic eel flesh by mongoose screening, when the liver extracts from the same eels prove to be ciguatoxic by the mouse injection test.

Vernoux et al.[46,62] stated that the sensitivity of chicks to ciguatera toxins, as well as their capacity to accumulate toxin, are equivalent to those of the cat and superior to those of the mouse. The authors also found the use of chicks as a test animal to be more practical and beneficial as opposed to that of the cats (which regurgitate test meal, are subject to legal constraints and are unavailable) or to that of mongooses (which are subject to captivity). Also, chicks are as satisfactory as mice for intravenous or intraperitoneal bioassay to detect ciguatera toxins.[46]

Vernoux and Lahlou[62] compared the ratios of ciguatera toxicity potentials (LD_{50}) in both the chick and the mouse (LD_{50} in test-fed chick/LD_{50} in intraperitoneally injected mouse). The authors used partially purified liposoluble extract and showed that the chickens were three to five times more sensitive to ciguatera toxin (from fish) than are mice.

Anderson[10] is of the opinon that all bioassay methods have at least the common disadvantage of lacking specificity for individual toxins. Banner et al.[25] cited authors who incidently tested fish, including snappers and moray eels, suspected to have caused human ciguatera intoxication. The mongoose test showed that all of the species tested caused a similar response in the test animals, and the reactions varied only with the toxicity of the sample. This would indicate that the toxin in moray eels and in the other fish may be the same as that of ciguatoxin.[63]

Yasumoto and Scheuer[13] conducted a study in which the toxicity of eel flesh obtained from different species from different areas, and fed to mongoose, was compared with the toxicity of their livers as extracts injected intraperitoneally in mice. The authors found higher toxicity of the liver in mice and raised the question of the nature of the relationship between ciguatera toxin levels in the flesh of the eel. They then suggested the possibility that the liver might serve as the major reservoir of toxin in ciguateric fish, might be the site where the modification of a biologic precursor takes place, or might facilitate both phenomena.

One objective of bioassays for ciguatera toxicity is to find an animal that would respond consistently with symptoms paralleling those found in humans. Cats and mongooses were reported to respond in such a manner.[7,25,33,40]

There seems to exist a high correlation of results between mouse interperitoneal injection and cat feeding, as well as published clinical records of human ciguatera intoxications.[1] Likewise, the reactions of mongoose to ciguatera toxins are similar in some respect to those observed for human ciguatera.[25]

V. ISOLATED TISSUES AND SYSTEMS USED FOR CIGUATERA TOXICITY STUDIES

Ciguatoxin from fish has been found to affect sodium movement in several preparations. Setliff and others[64] found that ciguatoxin increased passive sodium permeability in isolated frog skin. Using human erythrocyte ghosts, Rayner[65] concluded that sodium-potassium activated adenosine triphosphatase was inhibited by ciguatoxin.

Maitotoxin from *G. toxicus* cells was found to induce the acrosome reaction in mussel spermatozoa.[66] It was also reported by both Gomi[67] and Rayner[68] to inhibit sodium transport in frog muscle and by Miyamoto et al.[69] to inhibit calcium-channel transport in insect skeletal muscles.

Crude extracts of *G. toxicus* were found to first inhibit the synapse, then the nerve, and finally the muscle in a sciatic nerve-muscle preparation from frog.[70] The same extracts also inhibited crayfish nerve.[71] Legrand and others[72] also looked at the effects of extracts of both fish and *G. toxicus* on frog sciatic nerve. Boyarsky and Rayner[73] investigated the effects of fish extracts on *Aplysia* neurons.

Capra and others further investigated the effects of fish extracts on human,[74] mammalian,[35] and fish nerves.[75,76] They found, in patients who suffered intoxication and in animals that had fish extract administered, a change in nerve conduction parameters, such that there is lengthening of the relative refractory period. They investigated this by measuring the supernormal period. These authors came to several important conclusions: (1) the effect of the toxin on the supernormal period in humans can be detected by noninvasive means, (2) the effects on the supernormal period can be induced experimentally in laboratory animals, such as the rat tail nerve, and (3) the same effects are seen in intoxicated fish.

Several heart preparations have been utilized for assays. Maitotoxin inhibited calcium movement in the heart muscle of both the guinea pig and rat.[77-79] Concurrently, Ohizumi and others reported on the potent excitatory effects of maitotoxin on both cardiac and smooth muscle.[80] Quod and Legrand described the effects of ciguatoxin from the liver of *Gymnothorax javanicus* on isolated rat heart.[81] Seino and others discussed the inotropic[82] and cardiotonic[83] action of ciguatoxin on guinea-pig cardiac and atrial muscle, as did Lewis and others.[84,85]

Miyahara and others not only reported on the effects of ciguatoxin on isolated guinea-pig atria,[86] as did Oshika,[87] but Miyahara also compared it with the mouse bioassay and a radioimmunoassay.[88] Ohizumi compared the effects of ciguatoxin and maitotoxin on several tissue preparations.[89] Shimizu and others also looked at the effects of both maitotoxin and ciguatoxin from *G. toxicus* on heart muscle.[90] Shirai and others examined the effects of a low-dalton *Auricularia polytrichia* extract and ionophores on the inotropic response of ciguatoxin in guinea-pig atria.[91]

A variety of smooth-muscle preparations have been utilized for testing ciguatera-type toxins. Ohizumi and others examined the effects of ciguatoxin on guinea-pig vas deferens.[92-96] The smooth muscle of the large intestine was used as an assay system for ciguatoxin,[97] maitotoxin,[98] and scaritoxin.[96]

In 1981, Miller began using the guinea-pig ileum assay for ciguatera-type toxins. It has been found to be effective for extracts from *Scomberomorus cavalla*,[99] *G. toxicus*,[55] *Prorocentrum* sp., and *Ostreopsis*, in addition to scaritoxin[96] and palytoxin. The ileum preparation has been used by several authors to study the effects of ciguatera-type toxins.[70,92,100-105] The assay itself is further discussed in another chapter in this volume.

Cultured cells have been employed by many investigators. Freedman et al.[106] utilized cultured PC2A cells to assay a crude extract from *Gambierdiscus toxicus* and found that calcium-channel dynamics were altered. Seino et al.[83] used voltage-clamped cultured myocytes and found that CTX shifted the current voltage curve of sodium inward current 40 mV in the negative direction. Takahashi et al.[107] in 1982 found that maitotoxin activated voltage-sensitive calcium channels in cultured neuroblastoma cells. Later Yoshii et al.,[108] using cultured neuroblastoma cells, concluded that maitotoxin created a pore in the cell membrane with pharmacologic properties similar to those of a calcium channel. Hassan[109] has tested crude and semipurified extracts of *G. toxicus* on cultured (primary) cells of chick (liver and brain) and found that they induce a vacuolization in developing cells. These effects were both time and concentration dependent.

RIA and antibody tests for ciguatera-type toxins have been investigated. A series of publications since 1977 by Hokama and co-workers have dealt with the development of first a radioimmunoassay[26] for ciguatoxin, then an enzyme-linked immunoassay,[110] and over the succeeding 12 years the development of a enzyme immunoassay stick test for the detection of ciguatoxin and related polyethers.[27-29,111-114]

VI. *IN VIVO* VS. *IN VITRO* CIGUATERA TOXICITY ASSAYS

The use of intact animals as opposed to *in vitro* preparations allows examination of the effects of ciguatera toxins in conditions close to those of clinical presentation in humans.[12,35] Results from *in vivo* vs. *in vitro* assays for ciguatera toxicity have been reported as concurrent, conflictual, or controversial. Examples of correlation between *in vivo* vs. *in vitro* findings could be the demyelination of peripheral and central nerve tissue as an effect of ciguatoxin.[39,52,115] Another positive relationship between *in vivo* and *in vitro* results was that established in the assessment of ciguatoxin in fish tissues as follows: (1) using radioimmunoassay (RIA), guinea-pig atrium, and mouse bioassay;[34] (2) using RIA and the mongoose test;[26] and (3) using RIA and mouse assay expressed as the minimum lethal dose.[111]

A conflicting situation in the *in vitro* vs. *in vivo* assays might be illustrated by the subtle changes in nerve conduction parameters produced by even very low levels of ciguatoxin in the intact rat; such changes would not necessarily be manifest by isolated nerves *in vitro*.[35] Controversial results from *in vivo* vs. *in vitro* studies have surrounded the action of ciguatoxin on cholinesterase.[40,45,52,57,101,116,117]

Bagnis et al.[118] reported the relationship between the results from the cat, mouse, and mosquito bioassays to detect ciguatera toxicity in fish. The authors tentatively established the average amount of toxin per gram of fish that would make 50% of consumers sick. Subsequently, they defined ciguatera toxicity of fish in terms of cat units (CU) and *Aedes* mosquito units (AU), with the following correspondences: 1 mouse unit (MU) = 0.5 CU = 5.700 AU. The authors further placed the fishes roughly into three groups: (1) poisonous for at least 50% of the consumers, (2) safe for all the consumers, and (3) borderline (intermediate doses). Miller in this volume defines an ILU (ileum equivalent unit) and states that is equal to 0.0005 MU.

VII. SUMMARY

Bioassays for ciguatera toxins are progressing toward those systems that require less toxin for assay. What has not been addressed so far is the specificity of the assays for a particular toxin. Even the antibody-based assays are still nonspecific.

ACKNOWLEDGMENTS

This study was supported by U.S. Army Medical Research and Development Command, contract DAMD17-87-C-7002. The views, findings, and opinions expressed herein are those of the authors and should not be construed as those of the Department of the Army.

REFERENCES

1. **Halstead, B. W.,** *Poisonous and Venomous Marine Animals of the World*, Darwin Press, Princeton, NJ, 1988, chap. 10.
2. **Withers, N. W.,** Ciguatera fish toxins and poisoning, in *Handbook of Natural Toxins*, Tu, A. T., Eds., Marcel Dekker, New York, 1988,
3. **Banner, A. H.,** Ciguatera: a disease from coral reef fish, in *Biology and Geology of Coral Reefs*, Jones, O. A. and Endean, R., Eds., Academic Press, London, 1976, 177.
4. **Yasumoto, T., Nakajima, I., Bagnis, R. A., and Adachi, R.,** Finding of a dinoflagellate as a likely culprit of ciguatera, *Bull. Jpn. Soc. Sci. Fish.*, 43, 1021, 1977.
5. **Yasumoto, T., Oshima, Y., Murakami, Y., Nakajima, I., Bagnis, R. A., and Fukuyo, Y.,** Toxicity of benthic dinoflagellates found in coral reef, *Bull. Jpn. Soc. Sci. Fish.*, 46, 327, 1980.
6. **Taylor, F. J. R.,** A description of the benthic dinoflagellate associated with maitotoxin and ciguatoxin, including observations on Hawaiian material, in *Toxic Dinoflagellate Blooms*, Taylor, D. and Seliger, H. H., Eds., Elsevier North Holland, New York, 1979, 71.
7. **Bagnis, R. A.,** Clinical aspects of ciguatera (fish poisoning) in French Polynesia, *Hawaii Med. J.*, 28, 25, 1968.
8. **Bagnis, R. A., Kuberski, T., and Laugier, S.,** Clinical observations on 3,009 cases of ciguatera (fish poisoning) in the South Pacific, *Am. J. Trop. Med. Hyg.*, 28, 1067, 1979.
9. **Yasumoto, T., Raj, U., and Bagnis, R. A.,** Symposium on Seafood Toxins in Tropical Regions, Laboratory of Food Hygiene, Faculty of Agriculture, Tohoku University, Kagoshima, Japan, 1984.
10. **Anderson, D. M. and Lobel, P. S.,** The continuing enigma of ciguatera, *Biol. Bull.*, 172, 89, 1987.
11. **Scheuer, P. J., Takahashi, W., Tsutsumi, J., and Yoshida, T.,** Ciguatoxin: isolation and chemical nature, *Science*, 155, 1267, 1967.
12. **Hashimoto, Y.,** Ciguatera, in *Marine Toxins and Other Bioactive Marine Metabolites*, Japanese Scientific Societies Press, Tokyo, 1979, 91.
13. **Yasumoto, T. and Scheuer, P. J.,** Marine toxins of the Pacific — VIII. Ciguatoxin from moray eel livers, *Toxicon*, 7, 273, 1969.
14. **Yasumoto, T., Hashimoto, Y., Bagnis, R. A., Randall, J. E., and Banner, A. H.,** Toxicity of the surgeonfishes, *Bull. Jpn. Soc. Sci. Fish.*, 37, 724, 1971.
15. **Tindall, D. R., Miller, D. M., and Bomber, J.,** Culture and toxicity of dinoflagellates from ciguatera-endemic regions of the Caribbean and tropical Atlantic, in *Proc. Assoc. Island Mar. Lab. of Caribbean*, Mote Marine Laboratory, Sarosota, FL, 1988.
16. **Bagnis, R. A., Loussan, E., and Thevenin, S.,** Les intoxications par poissons perroquets aux Iles Gambier, *Méd. Trop.*, 34, 523, 1974.
17. **Chungue, E., Bagnis, R. A., Fusetani, N., and Hashimoto, Y.,** Isolation of the two toxins from a parrotfish, *Scarus gibberus*, *Toxicon*, 15, 89, 1977.
18. **Yasumoto, T., Nakajima, I., Chungue, E., and Bagnis, R. A.,** Toxins in the gut contents of parrotfish, *Bull. Jpn. Soc. Sci. Fish.*, 43, 69, 1977.
19. **Tachibana, K., Nukina, M., Joh, Y.-G., and Scheuer, P. J.,** Recent developments in the molecular structure of ciguatoxin, *Biol. Bull.*, 172, 122, 1987.
20. **Yasumoto, T.,** New results on marine dinoflagellate toxins, in *Toxic Marine Phytoplankton*, Graneli, E., Sundstrom, B., Edler, L., and Anderson, D. M., Eds., Elsevier Press, New York, 1989.
21. **Kodama, A. M., Hokama, Y., Yasumoto, T., Fukui, M., Manea, S. J., and Sutherland, N.,** Clinical and laboratory findings implicating palytoxin as cause of ciguatera poisoning due to *Decopterus macrosoma* (mackerel), *Toxicon*, 27, 1051, 1989.
22. **Murakami, Y., Oshima, Y., and Yasumoto, T.,** Identification of okadaic acid as a toxic component of a marine dinoflagellate *Prorocentrum lima*, *Bull. Jpn. Soc. Sci. Fish.*, 48, 69, 1982.
23. **Yasumoto, T.,** Recent progress in the chemistry of dinoflagellate and related toxins, in *Toxic Dinoflagellates*, Elsevier Science, New York, 1985.
24. **Gillespie, N. C., Lewis, R. J., Pearn, J. H., Bourke, A. T. C., Holmes, M. J., Bourke, J. B., and Shields, W. J.,** Ciguatera in Australia: occurrence, clinical features, pathophysiology and management, *Med. J. Aust.*, 145, 584, 1986.
25. **Banner, A. H., Scheuer, P. J., Sasaki, S., Helfrich, P., and Alender, C. B.,** Observations on ciguatera-type toxin in fish, *Ann. N.Y. Acad. Sci.*, 90, 770, 1960.
26. **Hokama, Y., Banner, A. H., and Boylan, D. B.,** A radioimmunoassay for the detection of ciguatoxin, *Toxicon*, 15, 317, 1977.
27. **Hokama, Y., Abad, M. A., and Kimura, L. H.,** A rapid enzyme immunoassay for the detection of ciguatoxin in contaminated fish tissues, *Toxicon*, 21, 817, 1983.
28. **Hokama, Y., Osugi, A. M., Honda, S. A. A., and Matsuo, M. K.,** Monoclonal antibodies in the detection of ciguatoxin and related toxic polyethers in fish tissues by a rapid poke stick test, in *Proc. Fifth Intl. Coral Reef Cong., Tahiti*, Antenne Museum-EPHE, Moorea, French Polynesia, 1985, 449.

29. **Hokama, Y., Honda, S. A. A., Uyehara, K., Shirai, M., and Kobayashi, N.,** Monoclonal antibodies to low dalton natural marine toxins, *Proc. ACS Rocky Mt. Regional Mtg., 8th*, 1986.
30. **Chungue, E., Bagnis, R. A., and Parc, F.,** The use of mosquitos (*Aedes aegypti*) to detect crude ciguatoxin in surgeon fishes (*Ctenochaetus striatus*), *Toxicon*, 22, 161, 1984.
31. **Bagnis, R. A., Chanteau, S., Chungue, E., Drollet, J. H., Lechat, I., Legrand, A.-M., Pompon, A., Prieur, C., Roux, J., and Tetaria, C.,** Comparison of the cat bioassay, the mouse bioassay and the mosquito bioassay to detect ciguatoxicity in fish, in *Proc. Fifth Intl. Coral Reef Cong., Tahiti*, Antenne Museum-EPHE, Moorea, French Polynesia, 1985, 4.
32. **Bagnis, R. A., Barsinas, M., Prieur, C., Pompon, A., Chungue, E., and Legrand, A.-M.,** The use of the mosquito bioassay for determining the toxicity to man of ciguateric fish, *Biol. Bull.*, 172, 137, 1987.
33. **Banner, A. H. and Boroughs, H.,** Observations on toxins of poisonous fishes, *Proc. Soc. Exp. Biol. Med.*, 98, 776, 1958.
34. **Kimura, L. H., Hokama, Y., Abad, M. A., Oyama, M., and Miyahara, J. T.,** Comparison of three different assays for the assessment of ciguatoxin in fish tissues: radioimmunoassay, mouse bioassay and *in vitro* guinea pig atrium assay, *Toxicon*, 20, 907, 1982.
35. **Capra, M. and Cameron, J.,** The effects of ciguatoxin on mammalian nerves, *Proc. Fifth Intl. Coral Reef Cong.*, 4, 457, 1985.
36. **Hoffman, P. A., Granade, H. R., and McMillan, J. P.,** The mouse ciguatoxin bioassay: a dose-response curve and symptomatology analysis, *Toxicon*, 21, 363, 1983.
37. **Kelley, B. A., Jollow, D. J., Felton, E. T., Voegtline, M. S., and Higerd, T. B.,** Response of mice to *Gambierdiscus toxicus, Mar. Fish. Rev.*, 48, 35, 1986.
38. **Laborit, H., Baron, C., Ferran, C., and Laborit, G.,** Biochemical and neurophysiological study of some fish toxins, *Agressologie*, 20, 81, 1979.
39. **Banner, A. H., Shaw, S. W., Alender, C. B., and Helfrich, P.,** Fish intoxication: notes on ciguatera, its mode of action and a suggested therapy, *South Pac. Commun. Tech. Pap. Nouvea, New Caledonia*, 141, 1, 1963.
40. **Bagnis, R. A. and Fevai, G.,** La ciguatera féline experimentale à Tahiti, *Rev. Méd. Vet.*, 122, 629, 1971.
41. **Legrand, A.-M., Galonnier, M., and Bagnis, R. A.,** Studies on the mode of action of ciguateric toxins, *Toxicon*, 20, 311, 1982.
42. **Larson, E. and Rivas, L. R.,** Ciguatera poisoning from barracuda, *Q. J. Fla. Acad. Sci.*, 28, 173, 1965.
43. **Banner, A. H., Sasaki, S., Helfrich, P., Alender, C. B., and Scheuer, P. J.,** Bioassay of ciguatera toxin, *Nature*, 189, 229, 1961.
44. **Li, K.-M.,** A note on ciguatera fish poisoning and action of its proposed antidotes (Ciguatera Fish Poisoning: A Symposium), *Hawaii Med. J.*, 24, 359, 1965.
45. **Kosaki, T. I. and Stephens, J.,** Pupillary miosis to ciguatoxin(s) (from *Gymnothorax javanicus*), *Fed. Proc.*, 26, 322, 1967.
46. **Vernoux, J.-P., Lahlou, N., Magras, L. P., and Greaux, J. B.,** Chick feeding test: a simple system to detect ciguatoxin, *Acta Tropica*, 42, 235, 1985.
47. **Vernoux, J.-P., Magras, L. P., Abbad el Andaloussi, S., and Riyeche, N.,** Contrôle biologique de la ciguatoxine chez le poussin: analyse des symptômes induits et de la toxicity d'extraits de poisssons ciguatoxiques, *Bull. Soc. Pathol. Exot.*, 79, 140, 1986.
48. **Hiyama, Y.,** Report on the research on poisonous fishes of the south seas, *Nissan Fish. Exp. Stat. Rep.*, 1943, 1, 1943.
49. **Halstead, B. W.,** Fish poisonings — their pharmacology, diagnosis, and treatment, *Clin. Pharmacol. Therap.*, 5, 615, 1958.
50. **Hessel, D. W., Halstead, B. W., and Peckham, N. H.,** Marine biotoxins I. Ciguatera poison: some biological and chemical aspects, *Ann. N.Y. Acad. Sci.*, 90, 788, 1960.
51. **Hashimoto, Y.,** A note on the poison of a barracuda, *Sphyrena picuda* Bloch and Schneider, *Bull. Jpn. Soc. Sci. Fish.*, 21, 1153, 1956.
52. **Kosaki, T. I. and Anderson, H. H.,** Marine toxins from the Pacific — IV. Pharmacology of ciguatoxin(s), *Toxicon*, 6, 55, 1968.
53. **Halstead, B. W. and Bunker, N. C.,** A survey of poisonous fishes of Johnston Island, *Zoologica*, 39, 65, 1954.
54. **Tachibana, K.,** Structural Studies on Marine Toxins, Ph.D. Dissertation, University of Hawaii, Honolulu, Hawaii, 1980.
55. **Dickey, R. W., Miller, D. M., and Tindall, D. R.,** Extraction of a water-soluble toxin from a dinoflagellate, *Gambierdiscus toxicus*, in *Seafood Toxins*, Ragelis, E. P., Eds., American Chemical Society Symposium Series 262, Washington, D.C., 1984, 257.
56. **Weil, C. S.,** Experimental design and interpretation of data from prolonged toxicity studies, in *Proc. Fifth Intl. Cong. Pharmacology*, Acheson, G. H., Eds., S. Karger, Basel, 1973, 4.
57. **Li, K.-M.,** Ciguatera fish poison: a potent cholinesterase inhibitor, *Science*, 147, 1580, 1965.
58. **Hahn, S., Capra, M., Miller, D. M., and Tindall, D. R.,** Unpublished data, 1989.
59. **Larsen, J. R., Miller, D. M., and Yamamoto, T.,** d-Tubocurarine chloride: effect on insects, *Science*, 152, 225, 1966.

60. **Granade, H. R., Cheng, P. C., and Doorenbos, N. C.,** Ciguatera I. Brine shrimp (*Artemia salina* L.) larval assay for ciguatera toxins, *J. Pharaceut. Sci.*, 65, 1414, 1976.
61. **Siger, A., Abbott, B. C., and Ross, M.,** Response of the housefly to saxitoxin and contaminated shellfish, in *Seafood Toxins*, Ragelis, E. P., Eds., American Chemical Society Symposium Series 262, Washington, D.C., 1984, 193.
62. **Vernoux, J.-P., Magras, L. P., Abbad el Andaloussi, S., and Riyeche, N.,** Evaluation of different-stage levels of ciguatera toxicity of the marine food fish chain found around Saint Barthelemy Island in French Antilles, *Bull. Soc. Pathol. Exot.*, 79, 275, 1986.
63. **Randall, J. E.,** A review of ciguatera, tropical fish poisoning, with a tentative explanation of its cause, *Bull. Mar. Sci. Gulf. Carib.*, 8, 236, 1958.
64. **Setliff, J. A., Rayner, M. D., and Hong, S. K.,** Effect of ciguatoxin on sodium transport across the frog skin, *Toxicol. App. Pharmacol.*, 18, 676, 1971.
65. **Rayner, M. D. and Szekerczes, J.,** Ciguatoxin: effects on the sodium-potassium activated adenosine triphosphatase of human erythrocyte ghosts, *Toxicol. Appl. Pharmacol.*, 24, 489, 1973.
66. **Nishiyama, I., Matsui, T., Yasumoto, T., and Yasumasei, I.,** Maitotoxin a presumed calcium channel activator induces the acrosome reaction in mussel spermatozoa, *Dev. Growth Differ.*, 28, 443, 1986.
67. **Gomi, S., Chaen, S., and Sugi, H.,** The mode of action of maitotoxin on the membrane system of frog skeletal muscle fibers, *Proc. Jpn. Acad., Ser. B*, 60, 28, 1984.
68. **Rayner, M. D. and Kosaki, T. I.,** Ciguatoxin: effects on Na fluxes in frog muscle, *Fed. Proc.*, 29, 548, 1970.
69. **Miyamoto, T., Ohizumi, H., Washino, H., and Yasumoto, T.,** Potent excitatory effects of maitotoxin on Ca channels in the insect skeletal muscle, *Pflügers Arch.*, 400, 439, 1984.
70. **Miller, D. M., Dickey, R. W., and Tindall, D. R.,** Lipid soluble toxins from a dinoflagellate, *Gambierdiscus toxicus*, isolated from a Caribbean region supporting ciguateric fish, *The Physiologist*, 26, a41, 1983.
71. **Miller, D. M., Tindall, D. R., and Tibbs, B.,** Ciguatera-type toxins: bioassay using crayfish nerve cord, *Fed. Proc.*, 45, 345, 1986.
72. **Legrand, A.-M., Benoit, E., and Dubois, J. M.,** Electrophysiological studies of the effects of ciguatoxin in the frog myelinated nerve fiber, in *Toxic Dinoflagellates*, Anderson, D. M., White, A. W. and Baden, D. G., Eds., Elsevier Science, New York, 1985, 381.
73. **Boyarsky, L. L. and Rayner, M. D.,** The effect of ciguatera toxin on *Aplysia* neurons, *Proc. Soc. Exp. Biol. Med.*, 134, 332, 1970.
74. **Cameron, J., Flowers, A. E., and Capra, M. F.,** The effects of ciguatoxin on nerve conduction parameters in humans and the laboratory rat, in *Proc. Ninth World Cong. on Animal, Plant and Microbial Toxins*, Intl. Soc. Toxicology, Stillwater, OK, 1988.
75. **Capra, M. F., Flowers, A. E., and Cameron, J.,** The effect of ciguatoxin on the rate of Na^+ efflux in unmyelinated olfactory nerves of teleosts, in *First Asia-Pacific Cong. on Animal, Plant and Microbial Toxins*, 1987.
76. **Flowers, A. E., Capra, M. F., and Cameron, J.,** The effects of ciguatoxin on nerve conduction parameters in teleost fish, in *Progress in Venom and Toxin Research*, Gopalakrishnakone, P. and Tan, C. K., Eds., First Asia-Pacific Congress on Animal, Plant and Microbial Toxins, Singapore, 1987.
77. **Kobayashi, M., Ohizumi, Y. and Yasumoto, T.,** The mechanism of action of maitotoxin in relation to Ca^{2+} movements in the guinea-pig and rat cardiac muscle, *Br. J. Pharmacol.*, 86, 385, 1985.
78. **Kobayashi, M., Kondo, S., Yasumoto, T., and Ohizumi, Y.,** Cardiotoxic effects of maitotoxin, a principle toxin of seafood poisoning, on guinea pig and rat cardiac muscle, *J. Pharmacol. Exp. Therap.*, 238, 1077, 1986.
79. **Kobayashi, M., Kondo, S., Yasumoto, T., and Ohizumi, Y.,** The mode of arrhythmogenic action of maitotoxin in relation to Ca^{2+} movements in cardiac muscle, *Jpn. J. Pharmacol.*, 46, 212, 1988.
80. **Ohizumi, Y., Kobayashi, M., Kajiwara, A., and Yasumoto, T.,** Potent excitatory effects of maitotoxin on cardiac and smooth muscle, in *Toxic Dinoflagellates*, Anderson, D. M., White, A. W., and Baden, D. G., Eds., Elsevier Science, New York, 1985, 369.
81. **Quod, J. P. and Legrand, A.-M.,** Effects of partially purified ciguatoxin from moray-eel, *Gymnothorax javanicus*, on action potential of isolated rat heart, in *Progress in Venom and Toxin Research*, Gopalakrishnakone, P. and Tan, C. K., Eds., First Asia-Pacific Congress on Animal, Plant and Microbial Toxins, Singapore, 1987.
82. **Seino, A., Kobayashi, M., Momose, K., Yasumoto, T., and Ohizumi, Y.,** The mode of inotropic action of ciguatoxin on guinea-pig cardiac muscle, *Br. J. Pharmacol.*, 95, 876, 1988.
83. **Seino, A., Momose, K., Yasumoto, T., Kobayashi, M., and Ohizumi, Y.,** The mode of cardiotonic action of ciguatoxin on atrial muscle, *Jpn. J. Pharmacol.*, 43, 173, 1987.
84. **Lewis, R. J.,** The cardiotoxic effects of ciguatoxin, in *Toxic Dinoflagellates*, Anderson, D. M., White, A. W. and Baden, D. G., Eds., Elsevier Science, New York, 1985, 379.
85. **Lewis, R. J. and Endean, R.,** Direct and indirect effects of ciguatoxin on the guinea-pig atria and papillary muscles, *Naunyn-Schmiedebergs Arch. Pharmacol.*, 1986.

86. **Miyahara, J. T., Akau, C. K., and Yasumoto, T.,** Effects of ciguatoxin and maitotoxin on the isolated guinea pig atria, *Res. Comm. Chem. Pathol. Pharmacol.*, 25, 177, 1979.
87. **Ohshika, H.,** Marine toxins from the Pacific — IX Some effects of ciguatoxin on isolated mammalian atria, *Toxicon*, 9, 337, 1971.
88. **Miyahara, J. T., Oyama, M., H., K. L., Honbo, K., Abad, M. A., Furuya, N., and Hokama, Y.,** Examination of three assays for ciguatoxin (CTX) determination: mouse toxicity, guinea pig atrium, and radioimmunoassay (RIA), *Fed. Proc.*, 40, 694, 1981.
89. **Ohizumi, Y.,** Pharmacological actions of the marine toxins ciguatoxin and maitotoxin isolated from poisonous fish, *Biol. Bull.*, 172, 132, 1987.
90. **Shimizu, Y., Shimizu, H., Scheuer, P. J., Hokama, Y., Oyama, M., and Miyahara, J. T.,** *Gambierdiscus toxicus*, a ciguatera-causing dinoflagellate from Hawaii, *Bull. Jpn. Soc. Sci. Fish.*, 48, 811, 1982.
91. **Shirai, L. K., Miyahara, J. T., Ching, N. P., and Hokama, Y.,** Effects of low dalton *Auricularia polytrichia* extract and ionophores on the inotropic response of ciguatoxin (CTX) in guinea pig atria *in vitro*, *Fed. Proc.*, 30, 812, 1986.
92. **Lewis, R. J. and Endean, R.,** Mode of action of ciguatoxin from the spanish mackerel, *Scomberomorus commersoni* on the guinea pig ileum and vas deferens, *J. Pharmacol. Exp. Therap.*, 228, 756, 1984.
93. **Ohizumi, Y., Kajiwara, A., and Yasumoto, T.,** Excitatory effect of the most potent marine toxin, MTX, on the guinea pig vas deferens, *J. Pharmacol. Exp. Therap.*, 227, 199, 1983.
94. **Ohizumi, Y., Ishida, Y., and Shibata, S.,** Mode of the ciguatoxin-induced supersensitivity in the guinea pig vas deferens, *J. Pharmacol. Exp. Therap.*, 221, 748, 1982.
95. **Ohizumi, Y. and Shibata, S.,** Mechanism of the action of palytoxin and n-acetylpalytoxin in the isolated guinea pig vas deferens., *J. Pharmacol. Exp. Therap.*, 214, 209, 1980.
96. **Tatsumi, M., Kajiwara, A., Yasumoto, T., and Ohizumi, Y.,** Potent excitatory effect of scaritoxin on the guinea-pig vas deferens, taenia caeci and ileum, *J. Pharmacol. Exp. Therap.*, 235, 783, 1985.
97. **Miyahara, J. T. and Shibata, S.,** Effects of ciguatera toxin on the guinea-pig taenia caecum, *Fed. Proc.*, 35, 842, 1976.
98. **Ohizumi, Y. and Yasumoto, T.,** Contraction and increase in tissue calcium content induced by maitotoxin, the most potent known marine toxin, in intestinal smooth muscle, *Br. J. Pharmacol.*, 79, 3, 1983.
99. **Dickey, R. W., Miller, D. M., and Tindall, D. R.,** The extraction and effects of crude ciguatoxin from *Scomberomorus cavalla* upon acetylcholine and histamine receptor sites of the guinea pig ileum, *Fed. Proc.*, 41, 1562, 1982.
100. **Miller, D. M., Dickey, R. W., and Tindall, D. R.,** The effects of a lipid extracted toxin from the dinoflagellate *Gambierdiscus toxicus* upon nerve-muscle and intestinal preparations, *Fed. Proc.*, 41, 1561, 1982.
101. **Miller, D. M., Dickey, R. W., and Tindall, D. R.,** Lipid soluble toxins from a dinoflagellate, *Gambierdiscus toxicus*, in *Seafood Toxins*, Ragelis, R. P., Eds., American Chemical Society Symposium Series 262, Washington, D.C., 1984, 241.
102. **Miller, R. J., Freedman, S. B., Miller, D. M., and Tindall, D. R.,** Maitotoxin activates voltage sensitive calcium channels in cultured neuronal cells, *Proc. Intl. Cong. Pharmacol. (9th)*, 80, 1984.
103. **Miller, D. M. and Tindall, D. R.,** Physiological effects of HPLC-purified maitotoxin from a dinoflagellate, *Gambierdiscus toxicus*, in *Toxic Dinoflagellates*, Anderson, D. M., White, A. W., and Baden, D. G., Eds., Elsevier Science, New York, 1985, 375.
104. **Miller, D. M., Tindall, D. R., and Hassan, F.,** Effects of maitotoxin on guinea pig ileum, *Fed. Proc.*, 44, 1985.
105. **Miller, D. M. and Tindall, D. R.,** Factors interacting with the effects of the maitotoxin fraction from *Gambierdiscus toxicus*, *Fed. Proc.*, 46, 1987.
106. **Freedman, S. B., Miller, R. J., Miller, D. M., and Tindall, D. R.,** Interactions of maitotoxin with voltage-sensitive calcium channels in cultured neuronal cells, *Proc. Natl. Acad. Sci. USA*, 81, 4582, 1984.
107. **Takahashi, M., Ohizumi, Y., and Yasumoto, T.,** Maitotoxin, a Ca^{2+} channel activator candidate, *J. Biol. Chem.*, 257, 7287, 1982.
108. **Yoshii, M., Tsunoo, A., Kuroda, Y., Wu, C. H., and Narahashi, T.,** Maitotoxin induces a steady current which is inhibited by calcium channel blockers, *Neurosci. Soc. Abst.*, 10, 528, 1984.
109. **Hassan, F.,** Effects of Maitotoxin and Ciguatoxin on Primary Cell Cultures of Chick Brain and Liver, Ph.D. Thesis, Southern Illinois University, Carbondale, IL, 1989.
110. **Hokama, Y., Yoyo, B. S., Sasaki, R. R., and Monta, A. H.,** An enzyme-linked immunological assay for the detection of ciguatoxin from fish tissues, *Science*, 41, 1978.
111. **Hokama, Y., Okubo, C. M., Cripps, C., Matsukawa, L. A., and Kimura, L. H.,** The effect of purified ciguatoxin on mitogen responses of mouse spleen lymphoid cells, *Res. Comm. Chem. Path. Pharmacol.*, 29, 397, 1980.
112. **Hokama, Y., Kimura, L. H., Abad, M. A., Yokochi, L., Scheuer, P. J., Nukina, M., Yasumoto, T., Baden, D. G., and Shimizu, Y.,** An enzyme immunoassay for the detection of ciguatoxin, in *Seafood Toxins*, Ragelis, E. P., Eds., American Chemical Society Symposium Series No. 262, Washington, D.C., 1984, 307.

113. **Hokama, Y.,** A rapid, simplified enzyme immunoassay stick test for the detection of ciguatoxin and related polyethers from fish tissues, *Toxicon*, 23, 939, 1985.
114. **Hokama, Y., Honda, S. A. A., Kobayashi, M. N., Nakagawa, L. K., Asahina, A. Y., and Miyahara, J. T.,** Monoclonal antibody (MAb) in detection of ciguatoxin (CTX) and related polyethers by the stick-enzyme immunoassay (S-EIA) in fish tissues associated with ciguatera poisoning, in *Proc. 7th Intl. Symp. on Mycotoxins and Phycotoxins (IUPAC, Tokyo)*, Elsevier Press, New York, 1989,
115. **Kosaki, T. I. and Anderson, H. H.,** Marine toxins from the Pacific III comparative bioassay of ciguatoxin(s) in the mouse and chicken, *Proc. West. Pharmacol. Soc.*, 11, 126, 1968.
116. **Rayner, M. D., Baslow, M. H., and Kosaki, T. I.,** Marine toxins from the Pacific — ciguatoxin: not an *in vivo* anticholinesterase, *J. Fish. Res. Bd. Can.*, 26, 2208, 1969.
117. **Baslow, M. H. and Rayner, M. D.,** Ciguatoxin: lack of evidence for anticholinesterase activity *in vivo*, *Proc. Intl. Cong. Pharmacol. (4th)*, 180, 30, 1969.
118. **Bagnis, R. A., Bennett, J., Prieur, C., and Legrand, A.-M.,** The dynamics of three toxic benthic dinoflgellates and the toxicity of ciguateric surgeonfish in French Polynesia, in *Proc. Third Int. Conf. Toxic Dinoflagellates*, Anderson, D. M., White, A. W., and Baden, D. G., Eds., Elsevier, New York, 1985, 177.

Chapter 7

NMR OF MARINE TOXINS

Charles W. Venable and Donald M. Miller

TABLE OF CONTENTS

I. INTRODUCTION

The establishment of an absolute configuration of a given compound usually requires the complementary efforts of X-ray crystallography, mass spectroscopy, and nuclear magnetic resonance (NMR). NMR is playing an increasingly important role today in the study of marine toxins, as FT-NMR allows for signal averaging for small sample amounts. All NMR data must be satisfactorily assigned to determine an absolute molecular structure.

II. PARALYTIC SHELLFISH TOXINS

The first marine toxin to be established was saxitoxin (STX), a powerful neurotoxin isolated from shellfish but later identified as a product of the dinoflagellate, *G. tamarensis*.[1,2] Due to its noncrystalline, highly polar, and nonvolatile nature, 20 years were required to determine its structure. Two structures were initially proposed that seemingly satisfied the NMR data (Figure 1).

In structure A, the 4.77 ppm signal is assigned as H5 with small 1-Hz coupling to H6 and with the proprionic chain from N3 bridged at C4. The 1-Hz coupling indicates an axioequitorial alignment for H6 and H5. In structure B, the N3 propionic chain is bridged at C5 and the 4.77 signal is assigned to H4. This necessitates a long-range, 1-Hz coupling between H4 and H6, an effect not commonly seen in polar solvents such as D_2O used here. Structure A is the accepted STX configuration, with C12 existing in an equilibrium state between the ketone and the hydrated ketone, with the latter favored at physiologic pH.[2]

At present 12 analogs of STX have been isolated. Proton NMR data has been presented for 10[1-8] of these compounds and ^{13}C data for 5.[4,8-10] The first derivatives of STX to be found were extracted from *G. tamarensis*,[9] coded GTX-II and GTX-III, and thought to be the 11(a-b) hydroxy epimers. They were later shown, however, to be 11(a-b)OSO^{3-} epimers of STX[3], with a mouse lethality of 2500 MU/mg, about one half that of STX. Then the N1 hydroxy STX derivative was found and named *neosaxitoxin* (neoSTX),[4] having an LD_{50} of 5000 MU/mg, thus rivaling STX in toxicity at 5500 MU/mg. Next the 11(a-b) OSO^{3-} epimers of neoSTX were isolated and coded GTX-I and GTX-IV.[5] ^1H NMR data is given in Table 1 for these toxins, which reveal the influence of the various substituents on the core framework of STX.

The N1 hydroxy substituent on neoSTX is seen to produce a downfield shift for H5, H6, H13A, and H13B. Also the H6 signal was seen to undergo the greatest increase (upfield shift) in ppm as pH was varied from 5 to 8 in association with the 6.75 pKa for the N1 hydroxyl.[4] For the *Gonyaulax* toxins, the NMR data reveal a strong electron withdrawing substituent on C11. The 2.4 ppm multiplet in the STX and neoSTX spectra is replaced by a downfield signal near 5.0 ppm with one or two coupling constants.[3] Furthermore, the coupling patterns on 10A, 10B, and 11 are altered from those in STX and neoSTX.[5] In GTX-I and GTX-II, the large coupling of H10A and H10B to H11 is lost but regained in GTX-III and GTX-IV. With inorganic sulphate hydrolyzed from GTX-II at a 1:1 molar ratio,[3] these data established GTX-II and GTX-III as the C11 (a-b) sulpho epimers of STX, and GTX-I and GTX-IV as the C11 (a-b) sulpho epimers of neoSTX (Figure 2).

Other derivatives of the parent compounds STX and neoSTX have been found that involve substitution at O14[6-8,10] and reveal some light on the nature of the toxicity of STX. Under strong hydrolysis conditions, the carbamyl group is removed and the resulting product decarbamyl STX (dcSTX) retains 60% of the original toxicity.[10] However, when the decarbamyl group is sulfonated with SO_3^-, the toxicity is reduced at least 15 times.[6,7] Six compounds of this type have been found.[7,8] The structures and accompanying ^1H NMR data of these are shown (Figure 3 and Table 2). The effect of the sulfonation of the carbamyl group is seen in GT-V, GT-VI, and GT-VIII by the downfield shift at H13A and H13B, while the effect of the OSO^{3-} substituent at C11 in GTX-VIII produces the identical shifts and couplings at H10A, H10B, and H11, as seen in GTX-III.

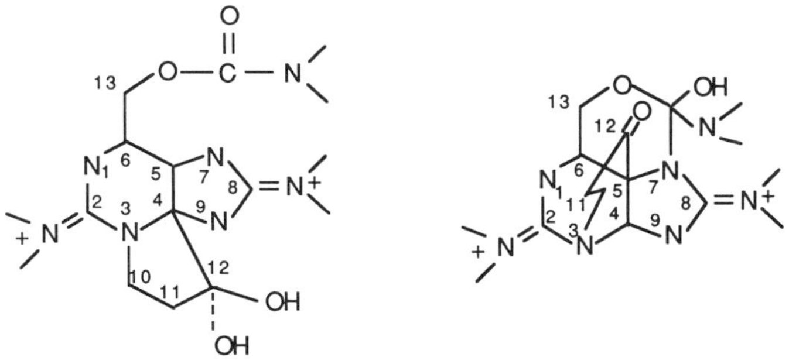

	4.77 (1)	3.87 (9,5,1)	4.27 (11,9)	4.05 (11,5)	3.87 M	3.57 M	2.37 M
A	H5	H6	H13A	H13B	10A	10B	11
B	H4	H6	H13A	H13B	10A	10B	11

FIGURE 1. Two initially proposed structures for STX fitted to existing ^{1}H NMR data. Signals observed in D_2O.

TABLE 1
^{1}H NMR Chemical Shifts and Coupling Constants (Hz) for STX, neoSTX, and GTX-I-IV in D_2O

	5	6	13A	13B	10A	10B	11
STX	4.77	3.87	4.27	4.05	3.85	3.57	2.37
	(1)	(9, 5, 1)	(11, 9)	(11, 5)	(2.5, 10, 11)	(8,10,11)	M
GTX-II					4.15	3.98	4.83
					(12)	(12, 5)	(5)
GTX-III					4.14	3.55	4.93
					(11, 9)	(11, 7)	(9, 7)
neoSTX	4.83	4.15	4.43	4.28	3.80	3.58	2.44
		(1, 6, 6)	(11, 6)	(11, 6)	(2.7, 10, 10)	(7, 10, 10)	M
GTX-I					4.15	3.97	4.85
					(11)	(5, 11)	(5)
GTX-IV					4.18	3.61	4.97
					(10, 8)	(7, 10)	(8, 7)

Note: Average values from sources cited in text have been listed. Only signals significantly different than STX for GTX-II and GTX-III are shown; likewise for neoSTX, GTX-I and GTX-IV.

For completeness we include the existing ^{13}C data presently available on the STX family (Table 3). These data were presented concurrently with various parts of the ^{1}H NMR data by different investigators[4,8-10] and utilized in establishing the configurations presented above.

III. BREVETOXINS

To date, eight neurotoxins have been isolated and identified for *Ptychodiscus brevis* (syn. *Gymnodinium breve*), the causative organism of massive fish kills along the Florida Gulf Coast. The six most potent toxins are cyclic polyether compounds with toxicities about 40 µg/kg. The other two toxins are novel phosphorus compounds with 1000-fold less toxicity. The most abundant polyether toxin, brevetoxin-B (BTX-B or GB-2), was the first to be determined.[11] It

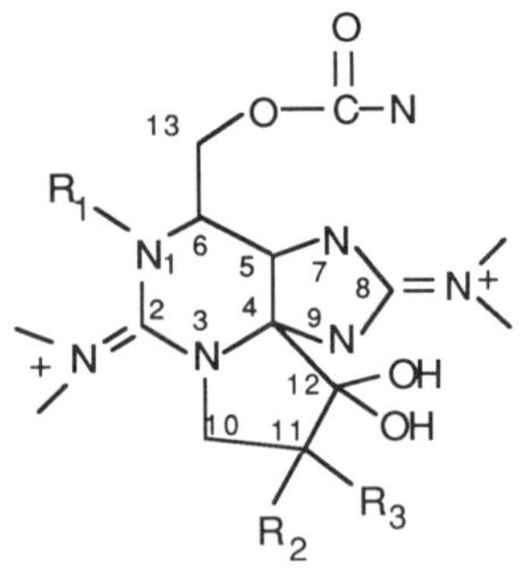

R_1	R_2	R_3	
H	H	H	STX
H	H	OSO_3^-	GTX-II
H	OSO_3^-	H	GTX-III
OH	H	H	NeoSTX
OH	H	OSO_3^-	GTX-I
OH	OSO_3^-	H	GTX-IV

FIGURE 2. Structural configurations for STX, neoSTX, and GTX-I to GTX-IV.

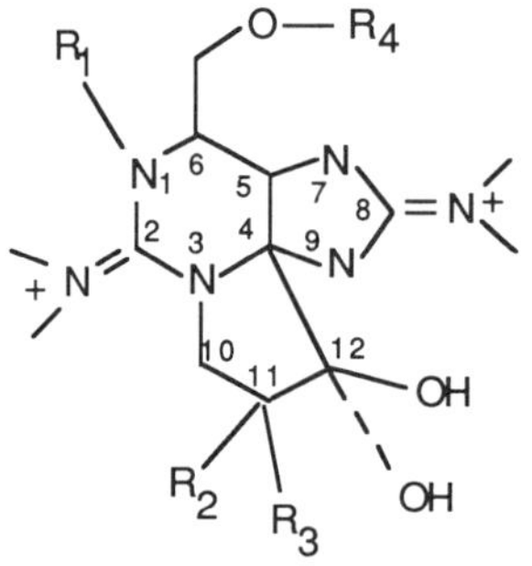

R_1	R_2	R_3	R_4	
H	H	H	H	dcSTX
H	H	H	$CONHSO_3^-$	GTX-XV, B_1
OH	H	H	$CONHSO_3^-$	GTX-VI, B_2
H	OSO_3^-	H	$CONHSO_3^-$	GTX-VIII, C_2
H	H	OSO_3^-	$CONHSO_3^-$	C1
OH	H	OSO_3^-	$CONHSO_3^-$	C3
OH	OSO_3^-	H	$CONHSO_3^-$	C4

	5	6	13A	13B	10A	10B	11
dcSTX	4.61	3.63M	3.63M	3.63M	3.77	3.54	
GTX-V	4.76	3.88 (9,5,1)	4.42 (12,9)	4.12 (12,5)	3.81	3.67	
GTX-VI	4.83	4.13 (6,6)	4.52 (11,6)	4.26 (11,6)	3.78 (10)	3.58 (10)	
GTX-VIII	4.78	3.81 (9,5)	4.32 (12,9,5)	4.11 (12,5)	4.12 (10,6,8)	3.54 (10,6,8)	4.91 (8,8)

FIGURE 3. Structural configurations for STX and neoSTX derivatives with O14 substituents.

TABLE 2
Available ¹H NMR Data for dc STX, GTX-V, GTX-VI and GTX-VIII

	5	6	13A	13B	10A	10B	11
dcSTX	4.61	3.63 M	3.63 M	3.63 M	3.77	3.54	—
GTX-V	4.76	3.88(9,5,1)	4.42(12,9)	4.12(12,5)	3.81	3.61	—
GTX-VI	4.83	4.13(6,6)	4.52(11,6)	4.26(11,6)	3.78(10)	3.58(10)	—
GTX-VIII	4.78	3.81(9,5)	4.32(12,9.5)	4.11(12,5)	4.12(10.6,8)	3.54(10.6,8)	4.91(8,8)

Note: In all but GTX-VIII, the C11 protons were unobservable due to deuterium exchange from D_2O solvent.

TABLE 3
¹³C Data for STX, neoSTX, and Related Derivatives

	STX	GTX-II	neoSTX	GTX-V	dcSTX
C14	159.0	159.1	159.0	154.1	—
C2	157.9	158.0	158.5	158.1	158.5
C8	156.1	156.2	157.4	156.1	156.7
C12	98.9	97.5	98.6	98.6	99.4
C4	82.6	81.5	82.2	82.6	83.1
C13	63.3	63.3	61.1	64.0	62.0
C5	57.3	57.9	56.9	57.2	57.3
C6	53.2	53.2	64.4	53.0	56.3
C10	43.0	50.9	43.9	42.9	43.6
C11	33.1	77.6	31.9	Unobserved	33.6

is a single carbon chain locked into a rigid planar ladderlike structure consisting of 11 contiguous transfused ether rings, a structure with no precedent or obvious plausable bioenergetic scheme. Four derivatives of BTX-B have since been identified and isolated: BTX-C, GB-3, GB-5, and GB-6, all minor compounds.[12-14] BTX-C and GB-5 have toxicities of about half that of BTX-B, and the toxicities of GB-5 and GB-6 are, as of yet, unknown. Recently the structure of a sixth polyether toxin, brevetoxin A(GB-1), the most potent of all the brevetoxins has been determined.[15] Its toxicity is tenfold greater than BTX-B, putting it in the class of the PSP toxins. Its structure is similar to that of BTX-B, but with significant differences. The structure of BTX-B and derivatives are shown in Figure 4.

While the seven ¹H NMR methyl signals and others are almost identical for BTX-B and its derivatives, the low field signals vary greatly.[12-14] Methyl signals are observed in CDC13 for BTX-B at $\delta 1.04^d$, $\delta 1.18^s$, $\delta 1.22^s$, $\delta 1.25^s$, $\delta 1.30^s$, $\delta 1.31^s$, and $\delta 1.97^s$. Other common ¹H signals are δ5.73 (H-2), δ4.17 (H-4), and δ5.78 (H-27, H-28). Low field signals that vary by derivative are shown in Table 4.[11-14] The ¹H spectrum for GB-5 and GB-6 is identical to that of BTX-B, except for the 36, 37 positions and 27, 28 for G-6.

The most potent of the brevetoxins, brevetoxin A(GB-1), has a similar but different polyether structure than the essentially planar BTX-B structure. The structure of brevetoxin A is shown in Figure 5.[15] It has ten ether rings, one less than BTX-B, with only four methyl groups, as contrasted to seven for BTX-B. Unusual peak broadings or disappearances of signals attributed to protons on or near ring G were experienced in the NMR studies, from which it is speculated that the BC form and the crown conformation exist simultaneously in solution. This and the presence of two double bonds in the larger central rings of the molecule may be additional factors contributing to the tenfold increase in toxicity of BTX-A over BTX-B and its derivatives. Reported ¹H and ¹³C NMR signals for BTX-A are shown in Table 5.[15]

The two phosphorus-containing toxins have structures that are very different from the

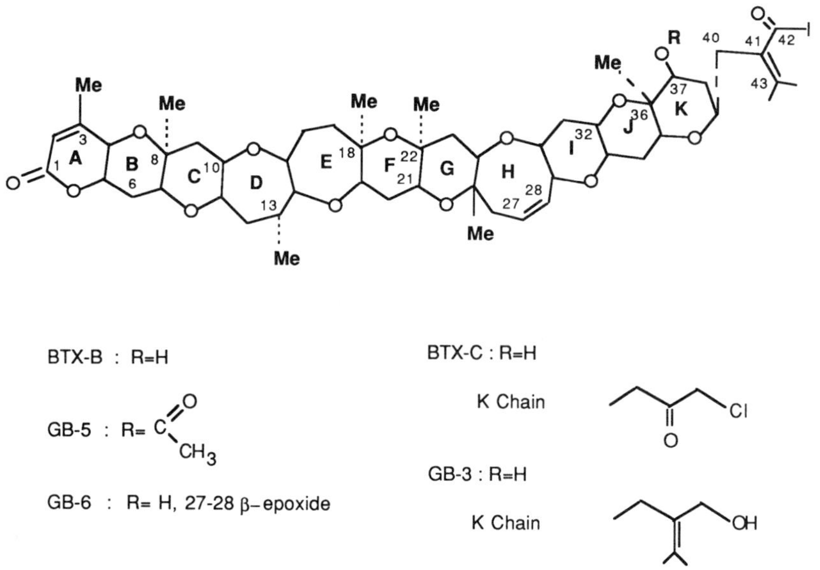

BTX-B : R=H

GB-5 : R= C(=O)CH3

GB-6 : R= H, 27-28 β-epoxide

BTX-C : R=H

K Chain

GB-3 : R=H

K Chain

FIGURE 4. Structure of BTX-B (GB-2) and derivatives.

TABLE 4
Low Field ^{1}H NMR Signals for BTX-B and Derivatives

	39H	40H-A	40H-B	42H	43H-A	43H-B	36Me	37H	R
BTX-B	3.92	3.16	2.49	9.53	6.32	6.09	1.22		
BTX-C	4.45	3.43	3.10	4.10					
GB-3	NA	NA	NA	4.09	5.11	4.95			
GB-5							1.30	5.10	2.12
GB-6				3.03(27H)	2.87(28H)		1.22	3.80	

polyethers. One of them, Gb-4, is a thiophosphonate with the structure shown in Figure 6 and the ^{1}H NMR data in Table 6.[16]

When the 1.70 ppm multiplet was irradiated, the absorptions at 3.97 and 4.02 collapsed into simple triplets, revealing the expected three-bond coupling between P and 1 HA, 1′ HA. The NOH signal was observed in DMSO at 8.39 ppm.[16]

The other phosphorus-containing toxin, PB-1, has been identified as O, O diphenyl-N-cyclooctyl phosphoramidate and has the structure illustrated in Figure 7.[17]

^{1}H NMR data for this compound reveal the signals listed in Table 7.

The three-bond coupling between P and H was also observed here. When the 3.45 ppm signal was saturated, and the 3.72 ppm signal collapsed to an 11-Hz doublet. As only a minimal sample amount for PB-1 was observed, a 2-d accumulation period with a 5-s relaxation delay and a 30° pulse width was necessary to resolve all the carbon signals.[17] The following assignments were made from the proton-decoupled ^{13}C spectrum (Table 8).

The long-range phosphorus coupling was again seen as the 151.1, 120.1, and 34.1 ppm signals all appeared as 6-Hz doublets.

IV. DIARRHETIC SHELLFISH TOXINS

The diarrhetic shellfish toxins (DSP) have been well studied and have been found to be polyether compounds. These compounds for which the toxicity has been completely determined

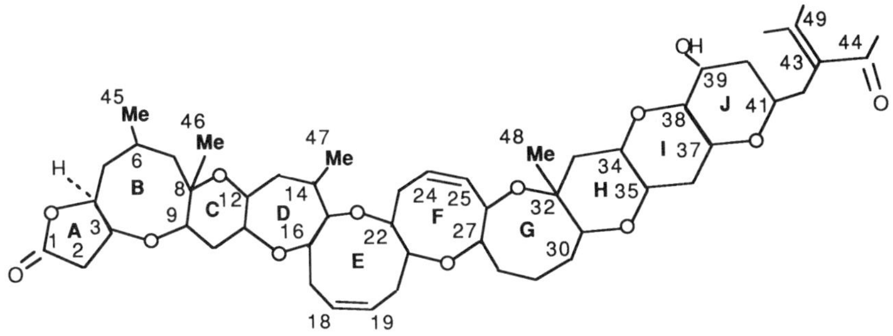

FIGURE 5. Structure of BTX-A.

TABLE 5
^{13}C and ^{1}H Signals for BTX-A (GB-1)

	2	3	4	9	18	19	24	25	
δ^{1}H	2.79, 2.61	3.95	4.10	3.24	5.53	5.53	5.53	5.66	
13C	38.1	85.2	85.3	87.2	129.7	126.8	124.7	138.9	
	26	27	37	38	39	41	42	44	49
δ^{1}H	4.40	3.37	3.86	3.06	4.14	3.92	3.16, 2.49	9.51	6.09, 6.36
13C	72.0	80.0	62.4	80.3	66.4	71.1	31.9	194.9	136.3
δ^{1}H	2.79, 2.61	3.95	4.10		3.24	2.60	5.53	5.66	
δ^{13}C	38.1	85.2	85.3	77.0	87.2	31.3	124.7	138.9	
	26	27	18	19	34	35	37	38	
δ^{1}H	4.40	3.57	5.53	5.53	3.25	3.06	3.86	3.06	
δ^{13}C	72.0	80.0	129.7	126.8	83.6	78.8	62.4	80.3	
	39	41	42	44	49				
	4.14	3.92	3.16, 2.49	9.51	6.09, 6.36				
	66.4	71.1	31.9	194.9	136.3				

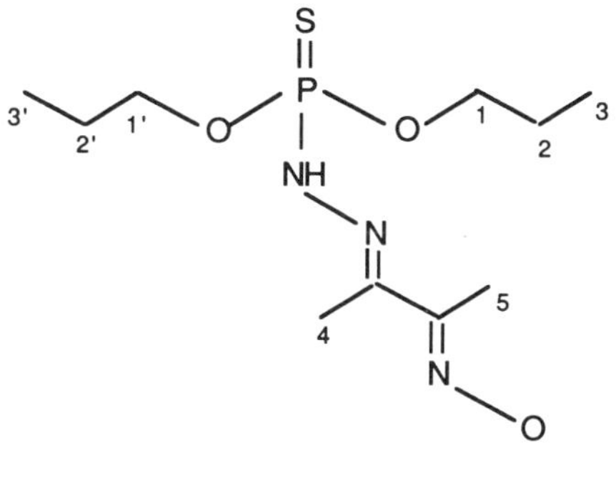

FIGURE 6. Structure of Gb-4.

were isolated from *Prorocentrum lima* [18] and also from two marine sponges.[19] Two derivatives of okadaic acid have been isolated from *Dinophysis fortii*,[20,21] designated DTX-1 (160 μg/kg) and DTX-3 (500 μg/kg). Furthermore, acanthifolicin, an episulfide derivative of okadaic acid, was isolated from the sponge *Pandorus acanthifolicin*,[22] but has not, as of yet, been shown to originate from dinoflagellates. The dinoflagellate *D. accumulata* [21] has also been assigned as a possible source of okadaic acid and also of two new novel polyether lactones named *pectenotoxins*, PTX-1 (250 μg/kg) and PTX-2 (260 μg/kg). Very recently, another novel polyether toxin, yessitoxin (100 μg/kg), was extracted from the scallop, *Patinopectin yessoensis*,[23] but a

TABLE 6
^{1}H NMR Signals for Gb-4

δ	Position	δ	Position
.94	6H	t,7.5 Hz	3Me, 3′Me
1.70	4H	M	2,2′ methylenes
1.94	3H	s	5Me
2.04	3H	s	6Me
3.21	2H	bs	1,1′HB
3.97—4.02	2H	M	1,1′HA
5.17	1H	bs	NH
8.39	1H	s	NOH

FIGURE 7. Structure of Pb-1.

TABLE 7
^{1}H NMR Signals for Pb-1

δ	Assignment	M, Δ	Position
7.0—7.4 ppm	1OH	M	Aromatic
3.72	1H	dd	NH, 11,11 Hz
3.45	1H	M	1H
1.9—1.7	4H	M	2,2′ CH2
1.6—1.3	1OH	M	3,3′, 4,4′, 5CH2

dinoflagellate origin has not yet been established. The okadaic acid structure for the toxic derivatives of dinophysis toxins is shown in Figure 8.

Near complete ^{1}H assignment for okadaic acid has been reported.[18,19] Chemical shifts δ (CDC13), multiplicity, and coupling constants Δ are given for reference and comparison in Table 9.

All 44 carbons of okadaic acid have been resolved. The spectrum shows 1 carboxylic singlet at 179.3, 6 olefinic carbons at 147.9 to 111.5, 3 ketal carbons at 105.7 to 95.6, 12 carbons bearing oxygen at 85.9 to 60.4, and 22 high field signals at 46.0 to 11.0 ppm.[19]

The first derivative of okadaic acid to be isolated was dinophysis toxin I (DTX-1) and was determined to be 35-s methyl okadaic acid.[20] The ^{1}H NMR spectrum showed a new methyl doublet at 0.92 ppm. When this signal was irradiated, the coupled methine proton (H35, d − 1.50) transformed into a sharp doublet by a doublet pattern with coupling constants of 11.2 and 3.2 Hz, typical for axial-equitorial and diaxial-vicinal protons on a 6-membered ring. If the new methyl doublet were attached at C36 or C37, a more complex multiplet was observed. The mass spectroscopy ion of 112 indicated that the new methyl was attached at either C-33 or some position on the last ring, while the ^{13}C spectrum definitely fixed the new methyl at C-35. All ^{13}C signals of carbons bonded to oxygen at 84.8 to 60.0 remained unchanged, which eliminated C-

TABLE 8
^{13}C Signals for Pb-1

Position	δ	Position	δ	Position	δ
C1	52.4 ppm	C4	25.5	C7	120.1
C2	34.1	C5	27.5	C8	129.4
C3	23.3	C6	151.1	C9	124.5

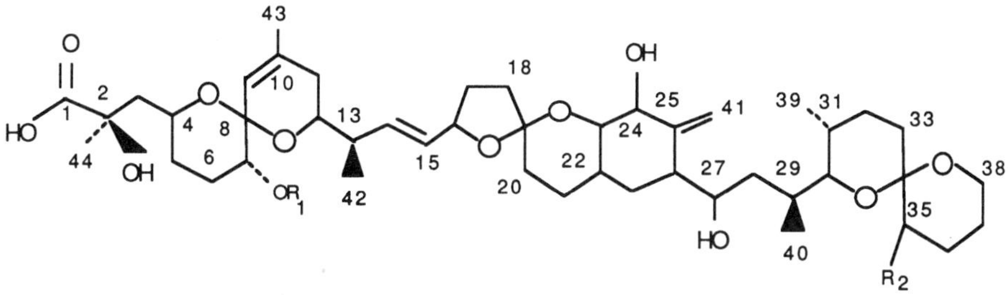

		R1	R2
I.	Okadiac Acid	R1 = H	R2 = H
II.	DTX-1	R1 = H	R2 = CH3
III.	DTX-3	R1 = Acyl	R2 = CH3

FIGURE 8. Structure of okadaic acid and derivatives.

TABLE 9
^{1}H Assignments for Okadaic Acid

Assign	δ	M, Δ	Assign	δ	M, Δ
H-14	5.65	dd 15.5, 8	H22	3.60	M
H-15	5.48	dd 15.5, 8	H 38-B	3.54	M
H-41A	5.42	s	H12	3.40	
H-9	5.31	q 1.5	H-7	3.35	
H-41B	5.06	s	H-30	3.27	dd 11, 2
H-16	4.53	d 9, 7	43 Me	1.73	s
H-24	4.10	bd 10	44 Me	1.37	s
H-27	4.07	t 10	Me	1.07	d
H-4	3.99	t, t11, 2	42 Me	1.04	d
H-26	3.93	d 10	Me	.93	d
H-38A	3.64	td 11, 3	*		

Note: Also various overlapping multiplets between 2.3 and 1.3 ppm.

38 as a possible attachment site. The 95.6 ppm hemiketal signal shifted to 97.9, indicating attachment at either C-33 or C-35. The ^{13}C off-resonance spectrum showed the 18.8 signal (t, C36) shifted downfield to 26.4, while the 30.3 signal (t, C-35) was shifted downfield as a doublet to 39.0 ppm. The 36.0 signal (t, C-33) was given a slight upfield shift to 34.6 due to a γ effect from the new methyl on C-35. If the new methyl had been on C-33, the signal from C-32 would have been shifted downfield to more than 40 ppm, a signal not observed in the ^{13}C spectrum of DTX-1.[20]

For DTX-3, the ^{1}H spectrum was the same as DTX-1, with the following changes.[21] The oxy methine signal at 3.40 (H-7) was shifted downfield to 4.76 ppm. Also, the following signals of a long unsaturated acyl chain were observed: δ 5.35 (5H, olefinic protons), δ 2.80 (6H,

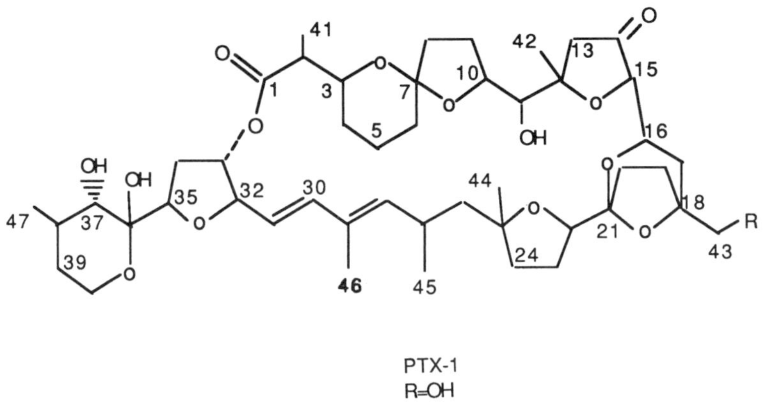

PTX-1
R=OH

FIGURE 9. Structure of PT toxins.

methylene between double bonds), δ 2.15 (2H, methylene adjacent to ester), δ 1.98 (2H, methylene adjacent to carbon double bond), δ 1.25 (25H, saturated methylene), and δ 0.88 (3H, terminal methyl). When samples of DTX-3 were frozen, saturation of the 7-O acyl chain was observed with loss of toxicity.

For acanthifolicin, the only difference in the ^{1}H spectrum from okadaic acid was an upfield shift of the 3.17 (H-9) ppm signal as the olefinic bond is replaced by the episulfide bridged across C-9 and C-10. The C-10 methyl singlet is still observed in the episulfide at 1.72 ppm.[22]

The PT toxins, novel polyether lactones, differ from the okadaic acid type toxins by having a longer carbon backbone (C40), a C-33 lactone ring, and a novel dioxabicyclo ring structure.[21] The PT toxin structures are shown in Figure 9.

Comparison of the ^{1}H NMR spectra of PTX-1 and PTX-2 showed the loss of d 3.56 and 3.61 ppm signals (C-43 H2) in PTX-2. The ^{13}C spectra showed a 65.8 (t, C43) signal in TX-1 changing to a 26.0 q in PTX-2. The R group does not appear to be a significant factor in producing toxicity, as the lethal doses to mice are very similar.

Recently a new polyether toxin has been isolated from the scallop *Patinopectin yessoensis*.[23] Named for the scallop of its origin, yessotoxin (YTX) has the highest toxicity of any polyether yet determined. ^{13}C NMR data obtained from a 60-mg sample revealed 6 methyls, 18 methylenes, 24 methines, and 7 quaternary carbons on a 55-carbon skeleton. The structure of YTX is shown in Figure 10.

Correlation spectroscopy, ^{1}H-^{1}H cosy, ^{1}H-^{1}H-relay, and ^{13}C-^{1}H Cosy were instrumental in assigning the basic skeletal framework of the toxin (Table 10).[23] The positions of the two sulfate esters was determined by chemical shift difference of H2-1, H2-2, Ch3-C3, H-4, and H-5 between the sulfated and desulfated compounds. The two hydroxyl groups were located by isotope shifts of ^{13}C NMR signals of C-32, C-41, and CH3-C41 between CD_3OD and CD_3OH solutions. The overall molecule or structure is very similar to the brevetoxins. It has a large backbone of 47 carbons, a terminal side chain of 9 carbons, and 2 sulfate esters, but has no carbonyl groups.

V. CIGUATOXIN AND MAITOTOXIN

The ciguatoxin (CTX) group of marine toxins possess the highest toxicity known to date. The first substantial progress toward the identification of this toxin was achieved about 10 years ago with the extraction of 1.3 mg of CTX from 50 kg of moray eel viscera.[24] Toxicity was established at 0.45 μg/kg. A molecular weight of 1111 Da and a chemical formula of $C_{53}H_{73}NO_{24}$ were determined. The ^{1}H NMR spectra revealed 4 carbon-carbon double bonds, 5 hydroxyl groups,

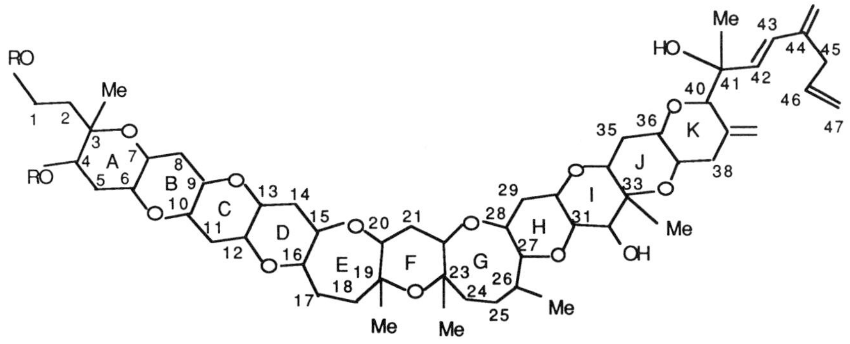

1. YTX: R = SO_3Na
2. Desulfated YTX R = H

FIGURE 10. Structure of YTX.

TABLE 10
Selected ^{1}H Resonances of YTX

Position	δ	Position	δ
H-1	4.24, 4.24	H-27	2.81
H-2	2.21, 1.99	H-28	3.34
CH3-3	1.31	H-29	2.32, 1.58
H-4	4.26	H-30	3.64
H-5	2.60, 1.77	H-31	3.22
H-6	3.09	H-32	3.89
H-7	3.36	CH3-33	1.25
H-9	3.18	H-34	3.80
H-10	3.16	H-35	2.14, 1.53
H-12	3.06	H-36	4.09
H-13	3.12	H-37	3.43
H-14	2.34, 1.47	H-38	2.75, 2.47
H-15	3.37	H-40	3.92
H-16	3.26	CH3-41	1.43
CH3-19	1.29	H-42	5.86
H-20	3.46	H-43	6.35
H-22	3.53	CH3-44	5.09, 5.01
CH3-23	1.20	H-45	3.00, 3.00
CH3-26	1.07	H-46	5.91
		H-47	5.12, 5.10

about 21 H's on carbons bonded to oxygen, and 5 methyl groups. A total of about 80 hydrogens were observed in the proton spectrum, including the 5 hydroxyl groups observable only in DMSO. Three resonances in the 2.95 to 2.60 ppm range gave the possibility of one or more nitrogen atoms in the molecule. Infrared spectra gave absorption peaks at 3450 cm^{-1} for hydroxyl groups and the 1080 cm^{-1} absorption is attributed to ether groups. While this early work was very informative, only partial structures were proposed for CTX; no complete molecular formula was set forth.[24]

In the intervening years CTX has been extracted from moray eel viscera and parrotfish, *Scarus sordidis*.[25,26] The chromatographic character of these toxins bear very close resemblance to okadaic acid, thus enhancing its existence as a polyether.

TABLE 11
Resonances of Tachibana's Partial Structures of CTX Fitted to the CTX Structure of Yasumoto

Position	δ (ppm)	J (Hz)	Position	δ (ppm)	J (Hz)
1	3.50	11, 5.5	23	3.78	m
	3.47	11, 6.5	24	3.35	m
2	4.12	6.5, 5.5, 5	31	2.07	m
2OH	4.79	s		1.84	m
3	5.82	16, 5	32	3.73	7.5, 1.5
4	5.85	16, 4.5	32OH	4.11	s
5	4.56	4.5	34	2.93	9.5, 9.5
6	5.71	m	39	2.08	m
7	5.79	4.5	40	1.80	m
8	2.59	16, 4		1.50	m
	2.38	16, 10	41	2.94	10, 5
9	3.22	10, 4	42	3.15	11.5, 10.5, 5
10	3.30	m	43	2.26	12, 5
14	2.29	12, 4.5		1.33	11.5
	1.60	m	44	3.80	11.5, 9.5, 5
15	3.35	m	45	2.81	9.5, 5
16	3.76	10, 2	46	1.94	7.5, 5
17	5.60	13, 2.5	46Me	1.10	7.5
18	5.68	13, 2	47	3.62	3.5, 1
19	3.95	9.5, 2	47OH	4.90	s
20	4.03	9.5, 2	53	1.55	m
21	5.50	13, 2.5	54	3.52	9.5, 1.5
22	5.83	m	54OH	5.08	s
			55	3.25	m

Recently a structure for CTX, isolated from moray eel and from the causative dinoflagellate, *Gambierdiscus toxicus*, has been presented.[27] This structure is a polyether with 13 alternating ether rings, 6 hydroxyl groups, 5 carbon-carbon double bonds, and 5 methyl groups. This proposed structure, $C_{60}H_{83}O_{18}$ has a molecular weight of 1096 Da. A proposed structure for CTX has been presented,[27] and it is interesting to note that the resonances of the partial structures of Tachibana[24] fit this CTX structure very closely. These assignments are given in Table 11.

Maitotoxin (MTX) is the most lethal of all known marine toxins to date. In mice, its lethality has been determined at 0.13 μg/kg,[28] three times stronger than CTX. The origin of this toxin is traced to the dinoflagellate *Gambierdiscus toxicus*. Progress toward the identification of its molecular structure has been achieved.[28] From 4000 l of cultures of *G. toxicus*, 20 mg of MTX was isolated and judged to be pure by TLC and HPLC standards. FAB mass spectra indicated a molecular weight of 3401 Da, with the first lower prominent peak of 3299, indicating desulfonation ($-SO_3Na + H$, 102). Solvolysis of the toxin further revealed a molar ratio of 1.85 mole of SO_4 per mole of toxin, indicating the presence of two sulfate esters in the molecule. The ^1H and ^{13}C NMR spectra further reveal the presence of a large number of oxygen atoms in the molecule. The ^{13}C spectrum indicated 160 ± 5 total carbons, 62 aliphatic carbons (δ 87.7 to 59.5), and 8 olefinic carbons (δ 155 to 110.7). No acetal/ketal or carbonyl carbons were observed. The proton spectrum indicated 225 ± 10 protons, including 5 doublet methyls (δ 1.01 to 0.86), 15 singlet methyls on oxygen/nitrogen-bearing carbons (δ 1.44 to 1.16), and a singlet methyl on an olefinic carbon (δ 1.82). The COSY ^1H NMR spectrum indicated a monosubstituted olefin (terminal) and an exomethylene conjugated with a trisubstituted olefin. Partial structures of MTX are shown in Figure 11, along with proton assignments. With a molecular weight of 3401

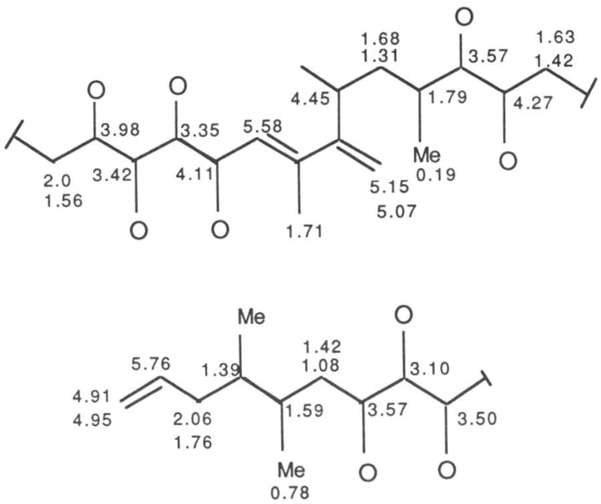

FIGURE 11. Partial structures of MTX.

TABLE 12
Comparison of Carbon Types in MTX and Those in Palytoxin

Shift range and type of group	Specific group	MTX	Palytoxin
δ 170—180	C=O	0	2
δ 155—110, olefinic	Quat	2	2
	CH	4	13
	CH_2	2	1
δ 110—100, hemi-ketal	R_2CO_2	0	2
δ 87.7—59.5, oxygenated or nitrogenated carbons	Quat	15	1
	CH	74	56
	CH_2	1	3
δ 52.4—10.6, aliphatic	Quat	0	0
	CH	5	5
	CH_2	36	37
	CH_3	21	7

(60 carbon atoms, 2 sulfate esters, 225 protons), and assuming no nitrogen atoms, a chemical formula of approximately $C_{160}H_{225}S_2O_{74}$ can be projected. It is suggested that the bulk of the oxygens are structured as hydroxyl and ether rings, reminiscent of palytoxin, a potent zooanthid toxin of similar toxicity comprised of a linear skeleton of 119 carbons substituted with 7 methyls and 1 exomethylene.[29] It is interesting to note the possible similarities between MTX and the known structure of palytoxin.[29] Table 12 shows a comparison of the type of carbon atoms in MTX, as given by Yasumoto's data and that expected of palytoxin. Several aspects are quite obvious. First, the number of methine carbons bearing oxygen are in direct proportion, 74 of the 160 carbons in MTX, as compared with 56 of the 127 carbons in palytoxin. Second, the degree of unsaturation is less in MTX. Third, MTX appears to be more highly methylated than palytoxin, thus increasing its lipid solubility. Fourth, the number of quarternary carbons bearing oxygen is quite drastically different in MTX. As these 15 carbons appear to be the backbone sites of the 15 methyl singlets, a spatial arrangement between hydroxyls and methyl groups may be a highly significant aspect of the toxic nature of MTX. Although at the present, the complete structure of MTX is still unknown, the proposed model does seem to satisfy most of the known chemical properties of MTX.

ACKNOWLEDGMENTS

This study was supported by U.S. Army Medical Research and Development Command, contract DAMD17-87-C-7002. The views, findings, and opinions expressed herein are those of the authors and should not be construed as those of the Department of the Army.

REFERENCES

1. **Wong, J. L., Oesterlin, R., and Rapport, H.,** The structure of saxitoxin, *J. Am. Chem. Soc.*, 93, 7344, 1971.
2. **Schantz, E. J., Ghazarossian, V. E., Schnoes, H. K., Strong, F. M., Springer, J. P., Pezzanite, J. O., and Clardy, J. C.,** The structure of saxitoxin, *J. Am. Chem. Soc.*, 97, 1238, 1975.
3. **Boyer, G. L., Schantz, E. J., and Schnoes, H. K.,** Characterization of 11-hydroxy saxitoxin sulphate, a major toxin in scallops exposed to blooms of the poisonous dinoflagellate, *Gonyaulax tamarensis*, *J. Am. Chem. Soc., Chem. Comm.*, 889, 1978.
4. **Shimizu, Y., Hsu, C., Fallon, W. E., Oshima, Y., Miura, I., and Nakanishi, K.,** Structure of neosaxitoxin, *J. Am. Chem. Soc.*, 100, 6791, 1978.
5. **Wichmann, C. F., Boyer, G. L., Diran, C. L., Schantz, E. J., and Schnoes, H. K.,** Neurotoxins of *Gonauylax excavata* and Bay of Fundy scallops, *Tetrahedron*, 1941, 1981.
6. **Koehn, F. E., Hall, S., Wichmann, C. F., Schnoes, H. K., and Reichardt, P. B.,** Dinoflagellate neurotoxins related to saxitoxin: structure and latent activity of toxins B1 and B2, *Tetrahedron*, 2247, 1982.
7. **Shimizu, Y., Kobayashi, M., Genenah, A., and Oshima, Y.,** Isolation of side chain sulfated saxitoxin analogs, *Tetrahedron*, 40, 539, 1984.
8. **Oshima, Y., Kotaki, Y., Harada, T., and Yasumoto, T.,** Paralytic shellfish toxins in tropical waters, in *Seafood Toxins*, Ragelis, E.P., Eds., American Chemical Society, Washington, D.C., 1984, 161.
9. **Shimizu, Y., Buckley, L. J., Alam, M., Oshima, Y., Fallon, W. E., Kasai, H., Miura, I., Gullo, V. P., and Nakanishi, K.,** Structures of gonyautoxin I and II from the east coast toxic dinoflagellate, *Gonyaulax tamarensis*, *J. Am. Chem. Soc.*, 98, 5414, 1976.
10. **Ghazarossian, V. J., Schantz, E. J., Schnoes, H. K. and Strong, F. M.,** A biologically active and hydrolysis product of saxitoxin, *Biochem. Biophys. Res. Commun.*, 68, 776, 1976.
11. **Lin, Y., Risk, M., Kay, S. M., Van Engen, D., Clardy, J. C., Golik, J., James, J. C., and Nakanishi, K.,** Isolation and structure of brevetoxin B from the "red tide" dinoflagellate *Ptychodiscus brevis* (*Gymnodinium breve*), *J. Am. Chem. Soc.*, 103, 6773, 1981.
12. **Golik, J., James, J. C., Nakanishi, K., and Lin, Y.,** The structure of brevitoxin C, *Tetrahedron*, 23, 2535, 1982.
13. **Chou, H. and Shimizu, Y.,** A new polyether toxin from *Gymnodinium breve* Davis (*Ptychodiscus brevis*), *Tetrahedron*, 23, 5521, 1982.
14. **Chou, H., Shimizu, Y., Van Duyne, G., and Clardy, J. C.,** Isolation and structures of two new polycyclic ethers from *Gymnodinium brevi* Davis (*Ptychodiscus brevis*), *Tetrahedron*, 26, 2865, 1985.
15. **Shimizu, Y., Chou, H., Bando, H., Van Duyne, G., and Clardy, J. C.,** Structure of brevetoxin A (GB-1 Toxin), the most potent toxin in the Florida red tide organism *Gymnodinium breve* (*Ptychodiscus brevis*), *J. Am. Chem. Soc.*, 108, 514, 1986.
16. **Alam, M., Sanduja, R., Hossain, M. B., and van der Helm, D.,** *Gymnodinium breve* toxins. 1. Isolation and X-ray structure of O,O-dipropyl (E)-2-(1-methyl-2- oxopropylidene) phosphorohydrazidothiolate (E)-oxime from the red tide dinoflagellate *Gymnodinium breve*, *J. Am. Chem. Soc.*, 104, 5232, 1982.
17. **Dinovi, M., Trainor, D. A., and Nakanishi, K.,** The structure of O,O-dipropyl (E)-2- (1-methyl-2- oxopropylidene phosphorohydrazidothiolate (E)-oxime from the red tide dinoflagellate *Gymnodinium breve*, *Tetrahedron*, 24, 855, 1983.
18. **Murakami, Y., Oshima, Y., and Yasumoto, T.,** Identification of okadiac acid as a toxic component of a marine dinoflagellate *Prorocentrum lima*, *Bull. Jpn. Soc. Sci. Fish.*, 48, 69, 1982.
19. **Tachibana, K., Scheuer, P. J., Tsukitani, Y., Kikuchi, H., Van Engen, D., Clardy, J., Gopichand, Y., and Schmitz, F. J.,** Okadaic acid, a cytotoxic polyether from two marine sponges of the genus *Halichondria*, *J. Am. Chem. Soc.*, 103, 2469, 1981.
20. **Murata, M., Shimatani, M., Sugitani, H., Oshima, Y., and Yasumoto, T.,** Isolation and structural elucidation of the causative toxin of the diarrhetic shellfish poisoning, *Bull. Jpn. Soc. Sci. Fish.*, 48, 549, 1982.
21. **Yasumoto, T., Murata, M., and Oshima, Y.,** Diarrhetic shellfish poisoning, *Tetrahedron*, 41, 1019, 1985.

22. **Schmitz, F. J., Prasad, R. S., Gopichand, Y., Hossain, M. B., van der Helm, D., and Schmidt, P.,** Acanthifolicin, a new eipsulfide-containing polyether carboxylic acid from extracts of the marine sponge *Pandaros acanthifolium*, *J. Am. Chem. Soc.*, 103, 2467, 1981.
23. **Murata, M., Kumagai, M., Lee, J. S., and Yasumoto, T.,** Isolation and structure of yessotoxin, a novel polyether compound implicated in diarrhetic shellfish poisoning, *Tetrahedron*, 28, 5869, 1987.
24. **Tachibana, K.,** Structural Studies on Marine Toxins, Ph.D. Dissertation, University of Hawaii, Honolulu, 1980.
25. **Nukina, M., Koyanagi, L. M., and Scheuer, P. J.,** Two interchangable forms of ciguatoxin, *Toxicon*, 22, 169, 1984.
26. **Tachibana, K., Nukina, M., Joh, Y. G., and Scheur, P. J.,** Recent developments in molecular structure of ciguatoxin, *Biol. Bull.*, 172, 122, 1987.
27. **Yasumoto, T.,** Marine microorganisms toxins, in *Toxic Marine Phytoplankton*, Graneli, E., Sundstrom, B., Edler, L., and Anderson, D. M., Eds., Elsevier Press, New York, 1989.
28. **Yokoyama, A., Murata, M., Oshima, Y., Iwashita, T., and Yasumoto, T.,** Some chemical properties of maitotoxin, a putative calcium channel agonist isolated from a marine dinoflagellate, *J. Biochem.*, 104, 184, 1988.
29. **Moore, R. E. and Bartolini, G.,** Palytoxin: a new marine toxin from a coelenterate, *J. Am. Chem. Soc.*, 103, 2491, 1981.

Chapter 8

THE GUINEA-PIG ILEUM: AN ASSAY SYSTEM FOR CIGUATERA-TYPE TOXINS

Donald M. Miller

TABLE OF CONTENTS

I. INTRODUCTION

The isolation and chemical resolution of toxins in general depends upon the methodology for detection. When extracting unknown toxins effective in the parts per billion range and that are only available in small quantities, it is essential to be able to assay small amounts of toxin. The mouse LD_{50} is considered the standard for the detection and quantification of toxins, nevertheless, it has disadvantages. It requires a large number of animals, it is nonspecific, and it requires an appreciable amount of toxin. Pharmacologic preparations that can serve as bioassays, therefore, are advantageous. They can be utilized to detect, and sometimes quantitate, the amount of toxin present. They can detect the toxin at very low levels. They can be utilized as prescreening mechanisms for mouse bioassays. Finally, they sometimes are more specific and provide some degree of pharmacologic information on the particular toxin.

The guinea-pig ileum has been utilized for many years as a pharmacologic preparation. It has been shown to respond to many agonists, such as acetylcholine, epinephrine, and histamine. Gaddum and Picarelli first reported that the direct action of 5-hydroxytryptamine on 5-HT receptors located on smooth-muscle cells in the guinea-pig ileum could be blocked by dibenzyline.[1] Later, Ochillo and others reported that the response to exogenously applied acetylcholine remained even after 5 d of cold storage of the ileum under nitrogen.[2]

The guinea-pig ileum preparation has been used by members of our group to clearly distinguish and semiquantitate nanogram levels of crude and purified toxins from dinoflagellates.[3-24]

II. METHODOLOGY FOR GUINEA-PIG ILEUM ASSAY

Guinea pigs (350 to 600 g) are sacrificed by a cervical dislocation. A 2- to 3-cm segment of the terminal ileum is removed and placed in physiologic saline solution at 37°C. The saline solution constituents are detailed in Table 1. If required, the intestinal lumen is evacuated by slowly flushing with saline solution. The dissected ileum is attached by a silver chain to the lever of an isotonic transducer with a tension of 2 g. The other end of the ileum is fixed in the bath. The apparatus utilized for studying the ileal response consists of a water-jacketed tissue bath, a 10-in. chart recorder, a circulating temperature bath, and an air pump (Figure 1). The protocol for an assay depends upon whether the toxin is reversible or irreversible.

A. ASSAY FOR REVERSIBLE TOXINS

Trial and error is utilized to determine a range of three or four doses of agonist (usually accomplished in triplicate), which will give full use of the 10-in. recorder. After a successful control run is accomplished with agonist (Figure 2), a second 15-min period may be utilized as a control. Upon completion of the controls, the physiologic saline rinse for the bath is switched to one containing the toxic extracts at a given concentration and allowed to bathe the preparation for the duration of the test period — 45 to 90 min. During this time, agonist trials are made at 15-min intervals. After each agonist trial, the preparation is washed with saline containing the toxin. At the end of the 90 min, physiologic saline containing the toxin is stopped, and regular physiologic saline is commenced, after which time a new set of control doses is accomplished. If the toxin is reversible, the values after the last wash should approximate the initial control values. (Figure 2).

Dose-response relationships for phasic contractions of ileal segments in response to agonist stimulation and methodology for conducting an assay have been detailed by Perry,[25] and more recently by Tallardia and Jacob.[26]

The line derived from points between 20 and 80% on the dose-response curve obtained during the toxin infusion is compared with the control curve obtained during the period before the infusion of the toxin to obtain a dose ratio. The above procedure is repeated at least three times in the concentration range that will result in dose ratios between 10 and 1000.

TABLE 1
Physiologic Saline Components

Chemical	mM	g/l	Stock g/ml	Amount/l
NaCl	136.9	7.014		Weigh out
KCl	2.68	0.372	186.37	2.0 ml
$CaCl_2$	11.84	0.277	55.5	5.0 ml
$MgCl_2$	1.03	0.095	23.8	4.0 ml
$NaHCO_3$	11.9	0.084	8.4	10.0 ml
KH_2PO_4	0.45	0.178	89.1	2.0 ml
Glucose	5.55	1.980		Weigh out

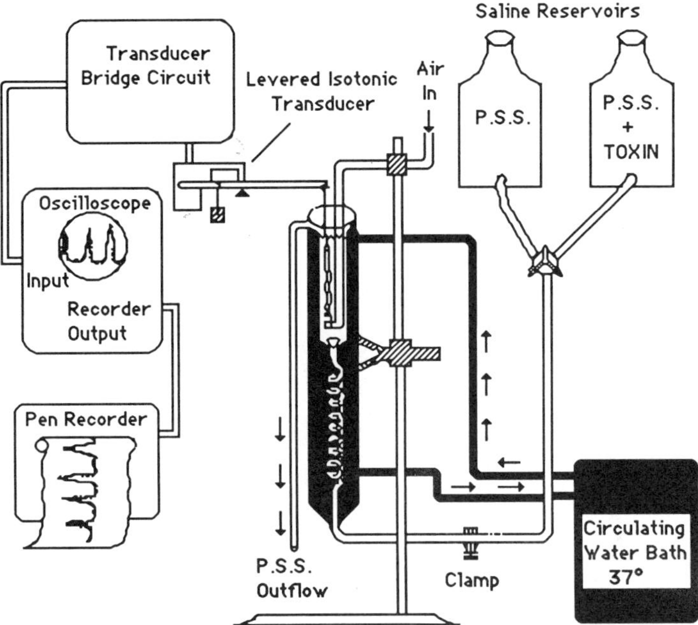

FIGURE 1. Diagram of the apparatus utilized for the ileum assay. The dissected ileum is attached by a silver chain to the lever of an isotonic transducer with a tension of 2 g. The other end of the ileum is fixed in the bath. The accessory equipment utilized for studying the ileal response consists of a water-jacketed tissue bath, a 10-in. chart recorder, a circulating temperature bath, and an air pump.

The theory of the dose-ratio calculation is as follows. Let

$$A + R \underset{K_{2a}}{\overset{K_{1a}}{\rightleftharpoons}} A - R$$

and

$$B + R \underset{K_{2b}}{\overset{K_{1b}}{\rightleftharpoons}} B - R$$

where A = agonist (ACH), B = antagonist (toxin), R = receptor site, and K = constant. At a given

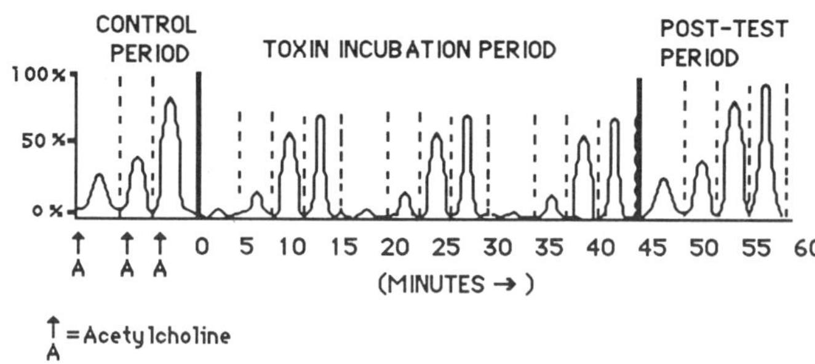

FIGURE 2. Diagram of a reversible assay. A control curve is established in the first part of the assay using varying doses of acetylcholine or histamine. The physiologic saline solution is then switched to one containing the toxin. After this, test doses of agonist is given at intervals. After 90 min, normal physiologic saline solution is resumed. Dashed lines indicate that a wash was performed with physiologic saline solution.

time T let X = A-R complexes, Y = B-R complexes, and Rt = total receptor sites. Then free sites = (Rt-X-Y), available ACH = A-X, and available toxin = B-Y.

As A >> X and B>>Y, then

$$A - X = ACH \quad \text{and} \quad B - Y = \text{Toxin}$$

Applying the mass action law to simultaneous equations for rate of formation,

$$\frac{dx}{dt} = K_{1a}A\left(R_t - X - Y\right) - K_{2a}X$$

$$\frac{dy}{dt} = K_{1b}B\left(R_t - X - Y\right) - K_{2b}Y$$

At equilibrium

$$\frac{dx}{dt} = \frac{dy}{dt} = 0$$

Therefore,

$$A\left(R_t - X - Y\right) = K_a X$$

where

$$K_a = \frac{K_{2a}}{K_{1a}}$$

and

$$B\left(R_t - X - Y\right) = K_b Y$$

$$K_b = \frac{K_{2b}}{K_{1b}}$$

$$Y = \frac{B(R_t - X)}{B + K_b}$$

substituted in the equation for X, gives

$$X = \frac{AR_t}{A + K_a\left\{1 + \frac{B}{K_b}\right\}}$$

If antagonist = B = 0, then

$$X = \frac{AR_t}{A + K_a}$$

If we add antagonist and then agonist (A′) to produce the same contraction

$$\frac{AR_t}{A + K_a} = X = \frac{AR_t}{A + K_a\left\{1 + \frac{B}{K_b}\right\}}$$

Then,

$$\frac{A'}{A} = 1 + \frac{B}{K_b} = \text{The Dose Ratio Equation}$$

The-dose ratio data can be easily plotted in Lineweaver Burke format as follows: Assuming E α X, and E_{max} α Rt, then, with no antagonist,

$$X = \frac{AR_t}{A + K_a} \longrightarrow E = \frac{E_{max}A}{A + K_a}$$

and the double reciprocal plot (L-B) is

$$\frac{1}{E} = \frac{1}{E_{max}} + \frac{K_a}{E_{max}}\frac{1}{A}$$

B. ASSAY FOR IRREVERSIBLE TOXINS

To assay for the irreversible toxins we have altered the procedure. Initially the determination of the standard doses of agonist is much the same as for a reversible assay. Once the controls have been established, the toxin containing saline is introduced into the bath and allowed to incubate for a period of 15 min. At the end of the 15-min incubation period, the preparation is washed with normal physiologic saline for 3 to 4 min. To test the effect of the irreversible toxin on the preparation, challenging doses of agonist are performed immediately after the postincubation wash and at 15-min intervals for a period of 90 min (Figure 3). At the end of the 90 min postincubation the run is terminated. If the response to the agonist at the end of the 90-min test period is not 50 ± 10%, then the concentration of toxin is adjusted and another ileal run is performed to achieve an approximately 50% inhibition. Once achieved, the dose for 50%

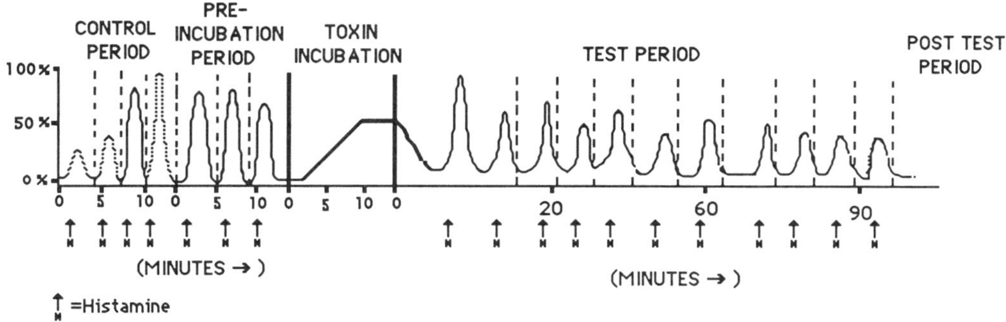

FIGURE 3. Diagram of an irreversible assay. A control curve is established in the first part of the assay using varying doses of acetylcholine or histamine. The dose closest to 80% of the maximum is then selected as the test dose. The preparation is then incubated with toxin for a period of 15 min. After this, a wash is performed and the test dose of agonist is given at intervals. Three doses are given after 90 min and the average is expressed as percent of the control value. Dashed lines indicate that a wash was performed with physiologic saline solution.

inhibition is defined as an ileum unit (ILU) for a irreversible toxin. Once obtained, the ileum unit is compared with the mouse LD_{50} (per kg mouse) or mouse unit (MU) (based on a 20-g mouse) value to arrive at an approximate ratio.

For example, the ratio for GT-4 from *Gambierdiscus toxicus* is

$$\text{Ratio}_{-\text{GT}-4} \cong \frac{\text{Mouse Unit}}{\text{Ileum Unit}} \cong 2000$$

Notice that once the ratio is obtained, it can be utilized to conserve animals and to shorten the assay of toxins when doing a mouse bioassay. In the case of GT-4 extract from *G. toxicus*, whatever concentration is used to obtain an ILU, when multiplied by 2000 is an approximate MU.

III. RESULTS WITH GT-1, A REVERSIBLE TOXIN

Prior to conducting an assay, a control run is accomplished to determine the effects of methanol on the ileum preparation (Figure 4). Methanol is used as a carrier for the toxin. Figure 5 is an example of an actual assay conducted upon the GT-1 fraction from *G. toxicus*, which is a reversible toxin. In the presence of the toxin, the agonist response is diminished by 70% from the control value. Notice that once the toxin is washed from the preparation, the control value of the agonist returns to its original value.

IV. RESULTS WITH GT-4, AN IRREVERSIBLE TOXIN

When, an irreversible toxin is applied to the ileum preparation for a period of 15 min (Figure 6), washing with fresh physiologic saline solution is not effective in restoring the control response to the agonist. Furthermore, once applied, the response of the isolated ileum decreases as a function of time. If the toxin is sufficiently dilute, then the time frame is extended and a stable end point can be determined at 90 min after application.

V. RESULTS WITH PC-2, A FAST-ACTING TOXIN, AND OKADIAC ACID

One toxin (PC-2) isolated from the toxic dinoflagellate, *Prorocentrum concavum*, is peculiar in that its action on mice is much faster acting, hence the name *fast acting*. When this toxin is

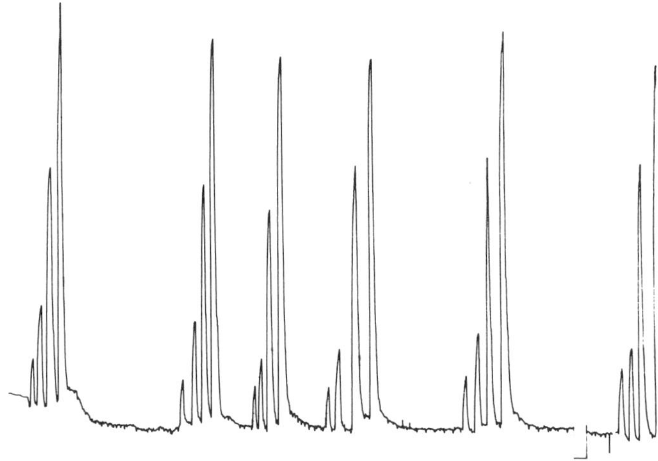

FIGURE 4. Effects of 400 μl of methanol introduced into the 10-ml bath of the ileum and allowed to incubate for 15 min. Notice that the average values of the agonist response are not affected.

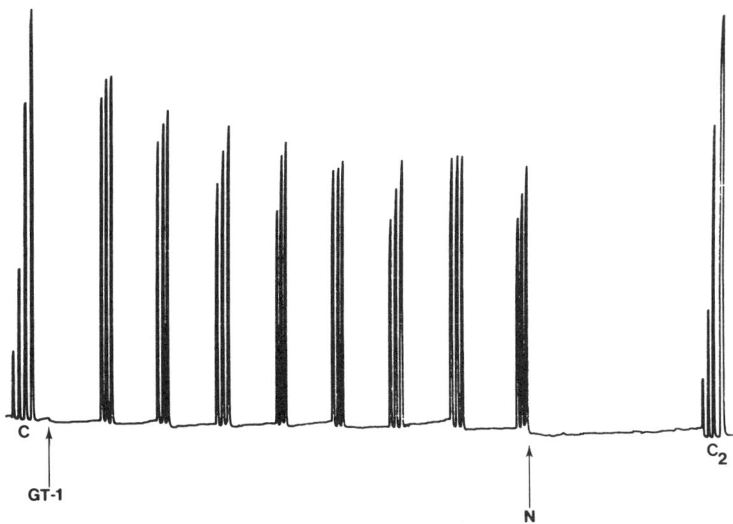

FIGURE 5. Actual record of an assay of GT-1. Control period is labeled C. Toxin is introduced at GT-1. Normal physiologic saline solution is resumed at N, at which time the agonist response has returned to normal.

applied to the ileum (Figure 7), the results at 15 min are much more significant than those at 90 min, just the reverse of GT-4 toxin. Okadiac acid from *P. concavum* has much the same effect as GT-4 (Figure 8).

VI. RESULTS WITH BREVETOXIN

Brevetoxin has very little irreversible effects upon the ileum preparation other than a small set of pertubations, which we interpret to be an action upon the neural elements in the ileum. This occurs, notwithstanding the fact that brevetoxin has been reported to operate at the same site on sodium channel as ciguatoxin.[27] This action of brevetoxin is exactly the same as the action of

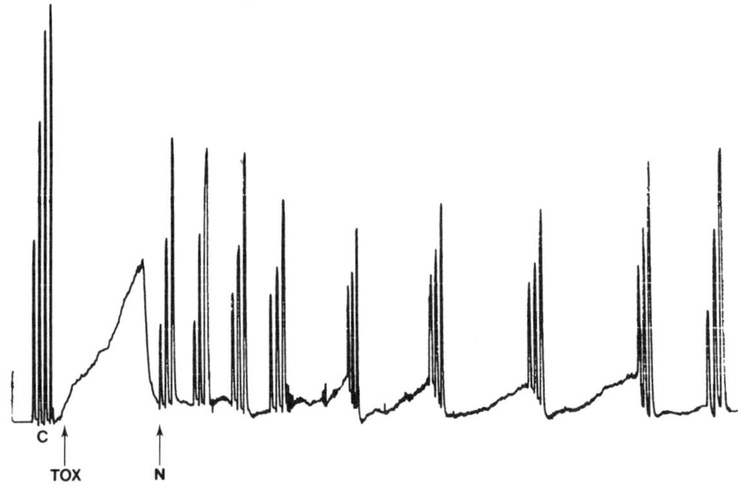

FIGURE 6. Actual record of an assay of GT-4. The control period is labeled C. Toxin is introduced at TOX. Normal physiologic saline solution is resumed at N. Notice that the agonist response decreases as a function of time. The approximate value of inhibition is read at 90 min into the assay.

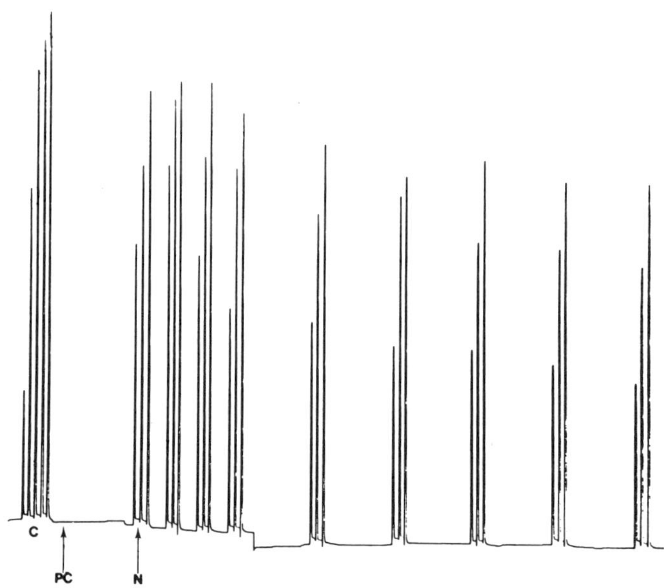

FIGURE 7. Actual record of an assay of PC Toxin. The control period is labeled C. Toxin is introduced at PC. Normal physiologic saline solution is resumed at N. Notice that the agonist response decreases as a function of time. The approximate value of inhibition is read at 90 min into the assay.

leptinotarsin, a presynaptic neurotoxin that stimulates the release of acetylcholine from synaptic terminals.[28,29] At much higher doses reversible effects are seen with brevetoxins.

VII. RESULTS WITH PALYTOXIN

The results with the application of palytoxin are shown in Figure 9. The effects of palytoxin are very similar to those that occur with GT-4 toxin.

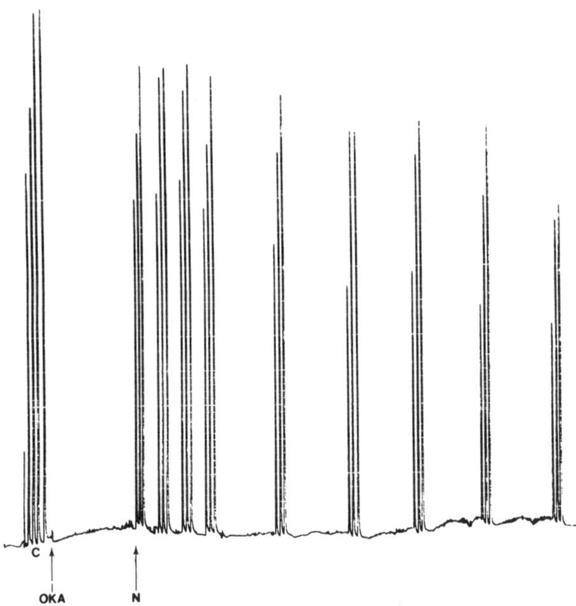

FIGURE 8. Actual record of an assay of brevetoxin. The control period is labeled C. Toxin is introduced at OKA. Normal physiological saline solution is resumed at N. Notice that there is no effect upon the agonist response.

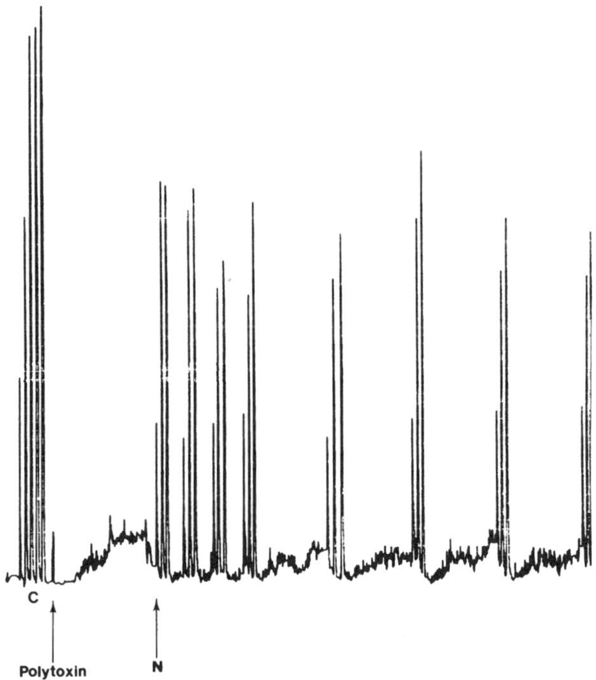

FIGURE 9. Actual record of an assay of palytoxin extract. The control period is labeled C. Toxin is introduced at palytoxin. Normal physiologic saline solution is resumed at N. Notice that the agonist response decreases as a function of time. The approximate value of inhibition is read at 90 min into the assay.

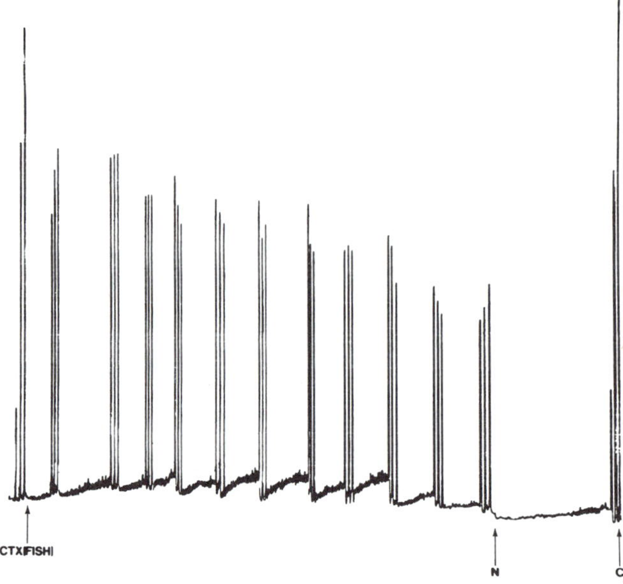

FIGURE 10. Actual record of an assay of fish extract (ciguatoxin). The control period is labeled C_2. Toxin is introduced at CTX(FISH). Normal physiologic saline solution is resumed at N. Notice that the agonist response decreases as a function of time. The approximate value of inhibition is read at 90 min into the assay.

VIII. RESULTS WITH TOXIC EXTRACTS OF FISH

The results that occur using fish extracts (Figure 10) are more complex than when using any of the purified toxins. There is an initial inotropic response, followed by an inhibition of the agonist response, and also a continued effect upon the ileum response to further agonist challenges. The interpretation that we make of the records obtained is that the toxic extract from the fish contains either modified toxins or a combination of toxins, which gives multiple effects on the ileum preparation.

IX. EXPERIMENTS WITH GT-4

For the following set of examples, GT-4 toxin (7.6 mg/kg mouse) from the dinoflagellate *Gambierdiscus toxicus* (SIU strain 350, harvests KL and 1a/87) from South Sound, Virgin Gorda, British Virgin Islands was utilized.[20] Detailed descriptions of the method of cultivation, extraction, and semipurification of GT-4 have been published.[20] Purification of GT-4 from this strain using high-pressure liquid chromatography was reported by Tindall and Miller.[21]

A. ETHANOL EFFECT

Ethanol, added as a pretreatment for the ileum preparation at dosages up to .001%, has no effect upon either the inotropic response or the agonist response. However, when ethanol of 0.00001% is added with the toxin, there is a 50% increase of both the inotropic effect and the percent inhibition at 90 min (Table 2). Many patients who recover from ciguatera intoxication report the reoccurrence of symptoms upon imbibing alcoholic beverages. Our results lend some credence to these claims of an "ethanol effect". Pretreatment of the tissues before the introduction of the toxin does not significantly change the toxic effects, but the presence of ethanol with the toxin or after the application of the toxin does augment the toxic effects. Ethanol

TABLE 2
Effect of ETOH Plus Toxin on the Ileum Preparation

	Incubation		Response Inhibition	
Pretreatment	**EtOH**	**Toxin**	**Inotropic**	**90 min**
None	2.0 ml	0	0	0
None	0	2.0 ml	5 mm	68%
2 ml	0	2.0 ml	7 mm	77%
None	1.0 ml	2.0 ml	28 mm	70%
None	1.5 ml	2.0 ml	46 mm	94%
None	2.0 ml	2.0 ml	52 mm	93%

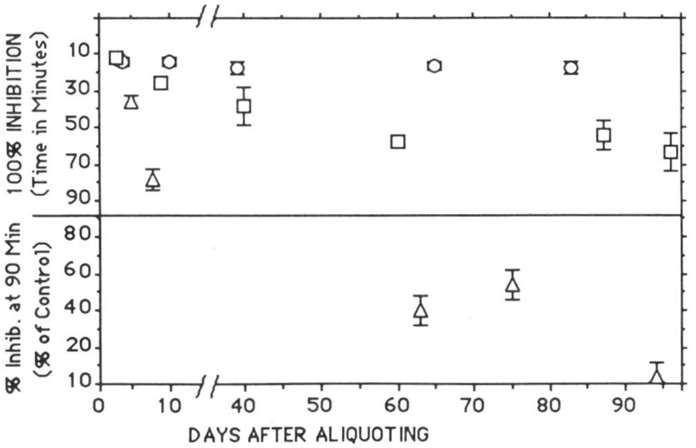

FIGURE 11. Effects of aliquots of MTX on guinea-pig ileum after storage in ethanol (O), methanol (¤), and a mixture of 50% methanol-50% water (Δ), all stored in the dark at 4°C. Each point is the mean of three tests with the range indicated. All doses of toxin applied to the ileum preparation were 2 ml per 500 ml of PSS for a period of 15 min. Note that the lower half of graph is inhibition of the agonist response 90 min after the preparation has been washed.

itself has been known to have an effect upon axonal sodium channels for more than 20 years.[30,31] Our results could be interpreted to implicate an effect upon sodium channels in the maitotoxin effect.

B. DEGRADATION OF TOXIN BY WATER

GT-4 stored in ethanol produced a greater inotropic effect and inhibited the ileum preparation significantly more than toxin stored in methanol. The inclusion of water (50%) in the methanol solvent system caused a progressive degradation of the toxin. In fact, the toxic activity deteriorated significantly after 8 d and was close to zero in 90 d (Figure 11).

C. SODIUM SALICYLATE EFFECTS

Sodium salicylate has been shown to increase the inhibitory potency of the diphenylalkylamines without changing the potency of nifedipine.[32,33] The mechanism for this is attributed to the fact that the inclusion of salicylate in the medium decreases the surface charge at the membrane. When increasing doses of sodium salicylate (40, 80, 160, 320, and 640 mg/ml) were included in the physiologic saline solution before during and after incubation with the same dose of toxin (Figure 11), both the inotropic response and the inhibition at 90 min were lessened, since increasing concentrations of salicylate tended to decrease the initial inotropic effect and the histamine inhibition. This is the same effect that salicylate has upon verapimil and diltiazem.

D. USE OF THE ILEUM TO ASSAY HPLC FRACTIONS

The ileum preparation has been utilized to assay HPLC fractions from the dinoflagellate *Gambierdiscus toxicus*.[3-8,10,11,13-16,19] Recently, Tindall and Miller[34] were able to assay fractions from HPLC peaks and to verify the presence of GT-4 toxins in amounts as small as 1.01 μg. The potency of the HPLC-purified toxin exceeded that of column purified material and less than 1 ng/ml of HPLC-purified toxin inhibited the toxin response in the guinea-pig ileum.

X. SUMMARY

The ileum preparation has been shown to react to most but not all ciguatera-type toxins. Nevertheless it has proven to be a very useful bioassay with many applications. Especially significant is its role in the reduction of the number of mice utilized in the mouse bioassay. Indeed, because of its greater sensitivity, it surpasses the mouse bioassay in the experimental area such as the assay of HPLC fractions.

Our experiments with the ileum preparation lead us to conclude that the inotropic effect may vary depending upon several factors (amplification of system, length of ileum segment, etc.) and is not as reliable a measure of toxicity as the reduction of agonist response. The experiment using 50% water and 50% methanol indicates clearly that the presence of water over long periods of time causes a degradation of the toxin in the case of GT-4. This has great significance for the extraction and storage procedures for this toxin.

ACKNOWLEDGMENTS

Brevetoxin was supplied by Dr. Mark Poli, USAMRIID, Fort Detrick, MD. Palytoxin and fish extract of ciguatoxin was supplied by Dr. Mike Capra, Queensland University of Technology, Brisbane, Australia. Leptinotarsin was isolated and supplied by Dr. Michael Koenig, Department of Biological Sciences, University of Southern California. This study was supported by U.S. Army Medical Research and Development Command, contract DAMD17-87-C-7002. The views, findings, and opinions expressed herein are those of the authors and should not be construed as those of the Department of the Army.

REFERENCES

1. **Gaddum, J. H. and Picarelli, Z. P.,** 5-HT receptors in the guinea-pig ileum, *Br. J. Pharmacol*, 12, 323-328, 1957.
2. **Ochillo, R., Rowell, P. P., and Rama Sastry, B. V.,** Effects of cooling on the levels of acetylcholine, cholinesterase, choline acetyltransferase and the intramural electrical stimulation on the guinea pig ileum, *Pharmacology*, 16, 121-130, 1978.
3. **Dickey, R. W., Miller, D. M., and Tindall, D. R.,** The extraction and effects of crude ciguatoxin from *Scomberomorus cavalla* upon acetylcholine and histamine receptor sites of the guinea pig ileum, *Fed. Proc.*, 41, 1562, 1982.
4. **Dickey, R. W.,** The Extraction, Purification and Characterization of Toxins from the Marine Dinoflagellates *Gambierdiscus toxicus* and *Prorocentrum concavum*, Ph.D. Dissertation, Southern Illinois University, Carbondale, IL, 1984.
5. **Dickey, R. W., Miller, D. M., and Tindall, D. R.,** Extraction of a water-soluble toxin from a dinoflagellate, *Gambierdiscus toxicus*, in *Seafood Toxins*, Ragelis, E. P., Ed., American Chemical Society Symposium Series 262, Washington, D.C., 1984, 257-269.

6. **Miller, D. M., Dickey, R. W., and Tindall, D. R.,** The effects of a lipid extracted toxin from the dinoflagellate *Gambierdiscus toxicus* upon nerve-muscle and intestinal preparations, *Fed. Proc.*, 41, 1561, 1982.
7. **Miller, D. M., Dickey, R. W., and Tindall, D. R.,** Lipid soluble toxins from a dinoflagellate, *Gambierdiscus toxicus*, isolated from a Caribbean region supporting ciguateric fish, *The Physiologist*, 26, a41, 1983.
8. **Miller, D. M., Dickey, R. W., and Tindall, D. R.,** Lipid soluble toxins from a dinoflagellate, *Gambierdiscus toxicus*, in *Seafood Toxins*, Ragelis, E. P., Ed., American Chemical Society Symposium Series 262, Washington, D.C., 1984, 241-255.
9. **Miller, R. J., Freedman, S. B., Miller, D. M., and Tindall, D. R.,** Maitotoxin activates voltage sensitive calcium channels in cultured neuronal cells, *Proc. Intl. Cong. Pharmacol. (9th)*, 80, 1984.
10. **Miller, D. M. and Tindall, D. R.,** Physiological effects of HPLC-purified maitotoxin from a dinoflagellate, *Gambierdiscus toxicus*, in *Toxic Dinoflagellates*, Anderson, D. M., White, A. W., and Baden, D. G., Eds., Elsevier Science, New York, 1985, 375-378.
11. **Miller, D. M., Tindall, D. R., and Hassan, F.,** Effects of maitotoxin on guinea pig ileum, *Fed. Proc.*, 44, 1642, 1985.
12. **Miller, D. M., Tindall, D. R., and Tibbs, B.,** Ciguatera-type toxins: bioassay using crayfish nerve cord, *Fed. Proc.*, 45, 344, 1986.
13. **Miller, D. M. and Tindall, D. R.,** Factors interacting with the effects of the maitotoxin fraction from *Gambierdiscus toxicus*, *Fed. Proc.*, 46, 957, 1987.
14. **Miller, D. M. and Tindall, D. R.,** Factors interacting with the effects of the maitotoxin fraction from *Gambierdiscus toxicus*, in *Conference on Natural Toxins from Aquatic and Marine Environments*, Woods Hole, MA, 1987.
15. **Miller, D. M. and Tindall, D. R.,** Identification of an acetonitrile-soluble toxic fraction from *Gambierdiscus toxicus*, *FASEB J.*, 2, A374, 1988.
16. **Miller, D. M. and Tindall, D. R.,** An acetonitrile-soluble toxic fraction from the dinoflagellate, *Gambierdiscus toxicus*, *Annual Meeting of the Association of Island Marine Laboratories of the Caribbean*, 1988.
17. **Miller, D. M. and Tindall, D. R.,** Preparative HPLC separation of maitotoxin from crude extracts of *Gambierdiscus toxicus*, *9th World Congress on Animal, Plant, and Microbial Toxins (IST)*, 1988.
18. **Miller, D. M.,** Dinoflagellates responsible for ciguatera food poisoning, USAMRIID contract DAMD17-87-C-7002, 1988.
19. **Tindall, D. R., Dickey, R. W., and Miller, D. M.,** Effects of a lipid soluble toxin from the dinoflagellate *Prorocentrum* cf. *lima* on mice and acetylcholine and histamine receptor sites in guinea pig ileum, *Fed. Proc.*, 41, 1561, 1982.
20. **Tindall, D. R., Dickey, R. W., Carlson, R. D., and Morey-Gaines, G.,** Ciguatoxigenic dinoflagellates from the Caribbean, in *Seafood Toxins*, Ragelis, E. P., Eds., American Chemical Society Symposium Series 262, Washington, D.C., 1984, 225-240.
21. **Tindall, D. R. and Miller, D. M.,** Purification of maitotoxin from the dinoflagellate, *Gambierdiscus toxicus*, using high pressure liquid chromatography, in *Toxic Dinoflagellates*, Anderson, D. M., White, A. W., and Baden, D. G., Eds., Elsevier Science, New York, 1985, 321-326.
22. **Tindall, D. R. and Miller, D. M.,** Bioassay of a fast-acting low molecular weight toxin from a dinoflagellate, *Prorocentrum concavum*, *Conference on Natural Toxins from Aquatic and Marine Environments*, Woods Hole, MA, 1987.
23. **Tindall, D. R. and Miller, D. M.,** Two potent toxins from *Ostreopsis lenticularis*, a dinoflagellate common to ciguatera-endemic regions of the Caribbean and tropical Atlantic, *Fed. Proc.*, 46, 3730, 1987.
24. **Tindall, D. R. and Miller, D. M.,** Toxins from *Ostreopsis lenticularis*, a dinoflagellate common to ciguatera-endemic regions of the Caribbean and tropical Atlantic, *Annual Meeting of the Association of Island Marine Laboratories of the Caribbean*, 1988.
25. **Perry, W. L. M.,** Use of the guinea-pig ileum preparation, in *Pharmacological Experiments on Isolated Preparations*, Churchill Livingstone, Edinburgh, 1970, 64-77.
26. **Tallardia, R. J. and Jacob, L. S.,** *The Dose Response Relation in Pharmacology*, Springer-Verlag, New York, 1979.
27. **Lombet, A., Bidard, J.-N., and Lazdunski, M.,** Ciguatoxin and brevetoxin share a common receptor site on the neuronal voltage-dependent Na^+ channel, *FEBS Lett.*, 2, 1987.
28. **McClure, W. O., Abbott, B. C., Baxter, D. E., Hsaio, T. H., Satin, L. S., Siger, A., and Yoshino, J. E.,** Leptinotarsin: a presynaptic neurotoxin that stimulates release of acetylcholine, *Proc. Natl. Acad. Sci. USA*, 7, 1219-1223, 1980.
29. **Yoshino, J. E., Baxter, D. E., Hsiao, T. H., and McClure, W. O.,** Release of acetylcholine from rat brain synaptosomes stimulated with leptinotarsin, a new neurotoxin, *J. Neurochem.*, 34, 635-642, 1980.
30. **Moore, J. E., Ulbricht, W., and Takata, M.,** Effect of ethanol on the sodium and potassium conductances of the squid axon, *J. Gen. Physiol.*, 48, 279-295, 1964.
31. **Armstrong, C. M. and Binstock, L.,** The effect of several alcohols on the properties of the squid giant axon, *J. Gen. Physiol.*, 48, 265-277, 1964.

32. **Spedding, M.,** Changing surface charge with salicylate differentiates between subgroups of calcium-antagonists, *Br. J. Pharmacol.*, 83, 210-220, 1984.
33. **Hille, W., Woodhull, A. M., and Shapiro, B. I.,** Negative surface charge near sodium channels of nerve: divalent ions, monovalent ions and pH, *Phil. Trans. R. Soc., Series B*, 270, 301-318, 1975.
34. **Tindall, D. R. and Miller, D. M.,** Purification and assay of two ciguatera toxins from the dinoflagellate, *Prorocentrum concavum, Proc. Amer. Symp. Animal Plant Microbial Toxins (2nd), Amer. Sect. I. S. T.*, II, 32, 1986.

Chapter 9

MORPHOLOGIC EFFECTS OF MAITOTOXIN ON LIVER AND BRAIN CELLS OF CHICK EMBRYOS: LIGHT MICROSCOPY AND ELECTRON MICROSCOPY STUDIES

Faiqa Hassan, Donald M. Miller, and Donald R. Tindall

TABLE OF CONTENTS

I. INTRODUCTION

Ciguatera was the name given to a food poisoning syndrome that affected Spanish people who settled in Cuba during the exploration of American continents. This serious human intoxication results from eating certain tropical and subtropical fishes associated with coral reefs and adjacent coastal waters. The disease is manifested in humans by a great variety of symptoms, including moderate to severe gastrointestinal disorders such as nausea, vomiting, diarrhea, and abdominal cramps. These disorders are of relatively short duration. There are, also, moderate to severe neurologic disorders, which may persist for days, weeks, or months, including headaches, severe pruritis, temperature reversal, arthralgia, paresthesia, myalgia, convulsions, muscular paralysis, audiovisual hallucinations, vertigo and loss of equilibrium, and, in some cases, death due to respiratory failure.[1] Ciguatera may be caused by over 400 species of marine fishes, including many that are highly prized for food.[2] Banner[3] provided a convincing argument that ciguatoxin, as defined by Scheuer and coworkers, was the principal toxin causing ciguatera. However, other authors have suggested that there is more than one primary toxin causing the disease.[4,5] The occurrence of maitotoxin and scaritoxin in association with ciguatoxin in fishes has been reported.[6]

It is now known that the main source of these toxins are several species of epiphytic/benthic algae called dinoflagellates, which comprise a significant portion of the food base in the tropical and subtropical latitudes. These dinoflagellates are consumed by herbivorous fishes. These in turn are eaten by carnivores, and the toxin is transmitted to many other fishes of higher trophic levels through the food chain, resulting in the biomagnification in the larger carnivorous fishes.[7]

Gambierdiscus toxicus was the first dinoflagellate that was linked to the formation of ciguatera-type toxins.[8] However, other investigations and observations have revealed that the presence of many additional toxic dinoflagellate species may contribute to ciguatera syndrome.[9,10] Tindall and coworkers have reported on similar toxins from ciguatera endemic region in the Caribbean.[11]

A specific water-soluble toxin from *G. toxicus*, referred to as *maitotoxin* (MTX or GT-4), has been purified using high-pressure liquid chromatography (HPLC) at SIU-C.[12,13]

Yasumoto and coworkers in their study on the toxins in the gut contents of parrotfish, found that the gut contents contained MTX and an acetone-soluble toxin besides ciguatoxin. This MTX was assumed to be a basic compound of small molecular size having a strong paralytic action.[8]

According to many reports on the action of MTX, it involves a direct stimulatory response on contact with the smooth-muscle preparation of the guinea-pig ileum,[14,15] produces an inhibitory effect on guinea-pig atrial muscles,[16,17] stimulates the release of norepinephrine from sympathetic neurons,[18] the release of prolactin from pituitary cultures[19] and has a positive inotropic effect.[16] It has been shown to interact with voltage-sensitive calcium channels in cultured neuronal cells.[20]

Numerous reports are available on the physiologic and pharmacologic actions of this toxin. A very few reports are available on its action on the morphology of stomach, heart, spleen, thymus, and adrenal glands of mice.[21,22] Except for one study, almost no evidence is available as to ciguatera-type toxins,[23] effects on the morphology of the liver and brain cells.

This chapter focuses on the morphologic effects of GT-4 on the liver and brain cells of chick embryos and discusses these effects relative to other morphologic effects.

II. LIGHT MICROSCOPICAL STUDIES

Light microscopic studies were performed on the liver and brain cells of adult chicks. Fertile chicken eggs (Rhode Island Reds or White Leg Horns) were purchased from a local farmer. For each set of experiments two dozen chicken eggs were incubated at 101°F in an incubator with relative humidity control. After 72 to 96 h of incubation, those eggs that showed development were divided into seven groups of three eggs each. They were cleaned with 70% ethanol and a very small hole was drilled in the broader end of the shell. Each egg was given a treatment of 2.015 mg/ml (LD_{50} = 151.125 µg) of crude GT-4 in methanol (MEOH) and 200 µl of 0.15 M NaCl in the following manner:

Group 1. Controls. No treatment, only 200 µl 0.15 M NaCl.
Group 2. Controls. Injected with 8 µl MEOH + 200 µl 0.15 M NaCl.
Group 3. Injected with 0.5 µl (5.0375 µg/ml) GT-4 + 7.5 µl MEOH + 200 µl 0.15 M NaCl.
Group 4. Injected with 1.0 µl (10.075 ng/ml) GT-4 + 7 µl MEOH + 200 µl 0.15 M NaCl.
Group 5. Injected with 2.0 µl (20.15 ng/ml) GT-4 + 6 µl MEOH + 200 µl 0.15 M NaCl.
Group 6. Injected with 4.0 µl (40.3 µg/ml) GT-4 + 4 µl MEOH + 200 µl 0.15 M NaCl.
Group 7. Injected with 8.0 µl (80.6 µg/ml) GT-4 + 200 µl 0.15 M NaCl.

The eggs were candled every day and allowed to incubate until they hatched. As the chickens hatched, they were removed to a brooder maintained at 90°F. They were watered, fed on starter feed daily, and observed for several days for their behavioral activities (gait, chirping) or any gross morphologic changes that might have occurred due to toxin treatment. They were then sacrificed and dissected. Their visceral cavities were examined for any kind of abnormalities. Intact livers and brains were removed and cut into small pieces separately (about 2 mm). They were then very quickly fixed in buffered 10% formalin, dehydrated, infiltrated with paraffin, and sectioned at 7-µm thickness. The sections were then stained with hematoxylin and eosin, and were studied under the light microscope. This procedure was repeated under the same conditions four different times.

A. BEHAVIORAL OBSERVATIONS

Eggs that had received 4 µl (40.3 µg/ml) and 8 µl (80.6 µg/ml) of toxin produced chicks that were severely affected. They appeared weak, had difficulty in walking, and collapsed after staggering. Their legs were flexed and they showed ataxia. They blinked their eyes more often and did not chirp as well as the controls (no treatment and 8 µl MEOH) and as chicks that had received 0.5 µl (5.0375 µg/ml), 1 µl (10.075 µg/ml), and 2 µl (20.15 µg/ml) of GT-4.

B. MORPHOLOGICAL CHANGES

The overall morphologic or histopathologic changes were roughly dependent on the doses that were injected to eggs during incubation. Livers that had received less than 40.3 µg/ml GT-4 did not show any discernable morphologic changes in the tissues. The parenchymal cells of the liver were surrounded by cell membranes, the blood cells were in the sinusoids, and the capillaries were intact and looked normal (Figure 1 control, other figures with less than 40.3 µg/ml treatment not shown). Histologically marked necrosis of the tissue was seen in the livers at 40.3 µg/ml and 80.6 µg/ml of toxin. Histopathologic examination of the liver revealed massive hemorrhaging of the entire tissue and the loss of characteristic architecture of the hepatic cells. They were congested with areas of perisinusoidal extravasation of blood into the liver parenchyma. The hepatocytes appeared to have lost cell-to-cell adhesion resulting in hepatocellular necrosis and collapsed parenchyma (Figures 2A and 2B).

In the brain tissue, similar observations were made. Here the untreated controls and those injected with 8 µl of MEOH, showed intact cells with very dense prominent nuclei (Figure 3, control untreated). Not many changes were observed at doses 5.0 µg/ml, 10.0 µg/ml, and 20.15 µg/ml. At 40.3 µg/ml and 80.6 µg/ml of GT-4, however, there were lesions and gross hemorrhaging of the tissue. The accumulation of blood cells was obvious and was a consistent histologic finding throughout the light microscope study. Only nucleated blood cells could be seen and cell to cell adhesion was lost (Figures 4A and 4B). The blood cells were counted using a micrometer of 16.9 $mm^2$and at the magnification of 400X (objective = 40X and ocular = 10X). The results are shown in Figures 5 and 6.

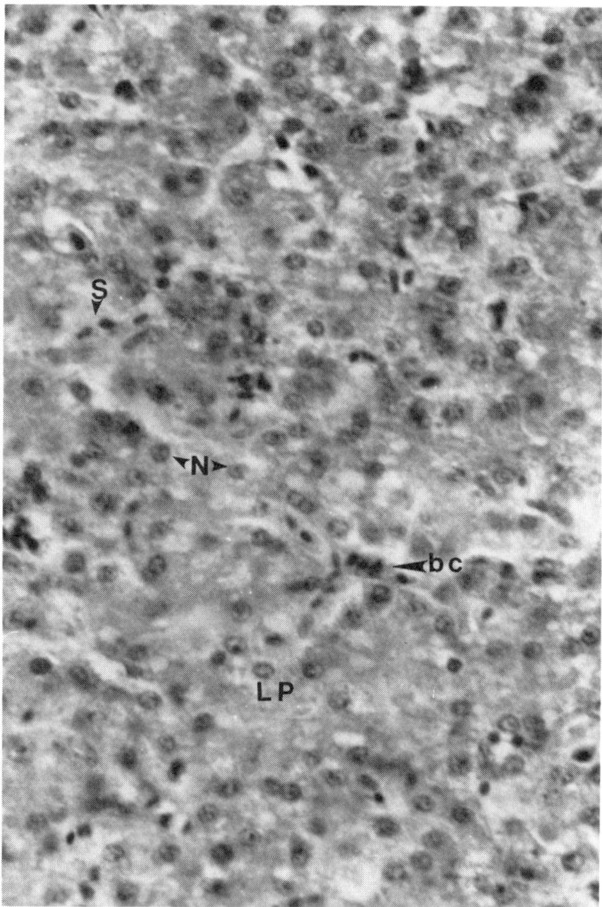

FIGURE 1. Liver cells from a control embryo, (received only 200 μl of 0.15 M NaCl). Here the parenchyma of the liver tissue (LP) is intact, but some clear spaces are visible. The large nuclei (N) represent the nuclei of the tissue; bc represents the blood cells that are within their capillaries or sinusoids (S). The cytoplasm is very dense. (Magnification × 1080.)

III. ELECTRON MICROSCOPICAL STUDIES

Fertile chicken eggs were incubated at 101°F for 10 days. Their livers and brains were removed aseptically, and the cells were cultured in medium 199 containing 5% calf serum and 1% antibiotic. After the formation of monolayers, the cells were treated with partially purified GT-4 at doses of 142, 284, and 568 ng/ml of medium for 15 min, respectively.

After toxin treatment the cell cultures were processed for electron microscopy using the same protocol as employed by Bozzola.[24] They were washed with phosphate buffer at pH 7.4, fixed in buffered 2% formaldehyde and glutaraldehyde, and rinsed three times for 1 h each in the same buffer at room temperature. They were then postfixed in 1% OsO_4, stained in uranyl acetate, dehydrated in graded ethanol series, infiltrated with ascending Epon:alcohol mixtures until monolayers were in pure Epon *in situ*. Gold to silver sections were cut using a diamond knife and stained with uranyl acetate and lead citrate. The sections were then studied by transmission electron microscope (TEM) operated at 50 kV. A qualitative analysis of the different organelles of the cells was made on the severity of the toxic effects as a function of dose. The mechanism

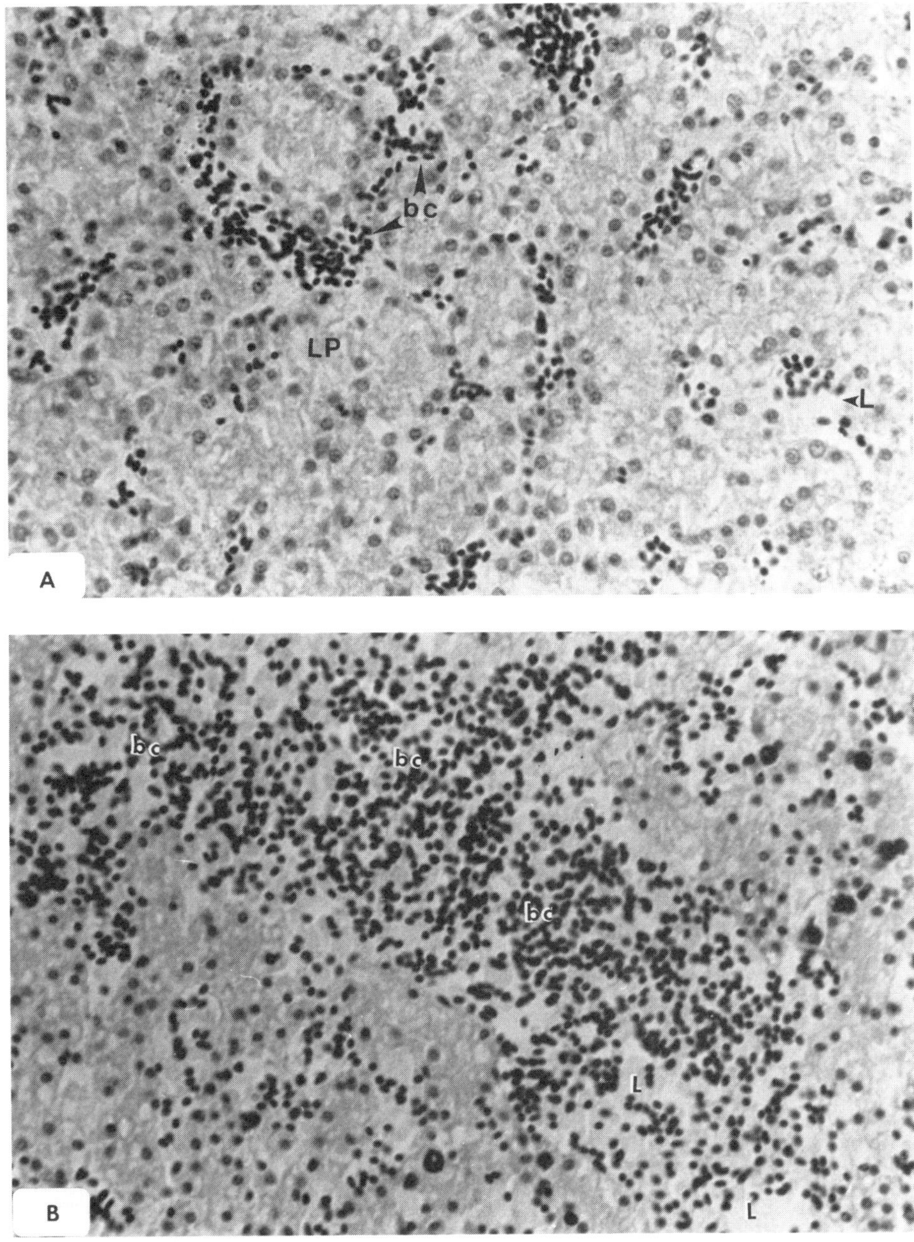

FIGURE 2. (A) Liver cells from an embryo treated with 40.30 μg/ml of crude GT-4. Here, the toxin shows a discernable effect. It shows hemorrhaging of some tissue, released blood cells (bc) into the liver parenchyma (LP), and lesions (L). (B) Liver cells from an embryo treated with 80.6 μg/ml of crude GT-4. There is a massive hemorrhaging of the entire tissue and loss of the characteristic architecture of the hepatocytes. The tissue is congested with areas of perisinusoidal extravasation of blood cells (bc) into the liver parenchyma (LP), causing lesions (L). (Magnification × 850.)

of the action of toxin was determined by taking into consideration the changes in the cell membrane, the nucleus, endoplasmic reticulum, polyribosomes, mitochondria, presence or absence of Golgi bodies, vacuoles, presence or absence of fibers or filaments, and electron density.

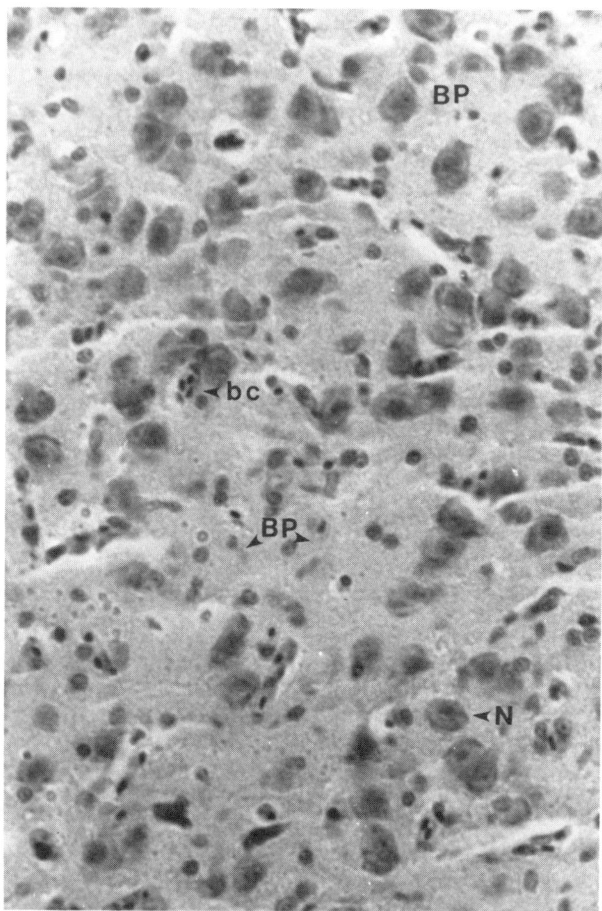

FIGURE 3. Brain cells from a control embryo (200 μl of 0.15 M NaCl). The brain parenchyma (BP) is smooth and intact, and the blood cells (bc) are within their capillaries. The cytoplasm is quite dense. The large nuclei (N) represent the nuclei of the brain parenchyma. (Magnification × 1080.)

Electron microscopic studies with control liver cultures showed polyhedral cells with intact plasma membranes, electron-dense cytoplasm, and fairly round electron-dense nuclei. The chromatin in some nuclei was concentrated to the periphery of the nuclei. There were numerous mitochondria of different shapes and sizes, and their cristae were extended into the mitochondrial matrices. There were many Golgi complexes in the cells. Endoplasmic reticulum was either tubular, segmented, or vesicular, and, in addition to these, there were many small membrane-bound vacuoles (Figure 7). With a treatment of 8 μl of MEOH, all the cellular organelles were very much like the untreated cells, except that there was a slight increase in the vacuoles.

Different doses of partially purified GT-4 on the liver primary cultures revealed the following. At the dose of 142 ng/ml, there was some fragmentation of the plasma membrane and the nuclei were slightly enlarged. The cytoplasm became electron lucent, and mitochondria became slightly rounded and increased in number. Endoplasmic reticulum (ER) segmented and accumulated around mitochondria. There was an increase in the number of vacuoles and their membranes began to disappear. The cytoplasmic integrity was not maintained as well as the controls (Figure 8). At 284 ng/ml of toxin, the plasma membrane in most of the cells was lost.

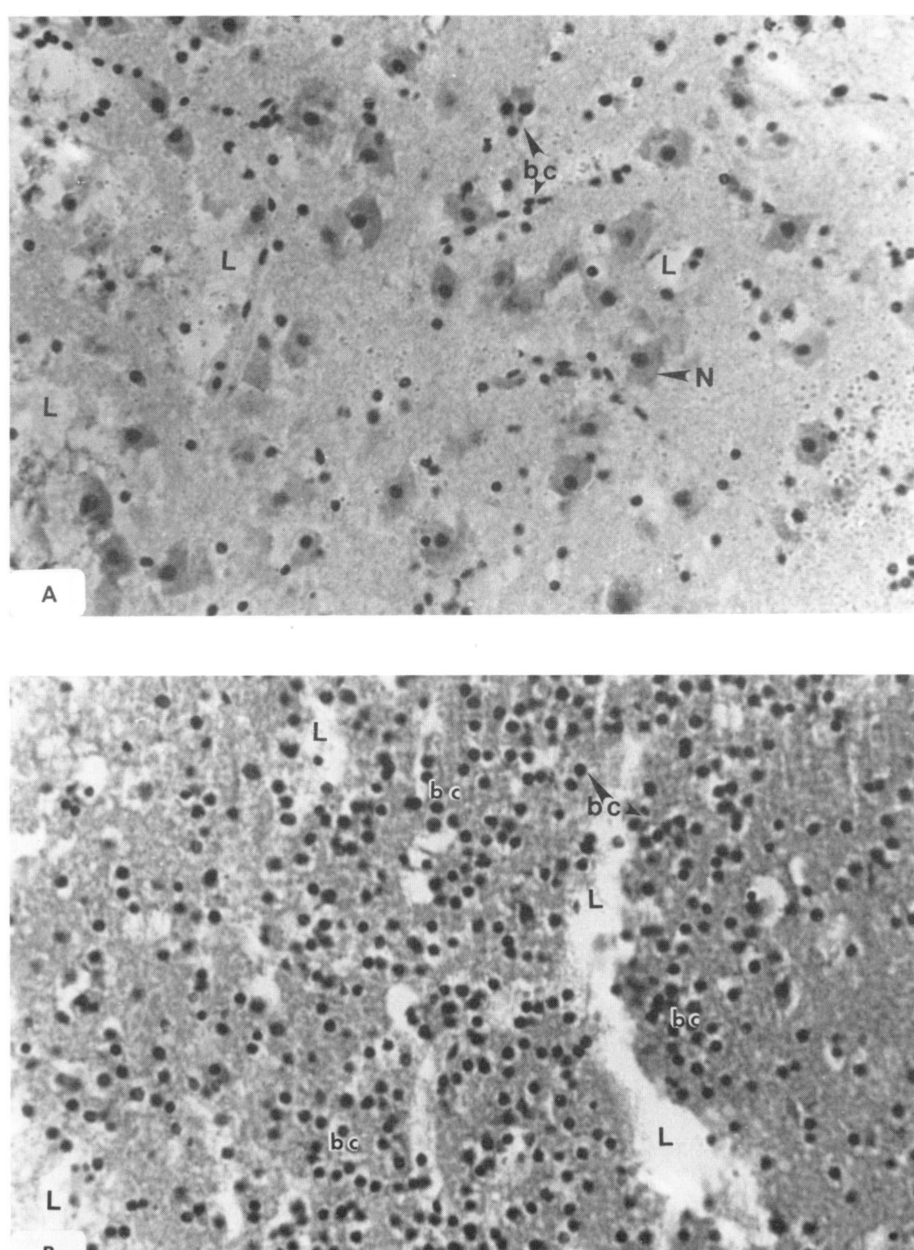

FIGURE 4. (A) Brain cells from an embryo treated with 40.3 μg/ml of crude GT-4. Here some of the capillaries ruptured, releasing the blood cells (bc) into the tissue causing lesions (L). N represents the nucleus of the brain cell. (B) Brain cells from an embryo treated with 80.6 μg/ml of crude GT-4. Here the brain tissue has completely lost its architecture. The blood cells (bc) dominate and no capillaries are visible. Lesions (L) have formed in the tissue. (Magnification × 850.)

The mitochondria became completely round, rough-surfaced endoplasmic reticulum (RER) decreased in number, Golgi complexes degenerated, and overall there was more cellular disintegration (Figure 9). At the highest dose of 568 ng/ml, there was a complete disintegration of the cells. Only large amounts of cellular debris, around swollen mitochondria with disorganized cristae, could be seen (Figure 10).

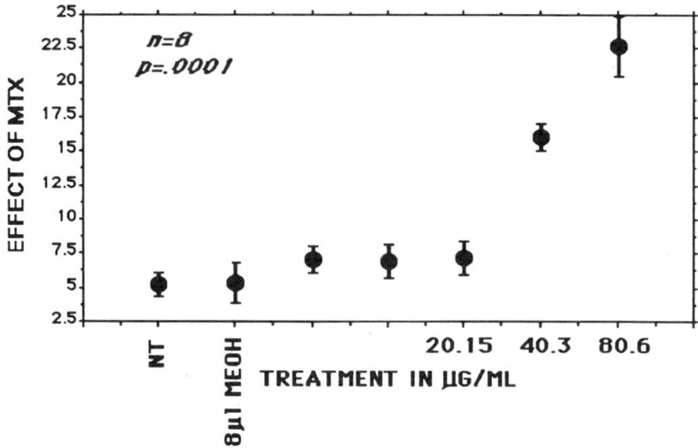

FIGURE 5. The effect of MTX on liver as a function of dose. The x axis represents the amount of toxin given in micrograms per milliliter. The y axis represents the effect of toxin in terms of blood cell count. n = 8 (total number of samples used per treatment). P is the probability for all the treatments using one way ANOVA across cell treatment.

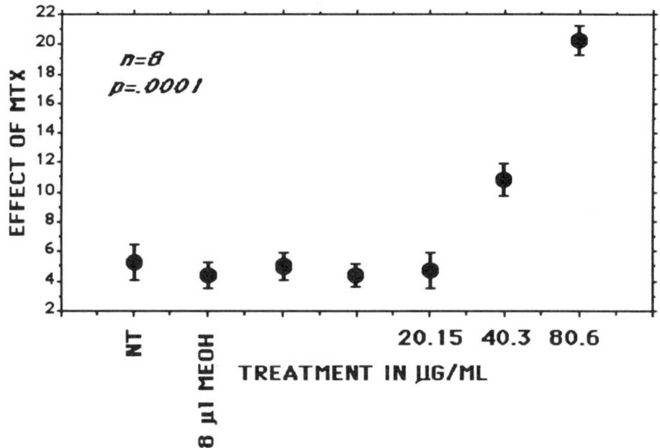

FIGURE 6. The effect of MTX on brain as a function of dose. The x axis represents the amount of toxin given in micrograms per milliliter. The y axis represents the effect of toxin in terms of blood cell count. n = 8 (total number of samples used per treatment). P is the probability for all the treatments using one way ANOVA across cell treatment.

With electron microscopic studies on brain cells, the control cultures showed very well-defined plasma membranes, electron-dense nuclei and cytoplasm, well-defined nuclei with intact nuclear membranes, and an evenly distributed chromatin. Mitochondria were small in size but were of different shapes and their matrices were dense. Cisternae of RER were of different shapes (Figure 11). With 8 µl treatment of MEOH, the brain cells had intact membranes of all the organelles, except that there was some increase in the number of vacuoles.

At 142 ng/ml of toxin treatment, the cytoplasm became electron lucent. There was a decrease in the number of polyribosomes. Mitochondria were small and their matrices were dense. Plasma membrane became discontinuous and there was an increase in the microfilaments (Figure 12).

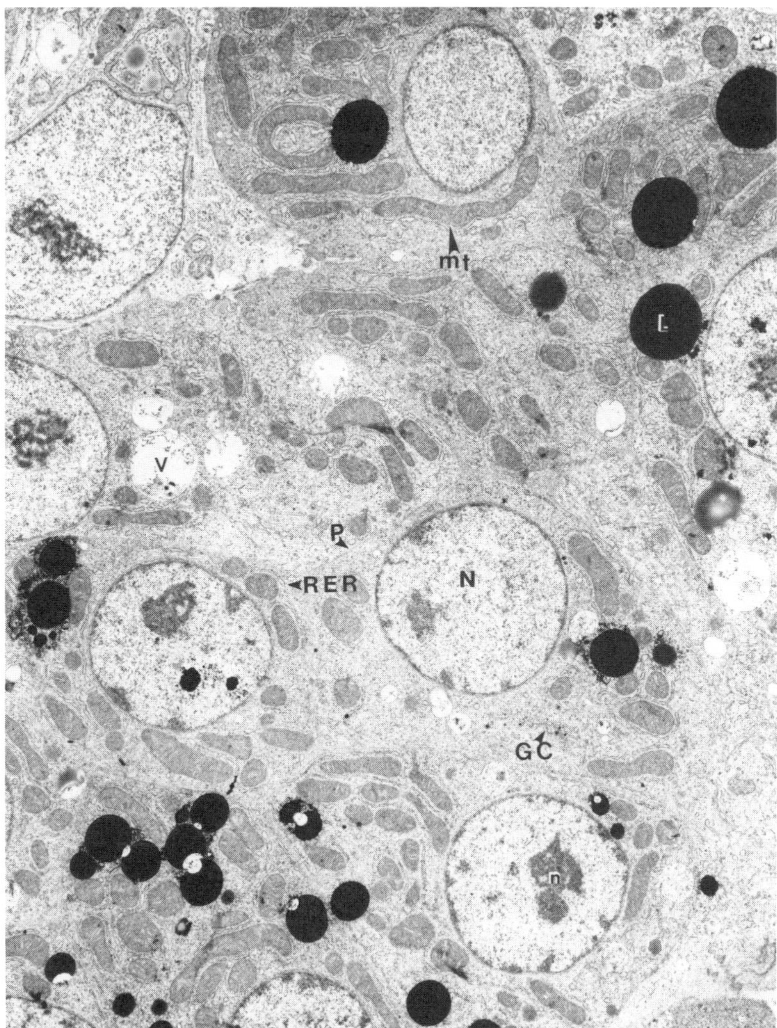

FIGURE 7. Untreated cultured liver cells. Though the cells have different electron densities, they all have very distinct and intact plasma membranes (P). Nuclei (N) are round or oval. Cell chromatin is unevenly distributed and is more concentrated towards the periphery of the nuclear membranes. Mitochondria (MT) are numerous and are of different shapes and sizes. They are round, oval, or elongated. Their cristae are well packed and form incomplete septa in the mitochondrial matrices. The cells that are less dense contain many active Golgi complexes (GC). There are many small clusters of polyribosomes. RER is either elongated, segmented, tubular, or vesiculated, and surrounds mitochondria. There are many dark lipid droplets (L) of different sizes. Many small vacuoles (V) with intact membranes can be seen. Some SER is also visible. (Magnification × 6500.)

At 284 ng/ml of GT-4 the brain cells lost their plasma membranes completely. There was a decrease in RER and smooth-surfaced endoplasmic reticulum (SER). There was an increase in the number of vacuoles. Many collagen fibers could be seen outside the cells (Figure 13). At 568 ng/ml of toxin, there was almost a complete destruction of cells. Only cellular debris with irregularly shaped nuclei and round mitochondria with disorganized cristae remained (Figure 14).

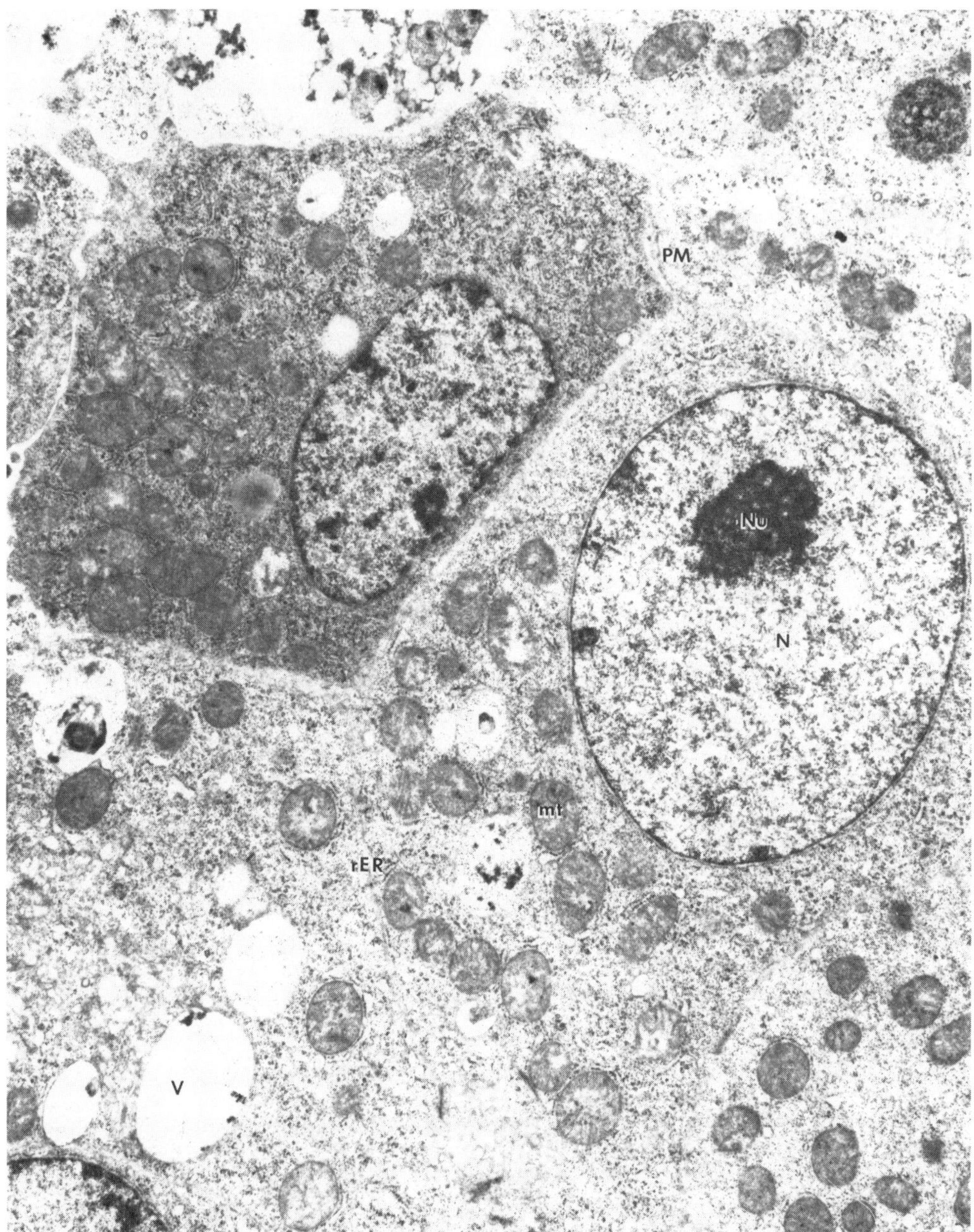

FIGURE 8. Liver cells treated with 142 ng/ml GT-4. Here the plasma membrane (pm) is fragmented in places. The nuclei (N) are becoming electron lucent, but the nucleolus (n) looks normal. The cytoplasm is becoming electron lucent at places. Mitochondria (mt) are becoming round and show disorganized cristae. Rough-surfaced endoplasmic reticulum (rer) is also increasing in number, because it is becoming segmented, tubular, and vesicular. Vacuoles (v) are increasing in number and their membranes have disappeared. Golgi complex is not visible. The cytoplasmic membrane integrity is not being maintained as well. No lipid droplets are present here. (Magnification × 10,500.)

IV. DISCUSSION

Crude GT-4 at doses of 5.037, 10.075, 20.15, 40.3, and 80.6 μg/ml was injected into the air sac of developing eggs. After the chicks hatched, the liver and the brain tissues were studied using light microscopy. This study showed that these tissues were severely affected at the two

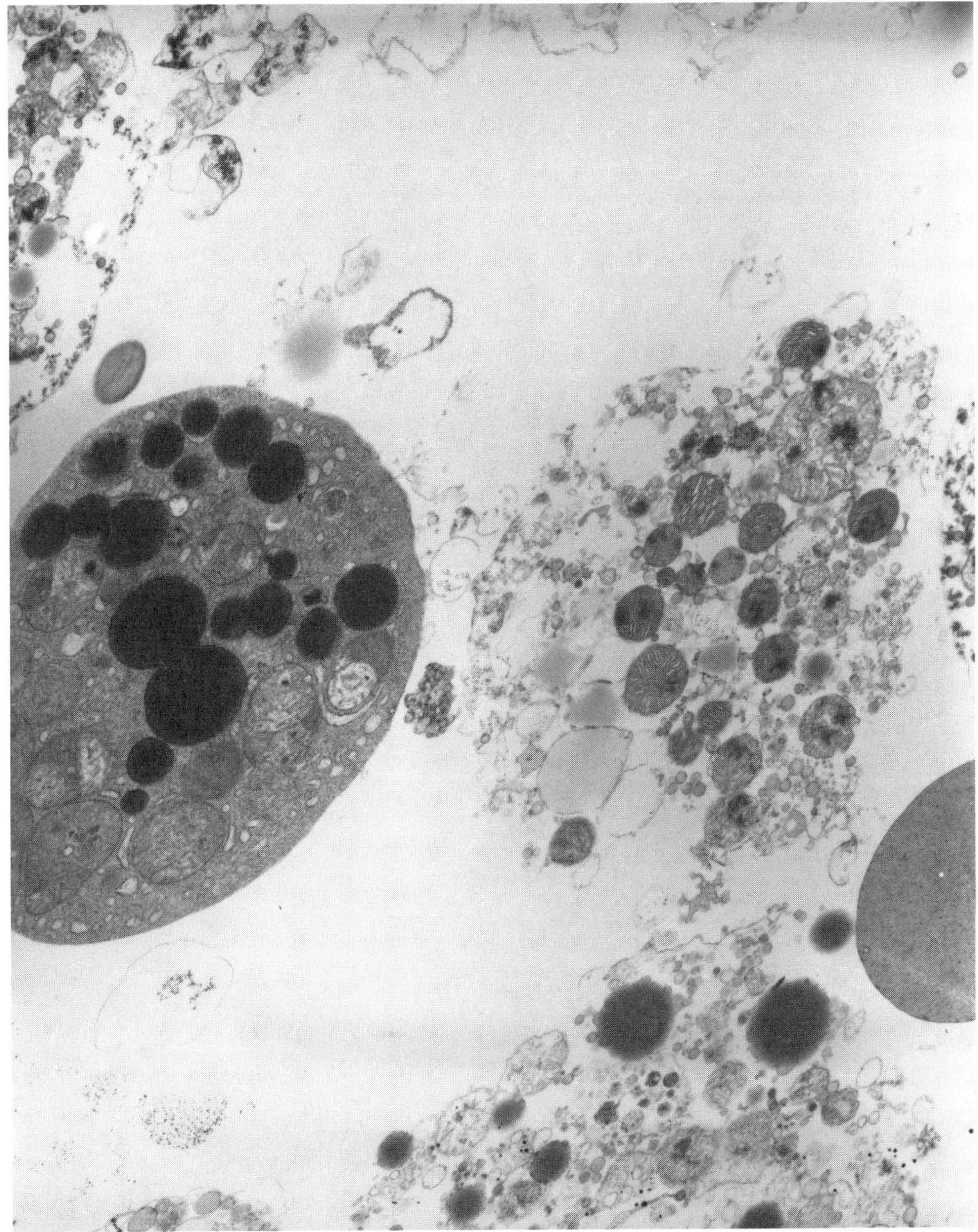

FIGURE 9. Liver cells treated with 284 ng/ml GT-4. Only two cells seem to have most of their plasma membranes (P). The other cells are disintegrated. Only a few lipid droplets and rounded mitochondria (MT) are left. ER is segmented or vesicular. Round mitochondria and few lipid droplets are present in two cells. (Magnification × 10,500.)

highest doses (40.3 and 80.6 μg/ml). Doses lower than these did not seem to have a discernable effect. This demonstrates that the toxin was able to pass through the shell membrane, through the albumin, through the yolk sac, and finally through the membranes of the embryos to reach these organs. It can be inferred from this that these organs are two of the target organs for the action of GT-4.

Both liver and brain as intact organs have revealed similar types of results, i.e., resulting in necrosis and lesions (Figures 2 and 4). Injuries to the brain cells particularly correlate with the

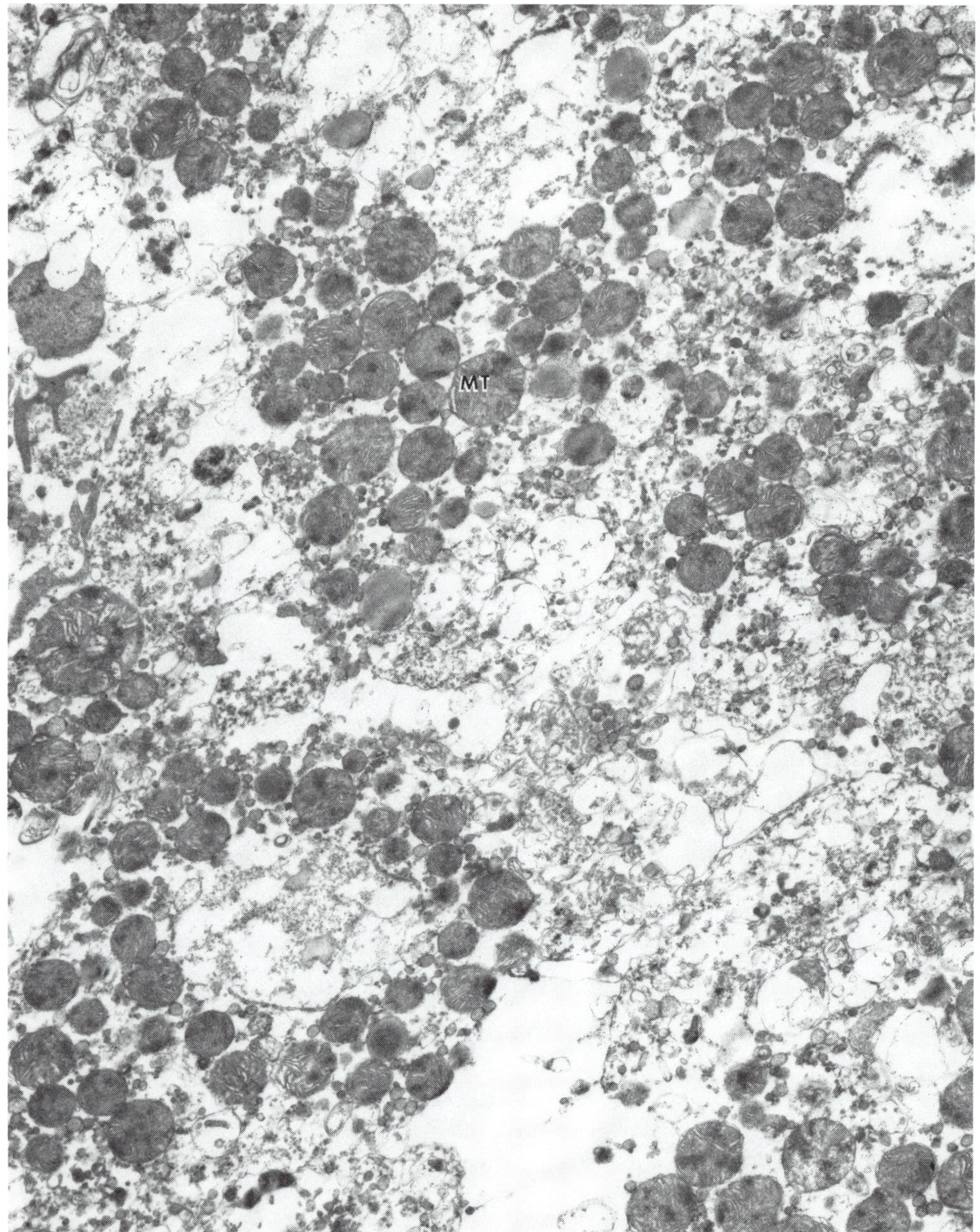

FIGURE 10. Liver cells treated with 568 ng/ml GT-4. The cells are disintegrated completely, leaving a large amount of cellular debris and a portion of a dead cell. Only round numerous mitochondria (MT) with disorganized cristae are seen. (Magnification × 10,500.)

neurologic symptoms seen in the chicks hatched from the eggs receiving the two highest doses of GT-4 (40.3 and 80.6 μg/ml).

Overall very significant histopathologic changes in liver and brain were similar and occurred in a dose-dependent pattern (Figures 5 and 6). Light microscopy studies showed that hepatic cord architecture was broken down (at 40.3 and 80.6 μg/ml of GT-4) due to hepatocellular dissociation. This dissociation was found throughout the tissues. Membrane damage and

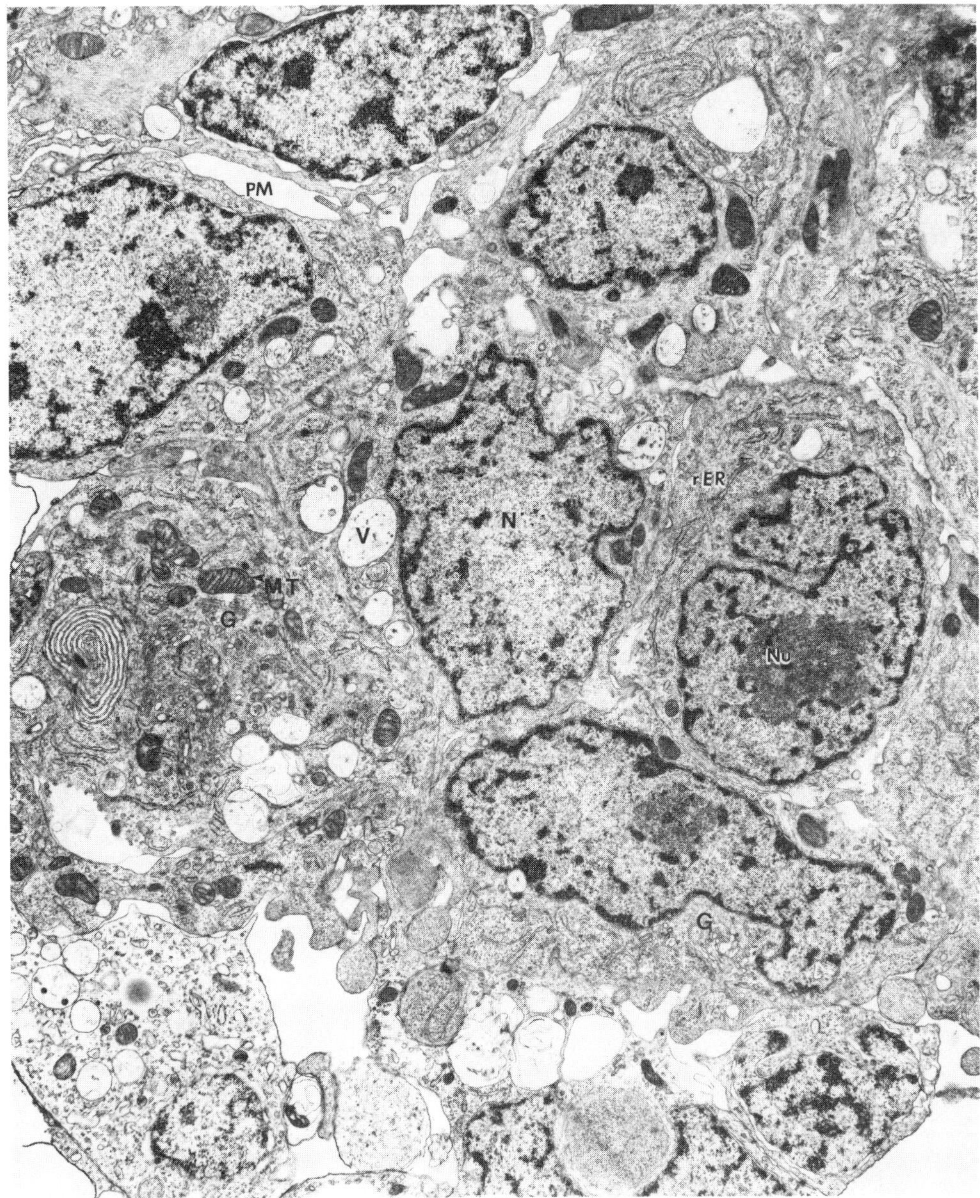

FIGURE 11. Untreated brain cells. Cells are electron dense and have very distinct and clear plasma membranes (PM). Nuclei (N) are of different shapes and sizes (due to the plane at which sectioned) with one or two nucleoli (n). Chromatin is almost evenly distributed. Mitochondria (mt) are small in size but variable in shape. At some places they are surrounded by ER. Their cristae are well organized. rER is segmented, tubular, or in the form of long channels. At some places the ER meets with the nuclear membranes. There are numerous microfilaments present, in addition to many small membrane-bound vacuoles (v). (Magnification × 6500.)

cytolysis were also found. The liver cell damage appears to be a direct effect of GT-4 on the cell membranes (Figures 2A and 2B). Similar observations were made in the brain tissue. With increasing doses, larger areas of the sections were affected and degenerative changes were widespread (Figures 4A and 4B).

At the electron microscopy level, the experiments reported in this study indicate that partially purified GT-4 produced histopathologic changes in the liver and brain primary cell cultures of

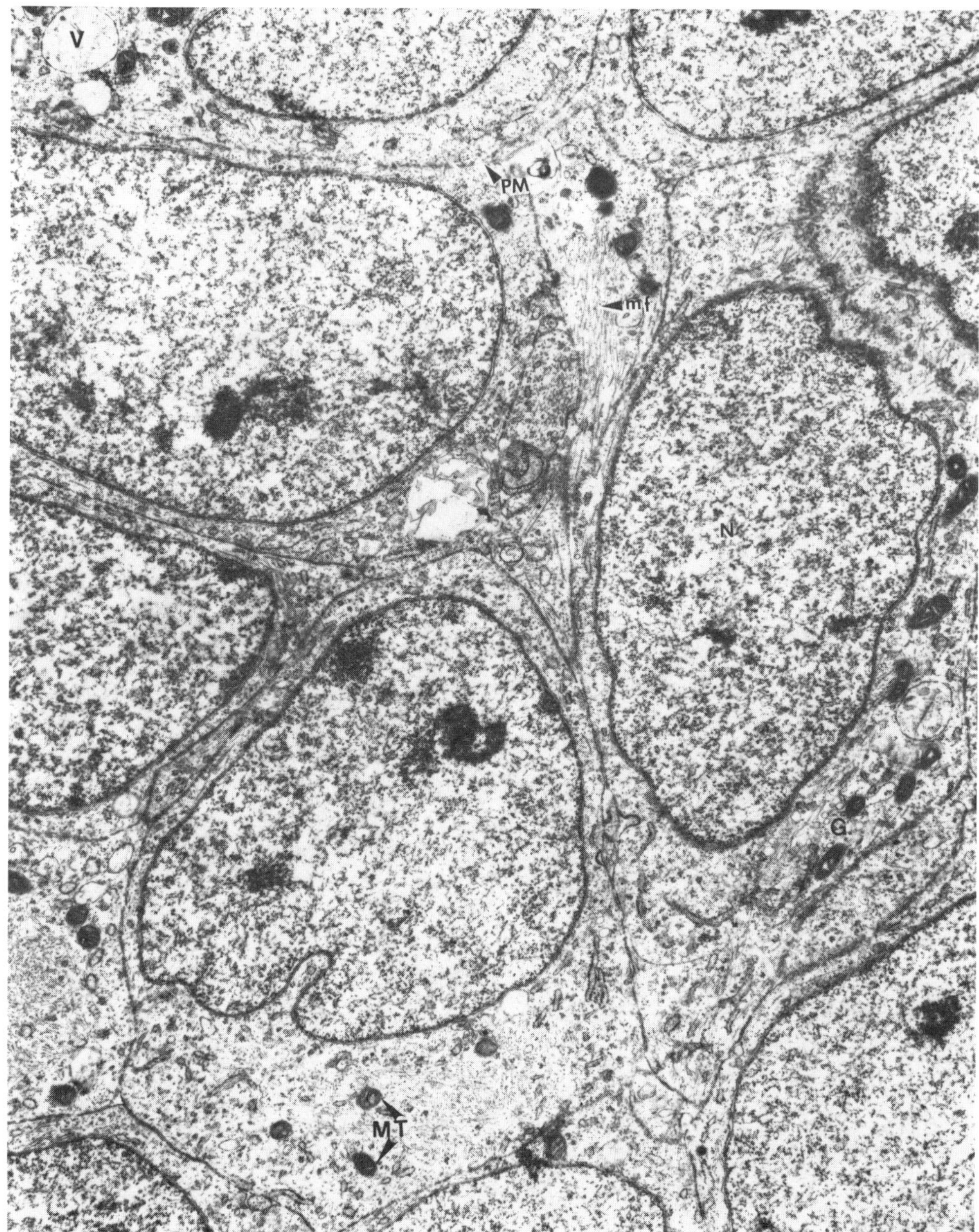

FIGURE 12. Brain cells treated with 142 ng/ml GT-4. Chromatin in the nucleus (N) is less dense compared to the normal cells. Discontinuity in the plasma membrane (pm) has started to appear at some places. Cytoplasm is electron lucent. Mitochondria (mt) are very small in size. Few elongated RER present. SER and many microfilaments also are present. (Magnification × 10,500.)

chick embryos. Samples for control and experimental cultures were obtained from the same growth clones to exercise a greater degree of uniformity and control in their sampling and preparation.

Hepatocytes and brain cells from control embryonic cell cultures revealed intact plasma membranes, a normal distribution of well-stacked ER, and tubular or branched ER. Dense

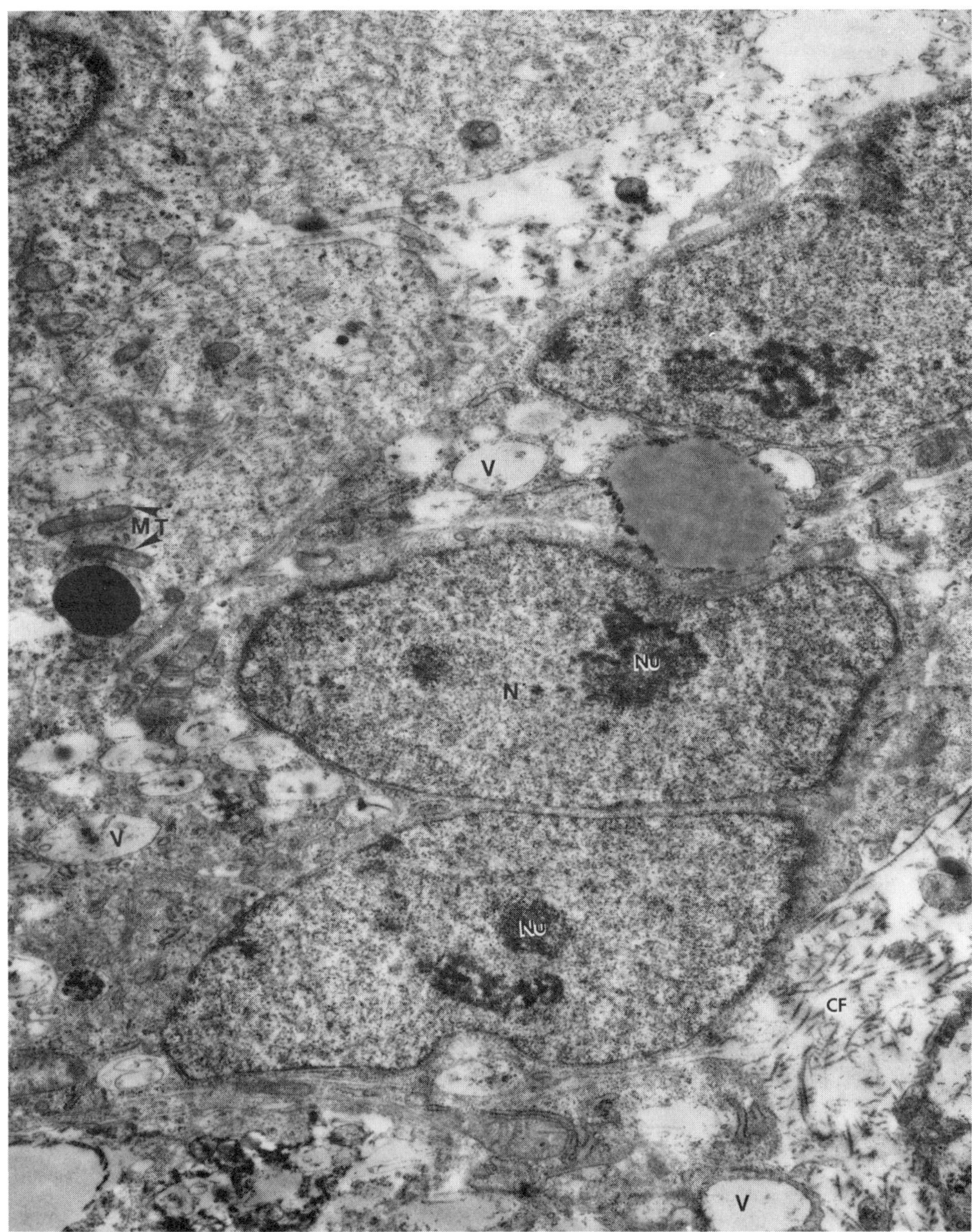

FIGURE 13. Brain cells treated with 284 ng/ml GT-4. The nuclei (N) are much elongated with one or two nucleoli (n) in them. The nuclear membranes are more distinct than the plasma membrane. Few mitochondria can be seen. There is a decrease in RER and SER, and vacuolization has taken place. Many collagen fibers (CF) are seen at the upper left corner. A few dark lipid droplets can also be seen. (Magnification × 10,500.)

mitochondria of different shapes and sizes with well-defined cristae were seen, in addition to small cytoplasmic vacuoles, many Golgi complexes, and lipid inclusions (Figures 7 and 11). The severity of the damage to the liver and brain cells appeared to be directly related to the dose concentration.

The treatment of cells with GT-4 for both liver and brain cell cultures brought about similar types of changes in the ultrastructure of the cells, such as fragmentation of the plasma

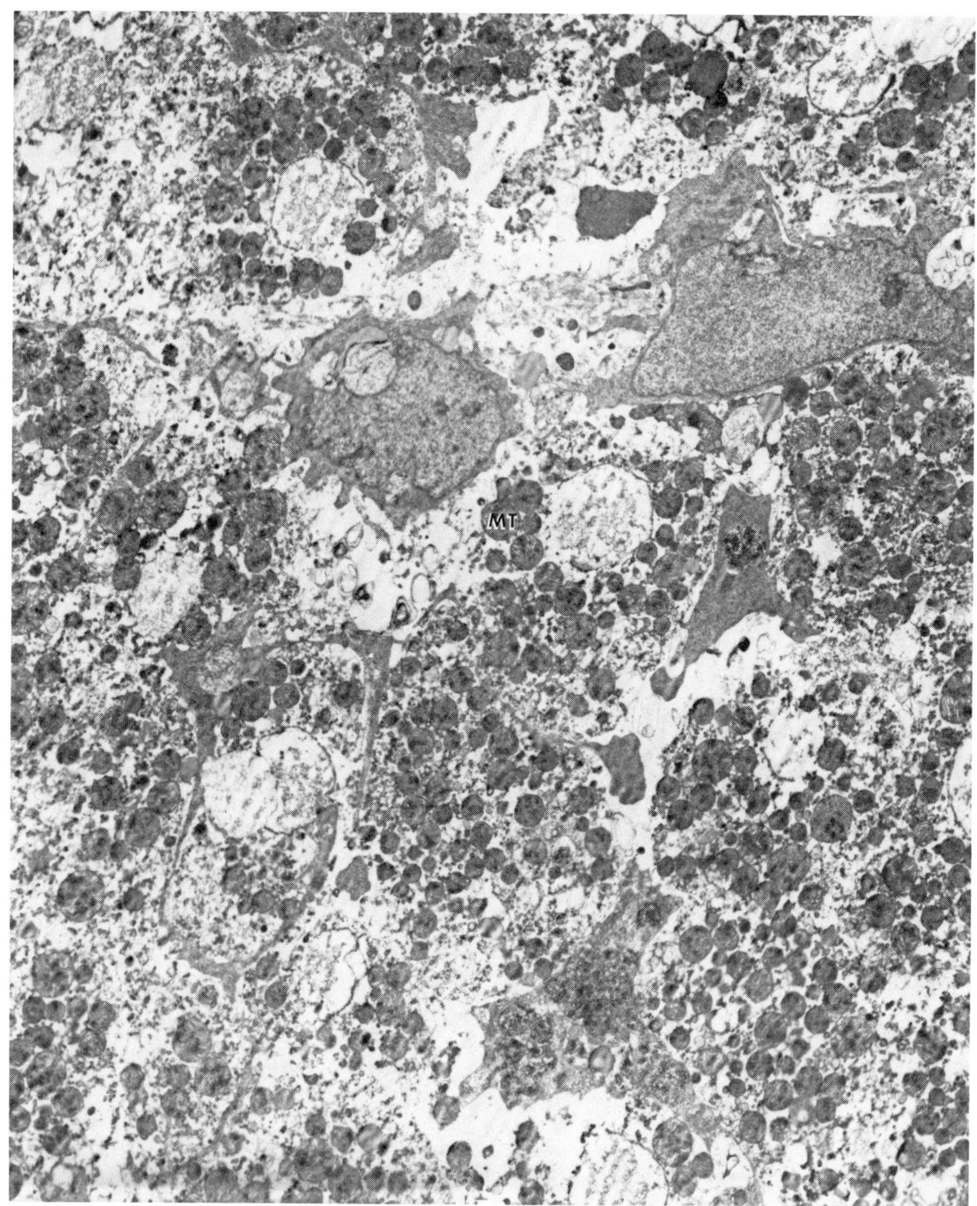

FIGURE 14. Brain cells treated with 568 ng/ml GT-4. No cell membrane is present. Only cellular debris with an irregularly shaped nucleus can be seen. Mitochondria (MT) have become round, swollen, and more dense, and their cristae are disorganized. ER has been changed into small vesicles. (Magnification × 10,500.)

membranes, segmentation or hypertrophy of ER, swelling or condensation and rounding of mitochondria, disintegration of Golgi complexes, and an increase in the number and size of vacuoles. The increase in the size of lipid droplets was variable. Very prominent changes were observed in most of the cellular organelles as a function of dose. Cells that were exposed to a smaller dose of toxin (142 ng/ml) showed less degeneration in their ultrastructures than those exposed to higher doses of 284 and 568 ng/ml, respectively.

Terao et al.[21,24] observed that stomach, heart, thymus, spleen, and adrenal glands of mice are the target organs for MTX in mice when the toxin is injected intraperitoneally. We, in our study, have demonstrated that liver and brain tissues are also affected morphologically when the toxin is injected into the chick embryos, and also when the primary cell cultures are incubated in the toxin for 15 min.

All normal and healthy cells maintain a calcium (Ca^{2+}) gradient across their outer membrane of 10,000-fold, and this only relatively small, but prolonged, change in this gradient would cause both disruption of cell metabolism and Ca^{2+} accumulation. It has been suggested by Farber and coworkers[25] that Ca^{2+} entry into cell is the common step in the death of cells injured by membrane toxins. The accumulation of Ca^{2+} can be in the mitochondria or the intracellular vacuoles, and can result in a decrease in ATP and other nucleotides, eventually causing cytolysis and cell death. Since GT-4 has been known to act on the voltage-sensitive calcium channels, resulting in an increase in the intracellular calcium.[20] It may be inferred that cellular membranes are the target sites for its action and that the morphologic changes described in this study seem to be directly related to GT-4-induced Ca^{2+} influx and accumulation in the cells, causing a depletion of ATP, which results in the arrest of the plasma membrane Ca^{2+} extrusion mechanism, along with a cessation of the Na^+-K^+ pump. This in turn results in necrosis and eventually cell death.

ACKNOWLEDGMENTS

This study was supported by U.S. Army Medical Research and Development Command, contract DAMD17-87-C-7002. The views, findings, and opinions expressed herein are those of the authors and should not be construed as those of the Department of the Army.

REFERENCES

1. **Regalis, E. P.,** Ciguatera sea food poisoning: an overview, in *Sea Food Toxins*, Regalis, E. P., Ed., American Chemical Society, Symposium Series 262, Washington, D.C., 1984, 25.
2. **Halstead, B. W.,** Poisonous and Venomous Marine Animals of the World, U.S. Government Printing Office, Washington, D. C, 1967, 1070.
3. **Banner, A. H.,** The biological origin and transmission of ciguatoxin, in *Marine Science. Bioactive Compounds from the Sea*, Humm, H. J. and Lane, C. E., Eds., Marcel Decker, New York, 1974, 15.
4. **Bagnis, R. A.,** Clinical aspects of ciguatera (fish poisoning) in French Polynesia, *Hawaii Med. J.*, 28, 25, 1968.
5. **Li, K.,** Ciguatera fish poison: a potent cholinesterase inhibitor, *Science*, 147, 1580, 1965.
6. **Chungue, E., Bagnis, R. A., Fusetani, N., and Hashimoto, Y.,** Isolation of the two toxins from a parrotfish, *Scarus gibberus.*, *Toxicon*, 15, 89, 1977.
7. **Randall, J. E.,** A review of ciguatera, tropical fish poisoning, with a tentative explanation of its cause, *Bull. Mar. Sci. Gulf. Caribb.*, 8, 236, 1958.
8. **Yasumoto, T., Nakajima, I., Bagnis, R. A., and Adachi, R.,** Finding of a dinoflagellate as a likely culprit of ciguatera., *Bull. Jpn. Soc. Sci. Fish*, 43, 1021, 1977.
9. **Yasumoto, T., Oshima, Y., Murakami, Y., Nakajima, I., Bagnis, R. A., and Fukuyo, Y.,** Toxicity of benthic dinoflagellates found in coral reef, *Bull. Jpn. Soc. Sci. Fish*, 46, 327, 1980.
10. **Nakajima, I., Oshima, Y., and Yasumoto, T.,** Toxicity of benthic dinoflagellates in Okinawa, *Bull. Jpn. Soc. Sci. Fish*, 47, 1029, 1981.
11. **Tindall, D. R., Dickey, R. W., Carlson, R. D., and Morey-Gaines, G.,** Ciguatoxigenic dinoflagellates from the Caribbean, in *Seafood Toxins*, Ragelis, E. P., Ed., American Chemical Society Symposium Series 262, Washington, D.C., 1984, 225.
12. **Dickey, R. W., Miller, D. M., and Tindall, D. R.,** Extraction of a water-soluble toxin from a dinoflagellate, *Gambierdiscus toxicus*, in *Seafood Toxins*, Ragelis, E. P., Ed., American Chemical Society Symposium Series 262, Washington, D.C., 1984, 257.
13. **Tindall, D. R. and Miller, D. M.,** Purification of maitotoxin from the dinoflagellate, *Gambierdiscus toxicus*, using high pressure liquid chromatography, in *Toxic Dinoflagellates*, Anderson, D. M., White, A. W., and Baden, D. G., Eds., Elsevier Science, New York, 1985, 321.
14. **Dickey, R. W.,** The extraction, purification and characterization of toxins from the marine dinoflagellates *Gambierdiscus toxicus* and *Prorocentrum concavum*, 1984.

15. **Miller, D. M., Dickey, R. W., and Tindall, D. R.,** Lipid soluble toxins from a dinoflagellate, *Gambierdiscus toxicus*, in *Seafood Toxins*, Ragelis, E. P., Ed., American Chemical Society Symposium Series 262, Washington, D.C., 1984, 241.
16. **Miyahara, J. T., Akau, C. K., and Yasumoto, T.,** Effects of ciguatoxin and maitotoxin on the isolated guinea pig atria, *Res. Commun. Chem. Pathol. Pharmacol.*, 25, 177, 1979.
17. **Shimizu, Y., Shimizu, H., Scheuer, P. J., Hokama, Y., Oyama, M., and Miyahara, J. T.,** *Gambierdiscus toxicus*, a ciguatera-causing dinoflagellate from Hawaii, *Bull. Jpn. Soc. Sci. Fish*, 48, 811, 1982.
18. **Takahashi, M., Ohizumi, Y., and Yasumoto, T.,** Maitotoxin, a Ca^{2+} channel activator candidate, *J. Biol. Chem.*, 257, 7287, 1982.
19. **Koike, K., Judd, A. M., Yasumoto, T., and MacLeod, R. M.,** Calcium mobilization potentiates prolactin release induced by protein kinase C activators, *Mol. Cell. Endocrinol.*, 40, 137, 1985.
20. **Freedman, S. B., Miller, R. J., Miller, D. M., and Tindall, D. R.,** Interactions of maitotoxin with voltage-sensitive calcium channels in cultured neuronal cells, *Proc. Natl. Acad. Sci. USA*, 81, 4582, 1984.
21. **Terao, K., Ito, E., Kakinuma, Y., Igarashi, K., Kobayashi, M., Ohizumi, Y., and Yasumoto, T.,** Histopathological studies on experimental marine toxin poisoning. Pathogenesis of experimental maitotoxin poisoning, *Toxicon*, 27, 979, 1989.
22. **Bozzola, J. J., Johnson, M. C., and Schechmeister, I. L.,** *In situ* multiple sampling of attached bacteria for scanning and transmission electron microscopy, *Stain Tech.*, 48, 317, 1973.
23. **Hassan, F.,** Morphological Effects of Maitotoxin on Liver and Brain Cells of Chick Embryos, Ph.D. Thesis, Southern Illinois University, Carbondale, IL, 1989,
24. **Terao, K., Ito, E., Sakamaki, Y., Igarashi, K., Yokoyama, A., and Yasumoto, T.,** Histopathological studies of experimental marine toxin poisoning. II. The acute effects of maitotoxin on the stomach, heart and lymphoid tissues in mice and rats, *Toxicon*, 26, 395, 1988.
25. **Farber, J. L.,** The role of calcium in cell death, *Life Sci.*, 29, 1289, 1981.

Chapter 10

TOXIGENESIS IN DINOFLAGELLATES: GENETIC AND PHYSIOLOGIC FACTORS

Jeff W. Bomber

TABLE OF CONTENTS

Within the infant rind of this small flower, poison hath residence, and medicine power, For this, being smelt, with that part cheers each part, Being tasted, slays all senses with the heart — Act 11, iii, Romeo and Juliet.

I. INTRODUCTION

Of course, William Shakespeare did not have dinoflagellate "flowers" in mind when he wrote the aforementioned words for the humble friar in Romeo and Juliet. Still, Shakespeare, and both Romeo and Juliet, were keenly aware of the powerful compounds hidden within plants. Interest in bioactive plant compounds dates back to our most primitive cultures, where dried plants and crude extracts were used for medicinal purposes.

Most of the more powerful compounds derived from plants are so-called secondary metabolites, i.e., those compounds not having a direct role in photosynthesis or respiration.[1] Consequently, the evolutionary significance of these compounds is not always clear. Why has their production been conserved? Do toxins have an ancillary role in metabolism and hence are suspect to linkage disequilibrium or pleiotropy, or, are they perhaps allelochemic? The definitive answers to these questions may never be known. Regardless, mankind is fortunate that these compounds have evolved, as they also have many applications in modern medicine and industry.[2]

Dinoflagellates are phylogenetically unique. For example, the fibrillar diameter of dinoflagellate chromatin, low level of chromosomal basic proteins, membrane attachment of chromosomes, and swirl pattern observed in sections of chromosomes suggest a prokaryotic affinity. Conversely, repeated and complex DNA, an S phase of DNA synthesis in the cell cycle, the presence of basic proteins, and possible extranuclear microtubules support eukaryotic status.[3] These data and fossil evidence verify that dinoflagellates are both an old and successful group of organisms dating back to the Precambrian in the Proterozoic era, 450 million years ago. They have been a dominant group since the Silurian in the Paleozooic era.[4-6] Have toxins helped foster the evolutionary success of the dinoflagellate algae? Given that dinoflagellates produce less than 10% of all polyether compounds known, for example, the question of why such a character has been conserved is intriguing indeed. Research with dinoflagellates supports hypotheses regarding both physiologic and allelochemical roles for their toxins.[7-14] In fact, more recent findings suggest that natural selection influences both quantitative and qualitative aspects of toxigenesis.[15]

At least 30 species of dinoflagellates are known to produce bioactive compounds (Table 1),[16-48] and this list is most likely incomplete. Relatively few dinoflagellates have actually been screened for toxicity by even the most basic techniques. Sometimes the results of such screenings are surprising. For example, Tindall et al.[39] recently detected toxicity in extracts of a Florida isolate of *Prorocentrum cassubicum*, a supposedly nontoxic dinoflagellate. In this work *P. cassubicum* was found to produce a powerful, fast-acting neurotoxin that is similar in effects to saxitoxin. Consequently, toxigenesis in dinoflagellates may be less rare than previously suspected.[49] As more species are screened via modern chemical methods, a clearer picture will hopefully emerge.

This chapter is not intended to supplant recent reviews regarding the genetics[50] and physiology[51] of the dinoflagellate algae. Rather, the objective here is to provide updates in these areas and to place ecologic, genetic and physiologic studies within the context of toxigenesis. To the best of the author's knowledge this type of synthesis has not been previously accomplished. Comments are made on the evolutionary significance of toxigenesis. It is intended that this synthesis will aid other scientists working in theoretic and empiric population genetics; dinoflagellate physiology; drug development, e.g., polyether antibiotics or molecular probes;

TABLE 1
Species of Dinoflagellates that Produce Bioactive Compounds

Species	Compound[a]	Type	Ref.
Alexandrium acatenella	U	Neurotoxin	16
Alexandrium catenella	Saxitoxin	Neurotoxin	17
Alexandrium cohorticula	Saxitoxin	Neurotoxin	18
Alexandrium monilatum	U	Ichthyotoxin	19
Alexandrium tamarensis	Saxitoxin	Neurotoxin	20
Amphidinium sp. (symbiont)	Amphidinolide A	Polyether macrolide	21
Amphidinium carteri	Hemolysins 1-5	Hemolytic	22
Amphidinium klebsii	U	Ichthyotoxin	22
Amphidinium rhycochepalum	U	Ichthyotoxin	23
Coolia monotis	U	Diatom inhibitor	24
		hemolytic	25
Dinophysis fortii	Methyl okadaic acid	Polyether	26
Gambierdiscus toxicus	Maitotoxin	Polyether	27
	Ciguatoxin	Polyether	28
		Antifungal compound	29
Goniodoma pseudogoniaulax	Goniodomin A	Polyether macrolide	30
		neurotoxin	31
Gonyaulax polyhedra	U	Undefined	32
Gymnodinium catenatum	U	Neurotoxin	33
Gymnodinium sanguineum	U	Ether soluble	34
Gymnodinium veneficum		Ichthyotoxin	35
Ostreopsis heptagona[b]	U	Mouse lethality	36
Ostreopsis ovata	U	Hemolytic	21
Ostreopsis siamensis	U	Hemolytic and mouse lethality	21
Peridinium polonicum	Glenodinine	Ichthyotoxin	37
Prorocentrum balticum	U	Fish kills	38
Prorocentrum cassubicum	U	Neurotoxin	39
Prorocentrum concavum	Okadaic acid	Polyether	40
Prorocentrum lima	Okadaic acid	Polyether	41
	Prorocentrolide	Nitrogenous macrocycle	42
Prorocentrum mexicanum	U	Hemolytic	24
Prorocentrum minimum	β-diketone	Norcarotenoid	44
Prorocentrum micans	U	Pigment inhibitor	45
			46
Ptychodiscus brevis	Brevetoxins	Polyethers	47
Pyrodinium bahamense	Saxitoxins	Neurotoxin	48

[a] U — unnamed or name unknown.
[b] Toxicity was not found in subsequent work by Bomber (unpublished).

fisheries programs; and in other basic research on aspects concerning this very old, successful, and fascinating class of microalgae. Regarding the use of thecal plate taxonomy and the cell cortex in dinoflagellate evolution and systematics/genetics, there are already a number of useful papers and reviews available.[3,52-59] Consequently, such variation will also not be discussed in detail herein. The chemistry of dinoflagellate toxins has also been explored in previous reviews[37,38,60] and in other chapters of the present volume. Therefore, discussions on toxin chemistry in this review are limited to evolutionary and physiologic consequences.

II. GENETIC VARIATION

A. CLASSIC GENETICS

At least 20 species of dinoflagellates are known to reproduce sexually.[49] Sexual reproduction in dinoflagellates is typically haplontic, commonly including a thick-walled (cyst) zygotic stage. Both homothallic and heterothallic reproduction are known, but homothallism is more common.[60] Classic breeding research with dinoflagellates is a major challenge. Difficulties inherent to such studies have been discussed in several papers.[31,38,49,50,61] Problems involve difficulties in manipulating and capitalizing upon sexual reproduction. In addition, dinoflagellates are fastidious and difficult to culture with consistent results.

Despite the inherent difficulties, breeding experiments with a heterotrophic dinoflagellate, *Crypthecodinium cohnii*, have been conducted by Beam and Himes.[62-65] Beam and Himes[62] determined that of 11 morphologically similar clones and 1 dissimilar isolate of *C. cohnii*, 5 reproduced sexually, 5 were incapable of conjugating, and the affinities of 2 others were uncertain. In this work, Beam and Himes also made comparisons of DNA profiles, radiation responses, drug sensitivities, and macroalgal associations, and all of these showed significant disparities. Based upon this research and later work,[63] Beam and Himes state that *C. cohnii* appears to be a species complex composed of many reproductively isolated sibling species.

Destombe and Cembella[66] have recently completed a study of mating type determination, gametic recognition, and reproductive success in *Alexandrium excavatum*. These authors determined that the frequency of gametic recognition in *A. excavatum* may not be clearly linked to the geographic origin of the isolates. In fact, the authors suggest no clear relationship exists between the frequency of gametic recognition and the rate of zygote formation. Among clonal isolates, there was a tendency for gametic recognition incompatibility to decrease with time in culture. Destombe and Cembella write that their results imply a polar complementarity model, with active gametic recognition sites at the cell surface.

Interestingly, the work by Beam and Himes with drift algal clones collected from the Florida region[63] revealed that a profusion of singly represented sibling species exists in this area. They suggest that the clones collected from drift algae in the Florida Keys could have originated from both the Bahamas or the Caribbean, creating what could be called a *genetically diverse mixing zone*. Bomber et al.[67] also determined that drift algal populations of the ciguatera-causing dinoflagellate *Gambierdiscus toxicus* may be more genetically heterogeneous than their benthic counterparts. Beam and Himes[63] suggest that the near-global distribution of *C. cohnii* is due to its rafting on macrophytes and distributing in tides and currents. Bomber et al.[67] contend that the same phenomenon is true for *G. toxicus* and other epiphytic dinoflagellates associated with it.

Due to the accessibility and "plasticity" of drift algal populations in space and time, they may be ideal habitats within which to study evolutionary theory. For example, dinoflagellate clones collected from these habitats can be used as models to explore genetic relatedness among sibling species distributed around the entire globe. These studies could lend insight towards understanding the radiation of algal species. In addition, given the diversity of habitats within which drift algae occur, these samples may help better understand which and how selective forces shape these populations.

In fact, dinoflagellates can be ideal models for studies of population genetics, due in part to most being haploid. Consequently, changes in a clonal line due to loss of heterozygosity,[68] for example, will not occur and adversely affect experiments in hypothesis testing. On the other hand, their haploid nature makes it difficult to extrapolate results to other groups of organisms. Nevertheless, dinoflagellates remain attractive models. With dinoflagellates one can be reasonably certain that as long as the magnitude of within-clone variation is known, in the absence of recombination all second-order differences are genetic. Stochastic problems can occur,[69] such as point mutations, which could cause variation among reproduction rates. Indeed, the complex phylogeny of dinoflagellates suggest that sexual mutation and/or sexual reproduction is

TABLE 2
Nuclear DNA Contents of *Peridinium volzii* Clones as Measured by Flow Cytometry

Clone	Number of nuclei counted	Nuclear DNA content (pg)	Coefficient of variation of peak (%)
MN-1	3000	161.3	2.4
MN-2	3000	173.8	3.5
MN-3	5000	196.5	3.4
MN-4	3000	159.1	3.7
MN-5	3000	138.3	4.0
MN-6	5000	139.9	4.6
MN-7	2500	167.4	4.0
MN-8	3000	160.0	3.7
MN-9	5000	171.0, (203.3)	4.2, (4.2)
OK-75	3000	131.9	5.3
OK-76	4000	163.3	4.9
NE-1	3000	172.1	3.9

From Hayhome, B. A., et al., *J. Phycol.*, 23, 573, 1987. With permission.

frequent. However, the overall effects of mutations within a clonal line are minimal when the results from millions of individuals are averaged.[69] Thus, barring laboratory mutations that result in a major genotypic change, genotypes in continuous batch culture should be consistent. This allows a genotype to be worked with for several years with consistency. Evidence for consistency has been found for a clonal line (350) of *G. toxicus* at Southern Illinois University, within which toxicity has remained unchanged for the past 10 years.[228]

It has been suggested that ciguatera-causing dinoflagellate *Gambierdiscus toxicus* also reproduces sexually.[70] Thus, the potential exists for creating hybrids that may be useful in drug development. For example, characters of rapid growth rate and biomass may be combined with high-level polyether production. In addition, clonal crosses could help improve our understanding of the induction of toxin synthesis and heredity, as suggested by Baden and Tomas.[71] However, in terms of applied research cross-breeding work may be bypassed by simply injecting the DNA from one clone into that of another.[72] A wide variation in nuclear DNA content does occur naturally among individuals in nature (Table 2).[73] The variation in DNA content is probably due to polyploidy and/or reduction aneuploidy. Considering these factors, foreign DNA injected into the nuclei of dinoflagellates has a high probability of resulting in establishing new, heritable character combinations.

B. MOLECULAR BIOLOGY AND IMMUNOCHEMICAL TECHNIQUES

Most genetic studies with autotrophic dinoflagellates consist of characterizing clonal lines through phenotypic assays. Many of these phenotypic studies have utilized electrophoretic studies of a variety of enzymes.[74-80] Other work has examined genetic variation by determining the amino acid composition of specific enzymes.[81] The advantages and disadvantages of the electrophoresis of isozymes technique, in general, was perhaps best explored by Avise.[82] Despite certain disadvantages, these enzymatic studies have done much to aid our understanding of genetic variation in dinoflagellates.

Research with dinoflagellate enzymes has resulted in establishing that three basic phenomena occur. First, dinoflagellates reproduce sexually and recombine frequently and/or are highly mutagenic, as stated earlier. This is evidenced by the work of Schmidt and Loeblich,[82] who found nearly every possible combination of the character traits examined in *Alexandrium* (=*Protogo-*

nyaulax) tamarensis and *A. excavata* (bioluminescence, toxicity, and the presence of a ventral pore). Consider also that Whitten and Hayhome[78] discovered that of 82 electrophoretic bands found in two dinoflagellates, only 28 were common to both species. However, it should be pointed out that the two species used in that study are binucleate.

Carrying variation one step further, some species may be more mutagenic than others. For example, Sako et al.[79] determined that *A. catenella* appeared to exhibit much more electrophoretic variation than both *Gymnodinium nagasakiense* and *Peridinium bipes*. The third phenomenon found is that populations within a site exhibit more homologous banding patterns than when compared to those from other geographic areas (see, for example, Hayhome et al.[73,74]).

Studies of dinoflagellate enzymes will most likely be replaced rapidly by work elucidating polymorphism in restriction enzyme fragments of dinoflagellate DNA. This is true for a wide range of organisms being used as models in studies of population genetics.[84] It will be interesting to see what new answers are generated to old questions by the use of this relatively new technique. However, all methods short of breeding experiments are still subject to speculation when defining a "biologic" species. For example, isozyme work, studies of thecal plate morphology, and other work indicated that sufficient genetic variation existed within the *A. catenella/tamarense* complex to warrant the designation of two different species.[85,86] However, Sako and colleagues[87] have recently been able to cross these two "species" and obtain a zygote. Consequently, these "species" are then possibly only varieties.

A review of the literature on dinoflagellate nuclei and chromosomes was compiled by Spector.[88] Basically, studies of DNA and restriction fragment polymorphisms in dinoflagellates are in their infancy. DNA contents have been compared among dinoflagellate genera.[3] On a finer scale, flow cytometry and a DNA stain have been used to examine G_1 and G_2 phase subpopulations in *Alexandrium tamarense*.[89] Other work has included quantitative comparisons of DNA content between clones as well (Table 2).[73,76] The study by Hayhome et al.[73] is one of the most comprehensive on the clonal level, and they were able to obtain data from a large number of replicates by using flow cytometry. Cembella and Taylor[76] also reported subclone variation in DNA content among *Alexandrium* isolates. Two isolates, 253 and 508, had about half the DNA content of all other isolates examined. Cembella and Taylor[76] suggested that their data indicate that isolates 253 and 508 may form the base of a ploidy series resulting from reduction aneuploidy.

Steele and Rae[90] determined that patterns of restriction endonuclease cleavage of ribosomal RNA in isolates of *Crypthecodinium cohnii* exactly paralleled their sexual compatibilities. This work represents the ideal balance in a study of *ecologic genetics*. The authors have combined both molecular and breeding studies and point out that neither can really stand alone. For example, breeding experiments help us define a species, but tell us nothing about genetic variation occurring at the subspecies level.

Immunochemical techniques offer still another way of examining genetic variation in dinoflagellates. Although immunofluorescent techniques have been used with algae as early as 1977,[91] this work has largely been restricted to the cyanobacteria, ("blue-green algae"). More recently, fluorescent antibodies have been used with natural populations of chroococcoid cyanobacteria. Campbell et al.[92] directed antisera against five strains and tested for cross-reactions. The antisera were relatively specific between strains isolated from similar oceanic environments. The antisera enabled Campbell et al.[89] to determine that different pigment types of *Synechococcus* dominated specific seasons.

Progress in immunofluorescent research with dinoflagellate systematics has lagged behind the level of sophistication achieved by bacterial microbiologists. For example, consider the intricacy of one bacterial study,[93] where the enzyme malate dehydrogenase was purified from *Rhodobacter capsulatus* and antibodies were raised against the enzyme. The amount of cross-reactivity between malate dehydrogenases from different strains and with other species (*R. sphaeroides*) was then quantified via an enzyme-linked immunoabsorbant assay (ELISA) test.

Nevertheless, immunofluorescent studies with dinoflagellates are underway. Sako et al.[87] have tested for cross-reactivity among *Alexandrium* varieties with a polyclonal antibody raised against whole cell antigens. The relative degree of antibody binding in this study roughly correlated with genetic distance determined by corollary electrophoretic work. Campbell et al.[94] have used a monoclonal antibody raised against polyethers to explore fish gut contents for the compounds. In doing so, Campbell et al.[94] turned up preliminary evidence suggesting cell wall localization of toxins in *Gambierdiscus toxicus*. In addition, a similar method was used to study toxigenesis in *Alexandrium*,[8] where toxin localization at the nucleus was found. Baden et al.[95,96] have raised antibodies to brevetoxins; perhaps this and other probes will find their way into future systematic and physiologic studies with toxic dinoflagellates.

Ideally, immunofluorescent studies will be coupled with flow cytometry,[97,98] which will enable the analysis of thousands of single-cell replicates of different clones. Without flow cytometry or a similar fluorescence-based means of numerically quantifying fluorescent antibody binding, we will only be able to report relative fluorescence based on a visual analysis (e.g., +, ++, +++, etc.). Statistical tools used in population genetics demand a more substantial data base.

Most studies of the population genetics of dinoflagellates have used relatively few clones, usually less than 30.[12,15,70,75,77,79] This is largely due to their fastidious nature. Consider, for example, a pioneering study of the population genetics of the diatom *Skeletonema costatum*, where Gallagher[99] examined 457 clones from two distinct populations by electrophoresis. Regardless of the molecular method of analysis used in assessing variation, the number of clones of dinoflagellates utilized will need to increase in the future. Wood[100] points out that much of the genetic variation encountered in phytoplankton populations is expressed as ecologically important characters. Therefore, it seems likely that microevolutionary processes, that is, changes in gene frequencies within populations, are an important part of the adaptive strategy of many microalgal species. The key word here is *frequency*, and in accord with Wood, we must shift from looking at means to looking at variances. Using small numbers of clones makes it difficult to obtain a realistic estimate of frequencies and the variation within and among populations.

C. OTHER METHODS IN QUANTITATIVE GENETICS

A number of studies have explored character variation among populations of microalgae isolated from different environments. These studies have explored differences in the uptake rates of silica[101] and phosphate,[102] differences in temperature and salinity tolerance,[103] and variation in trace metal tolerance,[104,105] and nutrient uptake rates.[106] The use of quantitative characters in genetic studies of crop plants and domesticated animals is well established.[107,108] However, not until recently have quantitative characters been used to assess genetic heterogeneity in microalgal populations using statistical analyses.

Brand,[109] Brand et al.,[110,111] Bomber,[9] and Bomber et al.[15,112] have utilized total fitness (reproduction rates) and analysis of variance techniques in studies of the quantitative genetics of dinoflagellates and other algae. Measurements of total fitness are easily obtained for most algae and bacteria but are difficult, if not impossible, to achieve with most other organisms.[113] The monitoring and subsequent achievement of acclimated reproduction rates (total fitness) enables one to filter out microenvironmental and developmental sources of noise in it and most other characters of interest. Consequently, the subsequent differences detected should represent true genetic differences. These factors argue even more convincingly for the use of algae as models for studying evolutionary processes.

Wood et al.[114] also used reproduction rate as an indicator of acclimation in their award-winning paper on the quantitative genetics of *Thalassiosira tumida*. In this work, differences in valve morphology were only analyzed for genetic variation after the acclimation process was completed. The importance of complete acclimation cannot be overemphasized. For example,

TABLE 3
Pre- and Postacclimation Potency Differences Among Six Clones of *Gambierdiscus toxicus*

Clone	Source	Potencies (MU/mg dried cells)	
		Preacclimation	Postacclimation
175(MQ-1)	Martinique, Caribbean	55.06	102.25
350	Virgin Gorda, Caribbean	3.84	18.33
177(T-39)	Hawaii	5.40	26.90
199	Knight Key, Florida	4.22	17.48
169	Drift Algae, Gulf Stream	4.09	4.40
163	Gingerbreads, Bahamas	4.52	8.84
Total		77.13	178.20

Note: The data presented below is related to previous work,[15] but has not previously been presented in this format.

Bomber et al.[15] determined that significant genetic differences in total potencies exist among 17 clones of *Gambierdiscus toxicus.* The potencies of these clones were assayed only after the clones had been completely acclimated to their environment (according to their reproduction rates). In this work, pre- and postacclimation potency differences within a clone were as large as the genetic differences between clones (Table 3). Had these clones not been completely acclimated, the authors' conclusions on the potencies of these clones may have been much different.

The total fitness of microalgal clones can lend insight into the nature of the selective forces shaping their populations. Models of natural selection based upon an adaptive topography for phenotypes have been developed by Lande,[115,116] based in part upon work by Wright.[117] With such models it is possible to show that for most phenotypic characters under natural selection, the evolution of the average phenotype in a population is usually towards an adaptive zone of high mean fitness. Lande states further that if significant treatment effects are found, this implies that natural selection was involved in producing genetic divergence. Consequently, measuring carefully selected characters in the laboratory may enable the assessment of relative fitness among genotypes and help determine which selective forces fostered genetic divergence.

Brand et al.[111] have conducted the type of study indicated above. In this work they were able to determine that populations of *Thalassiosira* were either r or k selected (sensu Pianka,[118] and MacArthur and Wilson[119]), as opposed to being adapted to specific light regimes. They based this determination on the absence of "crossing-over" of linear light intensity vs. reproduction rate plots. The term *crossing-over* in this regard is not directly related to recombination. Similar studies were conducted by Bomber et al.[15] with *Gambierdiscus toxicus* clones (Figure 1). In the case of *G. toxicus*, the slopes overlapped, indicating that the clones examined may be adapted to specific light regimes. The clones of *G. toxicus* utilized showed that significant variation (determined by analysis of variance, ANOVA) existed in reproduction rates at all four light intensities used. A significant clone or genotype x light interaction term was also detected in the ANOVA. The interaction further reinforces the role of natural selection in establishing these characters.

In the study by Brand et al.,[111] the clones examined were derived from similar latitudes and the lack of light adaptation could have been predicted. However, in the case of *G. toxicus*, clones were collected from between 14.50°N and 32.20°N. Over this large a geographic range the average annual light intensity varies tremendously, with more light present on average in lower latitudes. Consequently, low-latitude clones should be able to grow better in high light. In fact,

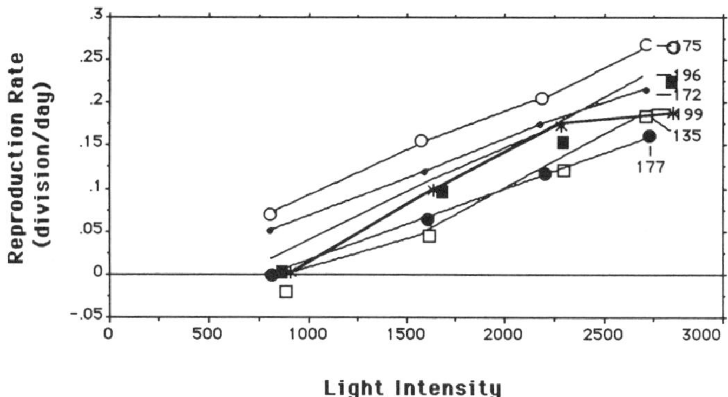

FIGURE 1. Reproduction rates at four light intensities for five clones of *Gambierdiscus toxicus*. (From Bomber et al., *J. Phycol.*, 25, 617, 1989. With permission.)

Figure 1 indicates this; note that the clone collected from the lowest latitude (175) also has the fastest reproduction rate in high light.

Some studies of the population genetics of microalgae have looked at variation among clones in other primary and secondary metabolites, including sterols[120,121] and pigments.[122] Monitoring differences in these molecular components via flow cytometry can easily be combined with analyzing differences in optical properties (light scatter) of dinoflagellate cells. Optical properties have been used to differentiate both intra- and interspecific single-cell variability.[97]

In thesis work conducted by Beseda,[120] two clones of *Coolia monotis* were compared for their percent composition of sterols. The two clones were similar and were composed of 67% vs. 64% cholesterol and 33% vs. 36% dinosterols. It would be interesting to see additional work done with more clones. However, sterols are effective species descriptors, using even a small number of clones. In the same study, Beseda determined that *Gambierdiscus toxicus* contained only 47% cholesterol and 20% dinosterol. Further, the sterols of *G. toxicus* were composed of 33% 24-methylcholesterol, which was not present in *C. monotis* or another species examined, *Ostreopsis ovata*. In addition, Withers[123] points out that sterols are phylogenetically useful and help place dinoflagellates at the base of eukaryotic lineage; that is, although they share certain sterols with prokaryotes, they have their own unique C_{30} sterols that are not found in prokaryotes or other eukaryotes. Withers also points out that another terpenoid class of dinoflagellate components, carotenoids, are also useful in this context. For example, consider that the C_{40} carotenoid peridinin is found only in the Dinophyceae.

In one pigment study, clonal lines of marine diatoms were shown to exhibit differences in cellular pigment content, even when grown in the same environment.[99] It is possible that this disparity may arise from genetic divergence into races that were selected based upon their indigenous light regimes. Bomber et al.[112] explored the pigment composition and low-light response of 14 clones of the ciguatera-causing dinoflagellate *Gambierdiscus toxicus*. In this study, 14 clones of *G. toxicus* were acclimated for 1 year in 500 ml and 1-l flasks in K medium[124] at 28°C and 1800 lux (Vitalite bulbs). The cultures were subsequently shifted to 900 lux and acclimated for up to 200 additional days. The authors found that *G. toxicus* required an unusually long acclimation period of up to 1 year for some isolates, although others acclimated within 16 weeks. This supports an earlier hypothesis set forth by Bomber et al.[125] that *G. toxicus* is accustomed to a relatively stable physicochemical environment and is not very adaptive to changes in these parameters.

Although the clones of *G. toxicus* examined by Bomber et al.[112] produced slightly more pigment at the lower light intensity, it is difficult to generalize. First, these authors did not

TABLE 4
A Comparison Between Low- and High-Latitude Clones of *Gambierdiscus toxicus*

Character	< 21°N	> 21°N
Chlorophyll *a* (pg/cell)	381.00 ± 136.00	662.00 ± 83.00
Chlorophyll c_2 (pg/cell)	122.00 ± 48.00	238.00 ± 67.00
Peridinin (pg/cell)	101.00 ± 28.00	228.00 ± 48.00
Reproduction rate (1800 lux)	0.19 ± 00.03	0.13 ± 00.02
Cell size (1800 lux, transdiameter)	71.60 ± 06.40	82.80 ± 02.50
Potency (1800 lux, mouse units per cell)	36.30 ± 00.16	10.00 ± 06.00

Note: Pigments are in picograms per cell and represent the mean from both light intensities (n = 8).

The potency data is from Bomber et al., *J. Phycol.*, 25, 617, 1989; all other data are from Bomber et al., in *Toxic Phytoplankton Blooms*, Elsevier, New York. With permission.

monitor changes in cell size between the different light intensities, and such changes could have affected the results. Secondly, significant "scatter" in pigment response was detected by a principal components analysis (Statview 512, BrainPower, Inc.). Two factors were extracted from the coded (observation — mean/standard deviation) data. The scatter indicated that a light × clone interaction exists, and again suggests that clonal lines of *G. toxicus* are adapted to specific light regimes. The clonal scatter was explained in part by the differences found between low- and high-latitude clones. The low-latitude clones 175, 177, and 350 had difficulty acclimating to low light and died during postacclimation transfers. These clones also had significantly different and lower pigment content than the high latitude clones (Table 4). A paired t test[126] comparison indicated that these groups have significantly different pigment concentration, even when the data are normalized to account for differences in cell size among clones (chlorophyll *a*, ts = 3.957; chlorophyll c_2 ts = 2.709, where $t.05_{[27]} = 2.052$).

In summary, work with quantitative characters also suggests that populations of dinoflagellates are composed of genetically distinct races. In some cases the data are consistent with the environments from which the clones were isolated. In the pigment study conducted by Bomber et al.,[109] the low-latitude clones would experience higher light intensities than the high-latitude clones due to their proximity to the equator. Thus, the low-latitude clones would require less pigment. Their lower pigment content was in fact observed in that study. In addition, mean cell size and potencies were also significantly different between the groups (Table 4).

D. TOXICOLOGY IN DINOFLAGELLATE SYSTEMATICS AND POPULATION GENETICS

1. Bacteria or Dinoflagellates?

The use of any biochemical as a genetic marker depends on its heritability as a trait linked to the genome of the organism under investigation. *De-novo* synthesis of dinoflagellate toxins cannot be assumed and is a matter of current debate (see also the review by Steidinger and Baden).[38] It has been suggested that "dinoflagellate" saxitoxin may in fact originate from a bacterial source.[127] It has also been suggested that toxin production may be linked to viral recombinant RNA.[38] Heritability of a trait is easy enough to test for, as there are adequate formulae worked out that can express the contribution of a trait as a numeric index.[107] However, these formulae were derived expressly for diploid organisms, and their extension to use with haploid organisms from primarily asexually producing populations is not necessarily valid or practical. Nevertheless, statistical tools (analysis of variance) can be used to estimate nongenetic contributions to total toxicity.[15] However, although these numeric techniques address problems of developmental and environmental "noise", they still cannot differentiate toxin production between an endosymbiont and its dinoflagellate host.

Determining the source of a toxin may at first seem an easy task; however, few topics have stimulated as much controversy among dinoflagellate researchers as the existence of *de-novo* synthesis of toxins, especially saxitoxin.[127] How does one go about solving this problem? Evaluating toxin production in bacteria present in dinoflagellate cultures would seem to be the first approach.[128] However, what if the data are negative? Does this mean that the bacteria do not synthesize the toxin or, conversely, perhaps they depend upon the stimuli of an associated alga? Or, as we have learned from Kodama et al.[127] (and personal communication), does a negative mean that the proper environment for toxigenesis has not yet been provided?

Axenic dinoflagellate cultures could be established and assessed for toxin production. However, if positive, the possibility of endosymbiotic bacterial production still exists. A so-called axenic culture defined by lack of bacterial growth from innocula from culture media or even algal extracts does not exclude the presence of endosymbionts. Thus, we are left looking for other biochemical or morphologic indicators. Sousa E Silva[129] was able to identify bacterial symbionts in samples of *Gymnodinium splendens* and *Glenodinium foliaceum* using transmission electron microscopy (TEM). Such an approach is valid, but again, what do negative data mean? Have a sufficient number of cells been sectioned? Has a given cell been examined from apex to antapex? Finally, the results of TEM are always subject to artifactual effects. Even if found, can the endosymbiont be isolated, cultured, and assayed? Perhaps fatty acid signatures may be the best way to determine the presence of bacterial symbionts. However, all techniques are subject to scrutiny, and it appears that this problem will remain with us for several years. Consequently, the present discussion, in fact most reports of dinoflagellate toxigenesis, should be considered in light of these limitations.

Most of the evidence accumulated to date tends to support *de-novo* synthesis. Carlson et al.[130] have demonstrated that axenic cultures of *Prorocentrum concavum* are toxic. Bomber et al.[15] demonstrated that axenic cultures of *Gambierdiscus toxicus* were capable of synthesizing the putative polyether maitotoxin. In this work crude extracts obtained from bacteria cultured from xenic (bacteria present) cultures of *G. toxicus* failed to kill mice at doses beyond 1 mg. Extracts from the bacterial source clone of *G. toxicus* (175) have killed mice at <2 μg. In addition, Bomber et al.[15] determined that reproductive rate and maitotoxin production (or total potency) are integrally linked (Figure 2). This suggests that pleiotropy or linkage disequilibrium exists within the dinoflagellate genome for other genes related to total fitness (reproduction rate) and maitotoxin synthesis. In addition, toxic clones of *G. toxicus* have been examined by TEM and no endosymbiotic bacteria were found.[128] Positive linkage between reproduction rate and toxigenesis has also been encountered for *Alexandrium* spp. and saxitoxin production under some circumstances.[13] However, another study has reported that the relationship between the inherent reproduction rate of a clone and toxin production presents no clear relationship.[12]

There is evidence to suggest, however, that toxigenesis is dependent on the bacterial composition of dinoflagellate cultures. Tosteson et al.[128,132] point out that inter- and intraspecific interactions of marine microbial cells and frequently mediated by macromolecular surface components. This, they assert, suggests the presence of specific receptor-ligand binding sites. Consequently, it follows that the stimuli of increasing numbers of associated bacteria would cause dinoflagellates to produce antibiotics, possibly polyethers. Tosteson et al.[132] have found toxicity in one bacterial strain, but only on one occasion. What was interesting about these studies, however, is that the only toxic isolate of *Gambierdiscus toxicus* encountered and the most toxic clone of *Ostreopsis lenticularis* shared the same *Pseudomonas* bacteria. *Pseudomonas* could not be detected in cultures of the nontoxic clones of *G. toxicus*.[128] Perhaps more

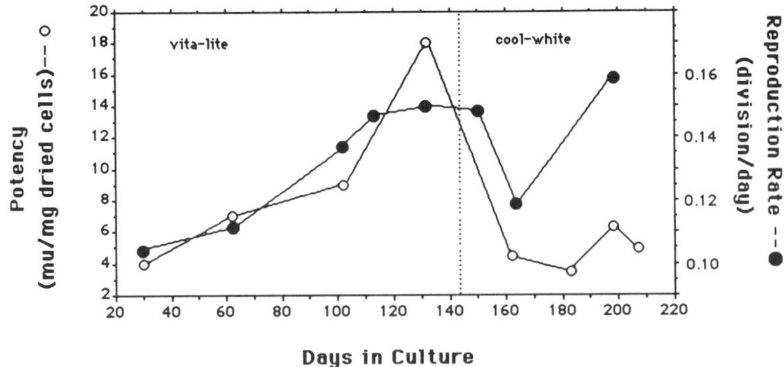

FIGURE 2. Potency (mu/mg dried cells) vs. number of days in culture for *G. toxicus* clone 350 (Caribbean). The first four potencies were determined under Vitalite bulbs and the last four under cool-white bulbs. (From Bomber et al., *J. Phycol.*, 25, 216, 1989. With permission.)

experimentation of this type can be conducted that will assay the effects of an array of dinoflagellate/bacterial combinations on toxin production, followed with the appropriate statistical tests.

It is surprising that the question of *de novo* synthesis of polyether compounds in dinoflagellates has not been as controversial as it has for saxitoxin production. This is because by far the greatest number of polyethers have been isolated from several species of soil-dwelling Actinomycetalean bacteria. *Streptomyces* spp. are most frequently found to produce the antibiotics,[130] whereas bacterial or bacterial production of saxitoxin has only been observed in isolated cases.[127,134]

In bacteria the polyethers often occur as a complex of closely related compounds, e.g., salinomycin is a major component of a nine-member complex in *S. albus*.[133,135] The homologs are typically present in small amounts. The same type of phenomenon is now being observed for dinoflagellate polyethers.[136] Polyether production is not present in the so-called higher dinoflagellates.[56] In addition, the molecular delineation between bacterial and dinoflagellate polyethers is not always clear. Consequently, this provides a good molecular argument for those who are convinced that bacterial exo- or endosymbionts actually produce the "dinoflagellate" polyethers. The rarity of polyether production in eukaryotes in general supports this argument.

However, there are some distinctions between the molecules in the bacterial vs. dinoflagellate polyethers. First, the most potent bacterial polyethers are A204, which has an LD_{50} of 8 mg/kg (po) and X-206, which has a potency of LD_{50} = 1 mg/kg (ip) and 17 mg/kg (po) (all values in mice).[85] Compare these to the potency in mice of the dinotoxins okadaic acid, LD_{50} = 0.2 mg/kg,[69,85] or maitotoxin, LD_{50} = 0.13 μg/kg.[89] To the best of the author's knowledge there no bacterial polyethers with more than seven fused rings. The dinoflagellate polyether from *Ptychodiscus breve*, brevetoxin B, has 11 fused heterocycles.[47] This suggests that dinoflagellates are capable of producing their own distinctive and more complex class of polyethers. In addition, most dinoflagellate polyethers have a molecular weight (mol wt) exceeding 1000 and most bacterial polyethers are below 800 mol wt. However, there are exceptions; for example, the bacterial polyether K-41B has a mol wt of 1083.3.[77]

A typical bacterial polyether is alborixin,[137] and this is shown with okadaic acid[138] and brevetoxin B[47] (Figure 3). Let us assume that polyether complexity is positively correlated with the phylogeny of the progenitor. If so, the molecular structures shown in Figure 3 may reflect phylogeny. Okadaic acid is produced by the more "primitive" dinoflagellates *Prorocentrum* and *Dinophysis*.[56] Therefore, based on our model we would expect their polyethers to be simpler than those produced by dinoflagellates that are further up the evolutionary ladder, e.g., brevetoxin

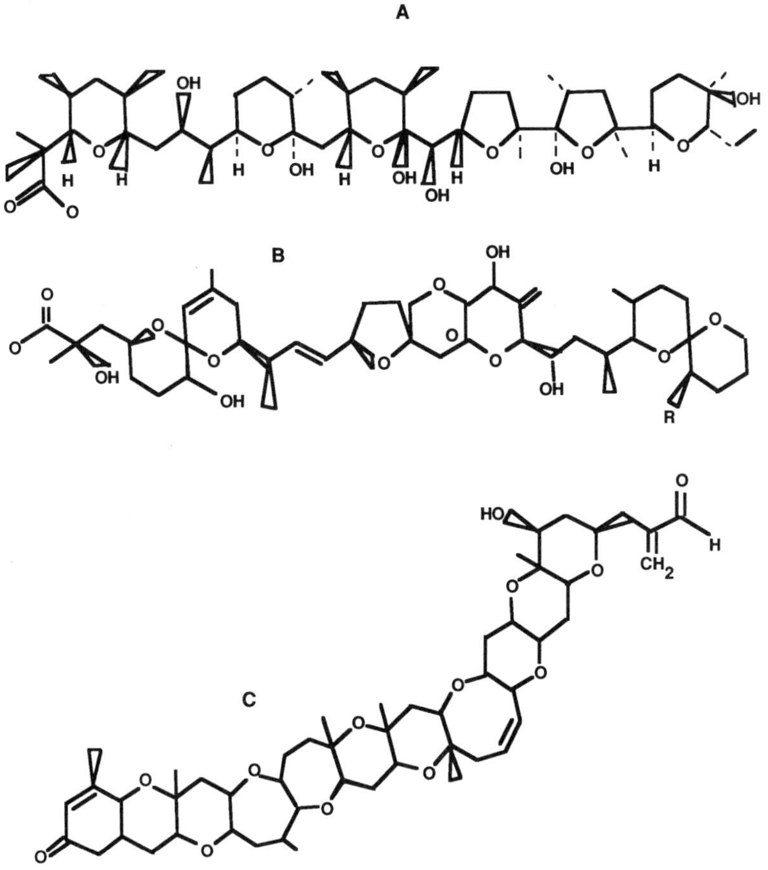

A

B

C

FIGURE 3. Molecular structures of (A) alborixin,[137] (B) okadaic acid,[138] and (C) brevetoxin.[47] (From Seto et al., *J. Antibiot.*, 32, 970, 1979; Tachibana et al., *J. Am. Chem. Soc.*, 103, 2469, 1981; and Lin et al., *J. Am. Chem. Soc.*, 103, 6773, 1981. With permission.)

and *Ptychodiscus brevis*. Ciguatoxin is now known to resemble brevetoxin and to originate in *Gambierdiscus toxicus*,[27] which is also more advanced than *Prorocentrum* spp. Of course, this model may dissolve if one considers that the most complex nonproteinaceous toxin known, palytoxin, may arise by a bacterium associated with the marine coelenterate *Palythoa*.[139] Then again, it has not yet been proved that palytoxin is not produced by *Palythoa*'s dinoflagellate endosymbiont.

2. Polyethers, Their Effects and Roles in Disease

The polyether class of antibiotics is a fascinating group of compounds, only three chemical structures of which were known in 1950.[140] However, since then research on these compounds has advanced rapidly, and over 100 new structures have since been elucidated. Polyethers are interesting because of their coccidiostat activity, their ability to improve food conversion in ruminant animals,[140] their role in human diseases,[41,141] and their usefulness as molecular probes.[142,143] For example, lasalocid and bromolasalocid (A23187) are widely used as probes in studies of Ca^{2+} transport in animal systems.[140] Polyethers are also used in studying the H^+-pumping ATPase in plant membrane vesicles; nigericin was used by Sze[144] to stimulate ATPase activity in microsomal vesicles of tobacco callus.

Estrada-O et al.[145] proposed that polyether antibiotics owe their biologic activity to interaction with alkali metal cations and their carrier mechanisms, which regulate the transport of K^+ across membranes. These molecules can assume a cyclic form, which concentrates their oxygen functions at the center of the structure, where they can complex a suitable cation.[146] Concurrently, the many-branched alkyl groups of these molecules are thrust outward over the surface and render the complex lipid soluble. Consequently, cations can be conducted across membranes by the so-called passive diffusion process.[147-149]

Polyether interactions with membranes and cations are thought to explain the antibiotic effects of these molecules. They are effective against gram-positive bacteria and a number of anaerobic bacteria,[130] fungi,[150] and viruses.[151] Harold and Baarda[152] showed that, like other classes of ionophorous antibiotics (valinomycin, gramicidin, and monactin), nigericin acts in *Streptococcus faecalis* by interacting with the cytoplasmic membrane and causing leakage of K^+. Harned et al.[153] reported that the inhibitory effects of the polyether nigericin against *Bacillus subtilus* could be reversed by the addition of excess K^+ to the medium. Considering that K^+ is critical for protein synthesis in bacteria,[156] this model would be sufficient to explain inhibition. This type of transport can also cause rapid acidification of the cytoplasm (pH 6.0 down to 3.5).

Relatively little is known about the molecular mechanisms by which polyethers cause human illnesses. Okadaic acid is involved in causing both diarrhetic shellfish poisoning[141] and ciguatera.[24,34,39,40] Diarrhetic shellfish poisoning (DSP) is a global health risk that is typically associated with blooms of *Dinophysis* spp. and the methyl-okadaic acid that these species produce.[141] In DSP, human gastrointestinal illnesses arise from consuming bivalves that have fed upon the toxigenic dinoflagellates.

Ciguatera is a debilitating, sometimes fatal human illness caused by consuming fish, typically reef dwellers, from the circumtropics. Both the symptoms and etiology of ciguatera are complex (see other chapters in this volume). Presently, most researchers agree that the observed multiplicity of the symptoms of this disease are due to several polyethers present in the fish.[21] Neurologic symptoms include dysesthesia, parasthesia, and arthralgia, sometimes leading to convulsions, paralysis and respiratory failure.[155] These indications suggest the role of powerful polyether neurotoxins, putatively attributed to ciguatoxin[156] and maitotoxin.[26] Elaboration of both of these toxins has been ascribed to the dinoflagellate alga, *Gambierdiscus toxicus,*[26,157] but its production of ciguatoxin is debated.[27,158]

There are also gastrointestinal symptoms associated with ciguatera, and these include nausea, vomiting, and diarrhea.[155] Consequently, other epiphytic dinoflagellates, *Prorocentrum lima* and *Prorocentrum concavum*, are thought to be involved in causing ciguatera because they produce the gastrointestinal toxin okadaic acid[40,41] and occur in close association with *G. toxicus in situ.*[159] Treatment of all ciguatera symptoms is presently symptomatic, but progress has been made in raising antibodies to ciguatera toxins.[160,161] However, the disease continues to have a profound negative impact on fisheries development worldwide.[155]

3. Exploring the Evolutionary Significance of Toxigenesis: Allelochemicals?

It is unfortunate that dinoflagellate polyethers effect humans, but it is unlikely that the synthesis of polyethers and other toxins evolved as a means of harming mammals. The bacterial literature discussed previously suggests that polyethers in dinoflagellates may serve as allelochemic[162] agents directed against closely competing or pathogenic organisms. Additionally, algal bioactive secondary metabolites may inhibit grazers,[30,163] which thereby help the progenitor sustain a bloom.[164] Dickey et al.[40] determined that okadaic acid extracted from *Prorocentrum concavum* inhibited the growth of *Candida albicans*. Trick et al.[165] bioassayed the effects of 1-(2,6,6-trimethyl-4-hydroxycyclohexenyl)-1,3-butanedione[166] (ß-diketone), an extracellular norcarotenoid of *Prorocentrum minimum*. The authors determined that ß-diketone had an inhibitory effect on the bacteria *Vibrio* sp. and *Flavobacter* sp. In addition, ß-diketone inhibited the growth of *Chromobacterium* sp. (Figure 4) that was isolated from cultures of *Scrippsiella sweeneyi*.

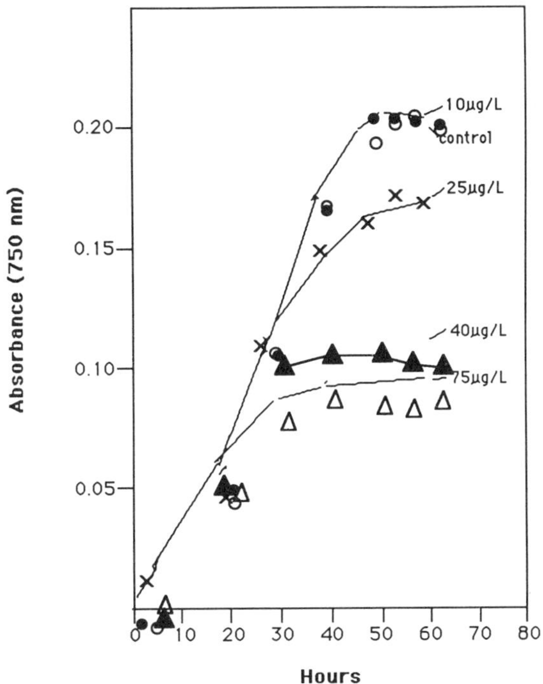

FIGURE 4. Influence of the addition of the ß-diketone on growth of *Chromobacterium* sp. Growth was measured by changes in absorbance at 750 nm. Cells were grown at room temperature in ISOL medium with varying concentrations of the ß-diketone. (Redrawn from Trick et al., *Can. J. Fish. Aquat. Sci.*, 41, 423, 1987. With permission.)

Freeberg et al.[7] assayed 28 species of phytoplankton in media preconditioned with *Ptychodiscus brevis*, the source of brevetoxins. The sensitivity of phytoplankton to these media appeared to be species specific and varied within a species. However, some dramatic effects were observed, including lysis of two dinoflagellate species when inoculated into the conditioned medium.

Carlson,[167] in bialgal and cross-cultures in dinoflagellate-conditioned media, determined that *Prorocentrum concavum* and *Gambierdiscus toxicus* were reciprocally inhibited. However, *Prorocentrum* spp. were mutually stimulated. Carlson suggested that the data revealing inhibition may indicate the presence of ectocrines. These ectocrines, he suggests, may enable the dinoflagellates to compete more effectively with other algae. It has been argued convincingly that two species with similar ecology cannot live together in the same place, the so-called competitive exclusion principle.[168] This principle may be particularly applicable to the epiphytic community, where space is a severely limiting factor, and Carlson's suggestion is highly reasonable. Alternatively, epiphytic algal species may simply occupy different temporal niches. An apparent seasonal niche specialization in population abundance has been detected between three closely competing "ciguatera species", *Gambierdiscus toxicus*, *Ostreopsis heptagona*, and *O. siamensis*.[9]

Preliminary studies using crude and semipurified extracts of *Gambierdiscus toxicus* also support the allelochemical hypothesis. Durand et al.[10] found that ciguatoxinlike extracts of *G. toxicus* inhibited the growth of the diatoms *Chaetoceros affinis* and *C. cantrans* and the chlorophytes *Dunaliella bioculata* (Figure 5) and *D. tertiolecta*. However, some algae were either unaffected or even stimulated by the extracts.

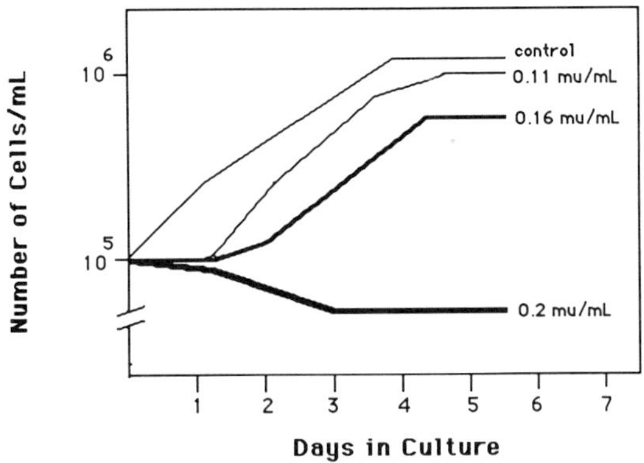

FIGURE 5. Ciguatoxin-like toxicity effects on *Dunaliella bioculata*. (Reproduced from Durand et al., *Proc. Fifth Intl. Coral Reef Cong*., Tahiti, 4, 483, 1985. With permission.)

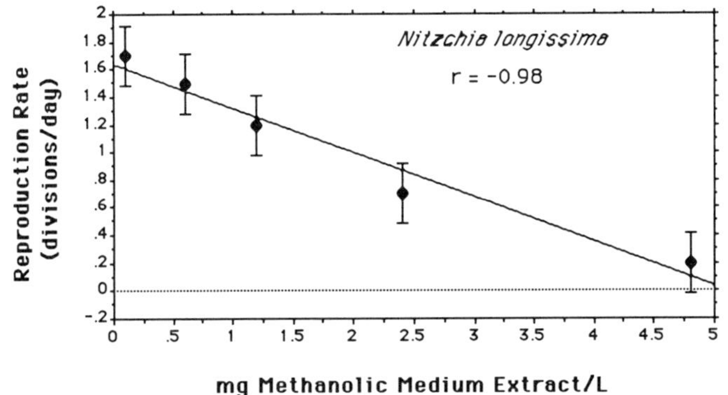

FIGURE 6. Growth rate of *Nitzchia longissima* in division/day vs. concentration of the aqueous fraction of the organic compounds extracted from spent *G. toxicus* medium. The means are for four replicates and the bars are 95% comparison intervals generated by the *T* method. The cultures were grown with Vitalite fluorescent tubes. The control is shown as the upper growth rate.

Work by Bomber[9] and Bomber et al.[169] supports the work of Carlson[164] and Durand et al.[10] In Bomber,[9] *G. toxicus* was shown to exude up to 2.6 mg/l of organic matter in axenic culture. The organics were extracted from the medium using XAD-2 (Mallinkrodt) resin. The organic extract was then eluted from the XAD-2 column with methanol and the eluate was assayed on two diatom species, *Nitzchia longissima* and *Amphora costatum*. Both of these diatoms occur with *G. toxicus in situ*. When added to a culture of *N. longissima* at 2.6 mg/l, the medium extract inhibited the diatom's growth rate 60% below the control (Figure 6). The same extract had inhibitory but reversible effects in a guinea-pig ileum assay,[170] and it was also toxic to mice. The water phase of an ether:water separation from the crude cell extract of the same axenic cultures of *G. toxicus* also had dramatic effects on the growth of the diatoms. Figure 7 shows the effects of this water-soluble cell extract on *A. costata*. *A costata* was also inhibited by the cell extract when it was supplied to cells grown on 2% agar.

Later experiments by Bomber and Tindall[229] show that the diatom inhibitor produced by *G. toxicus* could be maitotoxin. Crude extracts from *G. toxicus* were purified by a silicic acid column and thin-layer chromatography, and assayed with mice and *N. longissima*. The effects

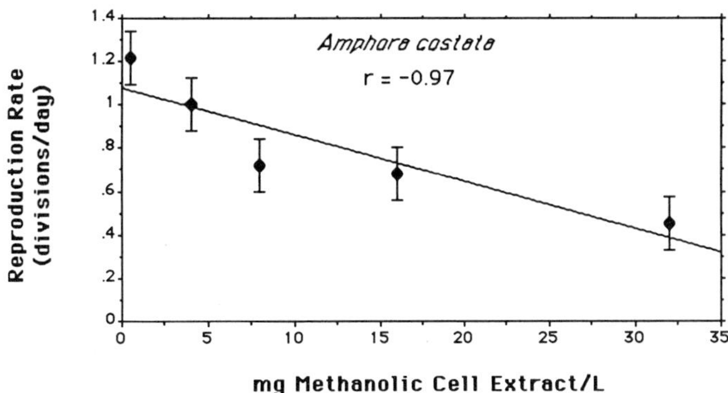

FIGURE 7. Growth rate of *Amphora costata* in division/day vs. concentration of the aqueous fraction (ether/water) of the organic compounds extracted from *G. toxicus* cells. The means are for four replicate and the bars are 95% comparison intervals generated by the *T* method. The cultures were grown with Vitalite fluorescent tubes. The control is shown as the upper growth rate.

TABLE 5
Effects of Semipurified Fractions of *Gambierdiocus toxicus* Extract on Yield of *Nitzchia longissima*

Band #	Identity (mg dry weight/ml)	Mean final yield
1	ß-carotene	0.36
2	Lipids	0.60
3	Chlorophyll *a*	0.64
4	Xanthophylls	0.62
5	Peridinin	0.67
6	Chlorophyll *c*'s	0.35
7	Chlorophyll *c*'s + toxin	0.08
Control	f/2 only	0.20

Note: All fractions were added to f/2 medium at 20 µg/ml and grown in duplicate.

of all eluates on *N. longissima* are shown in Table 5. The only eluate that killed mice or inhibited *N. longissima* was the green (chlorophyll c_2) maitotoxin-containing fraction. One has to wonder, however, if lysis of *G. toxicus* in nature would sometimes provide more beneficial results to diatoms than negative ones. Note that in Table 5 all but one eluate actually stimulated diatom growth. However, in all experiments conducted to date in the author's laboratory, crude extracts have always been inhibitory. Hopefully, research with purer toxins can be conducted to test the allelochemical hypotheses further. In the meantime, a physiologic role for the toxins should not be ruled out (see Physiology).

4. Variation in Toxigenesis

Research with genetic variation in genesis of sulfocarbamoyl, carbamate, and decarbamoyl toxins (e.g., saxitoxins and gonyautoxins) in *Alexandrium* spp. has progressed further than the work with toxigenesis of the ciguatera toxins. This is primarily because a concerted effort on elucidating the structure of saxitoxin began more than 20 years before the polyether work. *Gambierdiscus toxicus* was not known to be toxic until about 1977,[171] whereas Schantz et al.[172]

published on the isolation and purification of saxitoxin in 1957. Likewise, research on toxins from *Ptychodiscus breve* has progressed further due to the time factor.[96,173] The aforementioned research and several other studies have provided many exciting discoveries. These discoveries include that the content and composition of toxins can vary tremendously among clonal lines of *Alexandrium* spp. and *P. breve*.[12,19,71,76,83]

Yentsch and Mague[174] provided a rare glimpse of an apparent annual rhythm in the reproduction rate of *A. excavatum*. Although other studies have examined rhythms in dinoflagellates,[175] (Yentsch and Mague present data from an unusually long (5-year) laboratory study period. This study determined that reproduction rate follows a bell-shaped curve through a given year, with peak rates occurring in spring and summer. These changes occurred despite the fact that the cultures were maintained in a constant environment. Considering that reproduction rate and toxigenesis may be negatively and positively correlated (depending on the species and culture conditions),[12,13,15] does this imply that toxicity may vary during the year as a result of genetically based rhythms? Such a phenomenon could explain the unusually high toxin content of *A. excavatum* found in nature vs. laboratory cultures.[176,177] Rhythmicity in toxigenesis could also account for the presence of so-called nontoxic clones of *G. toxicus*.[128,132]

Ballantine et al.[178] provided an unusual view of toxicity variation over time in a natural population of *Ostreopsis lenticularis*. In this study the toxicity of *O. lenticularis* ranged from 182 μ/cell ($\times 10^{-6}$) in October to having no measurable toxicity in December. There are a number of explanations that could account for this variation, including a shift in genotypes within the population. However, among these explanations lies the existence of an endogenous toxicity "clock".

On a smaller time scale, at least three studies have detected some variation in toxigenesis in *Alexandrium* spp. during batch culture.[179-181] The most comprehensive studies of this type were conducted by Boczar et al.[181] and Boyer et al.[180] These studies report opposing results. Boczar et al.[181] state that both the amount of toxin produced and toxin profiles can change dramatically in batch cultures of *A. tamarense* and *A. catenella*. However, Boyer et al.[180] and other studies[12,76] have found toxin composition to be a fairly stable character.

Ogata et al.[12] randomly selected five clones of *A. tamarensis* from a pool of 17 clones. Of these, there was little variation in the mole percentages of gonyautoxins 1,4; 2; 3; and neosaxitoxin (Figure 8). Ogata et al.[12] concluded that total toxicity in their study reflected toxin content. In addition, the toxin profiles of eight subclones of a single clone (OF84423D-3) were largely homogeneous. Other populations of *Alexandrium* spp. (or varieties) are more variable. Consider the principal components plots of total toxin composition of several clones of *Alexandrium* varieties (tamarensoid and catenelloid) presented by Cembella and Taylor[76] (Figure 9). The ordination selected for presentation here from Cembella and Taylor[76] is only one of three shown in their work. The Cx and B2, carbamyl-N-sulfocompounds, were the two principal toxin components of most of the isolates they examined. These two components are readily hydrolyzed to their corresponding carbamates GTXx and NEO. The plot reveals a significant amount of scatter, in fact, the catenella-like isolates were not segregated as a single group. The spread of data points among at least three quadrants of the principal components plots suggests that the variation detected among clones is due to some factor other than microenvironmental noise in toxin composition. This variation can probably be attributed to genetic differences among clones.

Ogata et al.[12] have questioned the reliability of using the quantity of paralytic shellfish toxins produced as a chemosystematic tool. This is due to a large degree of subclone variability in cell potencies encountered by the authors. This work supports the study by Boczar et al.[181] Attention is now being focused on using the putative polyether maitotoxin in comparing clonal lines of *G. toxicus*,[15,182] and the subclone variation problem has been addressed in this species by Durand-Clement[183] and Bomber et al.[15] In both cases subclone variability in total toxicity was found to be nominal.

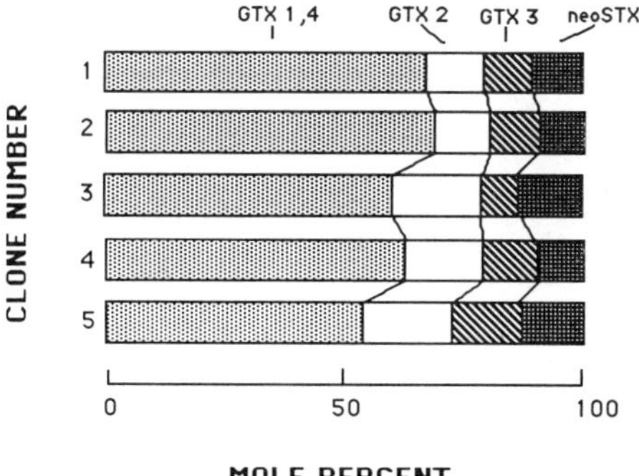

FIGURE 8. Toxin composition of five clones of *Alexandrium tamarensis*. The clones were selected randomly from a pool of 17 clones and analyzed by a liquid chromatographic analyzer of paralytic shellfish toxins. GTX = gonyautoxin; neoSTX = neosaxitoxin. (From Ogata et al., *Toxicon*, 25, 923, 1987. With permission.)

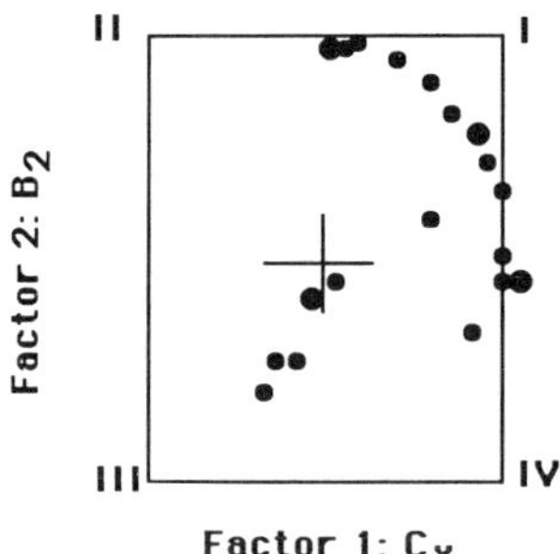

FIGURE 9. Ordination of *Alexandrium* isolates by principal components analysis, based on percent toxin composition. See text for explanation. (From Cembella, A. D. and Taylor, F. J. R., in *Toxic Dinoflagellates*, Elsevier, New York, 1985, 55. With permission.)

In the study by Bomber et al.[15] the continuous batch culture method with concomitant monitoring of reproduction rates was used to measure the total fitness of clones of *G. toxicus*. The cell potencies and cell yields of this species increased as the reproduction rate increased. The pattern of change in these characters was particularly striking when the data for a Hawaiian clone (177 or T-39) were compared over time. Despite the lag time between reproduction rate and potency increases, the two characters appeared to be associated (Figure 2).

Bomber et al.[15] argue that they eliminated environmental and developmental processes from genetic differences by comparing clones only in the acclimated cell condition. All cultures were harvested in the early stationary phase, where toxin content is relatively constant.[230] The results corroborated previous results closely. For example, Babinchak[281] found a value of 250 cells/mouse unit (MU) for acclimated cultures of clone 175, whereas Bomber et al.[15] calculated an acclimated cell potency of 183 cells/MU for this clone. The relative differences among clones were highly significant by statistical analyses and were different from one another, no matter

TABLE 6
Summary of Results for the Different Clones in the Potency Study

Clone	MU[a]/mg	MU/cell ($\times 10^{-6}$)	Cells/MU
		Caribbean	
175	120	55	183
350	18	27	368
		Hawaii	
177	30	27	372
		Florida Keys	
196	4.1	8.0	1263
199	17.5	16.7	601
200	2.6	3.9	2537
300	7.3	18.0	555
		Bahamas	
162	5.5	4.6	2170
163	8.8	19.8	504
170	5.1	19.2	522
171	3.0	5.5	1804
172	2.2	3.8	2605
		Drift Algae	
157	2.9	1.8	5512
158	5.6	6.6	1511
165	12.8	17.3	577
169	4.4	10.4	963
		Bermuda	
135	11.1	5.4	1861

[a] One mouse unit (MU) is defined as the amount of material required to kill 50% of a population of inoculated 20-g mice in 48 h. Alternatively, it is the LD_{50} dose for a 20-g mouse.

From Bomber et al., *J. Phycol.*, 25, 617, 1989. With permission.

how compared (Table 6). More recent evidence from Tindall et al.[184] suggests that clones of *O. lenticularis*, another epiphytic dinoflagellate, also exhibit significant differences in total toxicity.

G. toxicus may produce multiple toxins,[27,185] and this is still a matter for debate. Consequently, the potency differences observed by Bomber et al.[15] among clones may be due to the relative amount of maitotoxin produced or to other toxins. In fact, Bomber et al.[15] observed unusual lumbar contractions in mice inoculated with the methanolic extract of the Bermuda clone (135 of L1928B). Lumbar contractions in mice had not been previously observed from extracts of *G. toxicus* clones, and this supports contention that this species may produce several toxins. Therefore, the matter needs to be resolved at the molecular level. Variations in the molecular

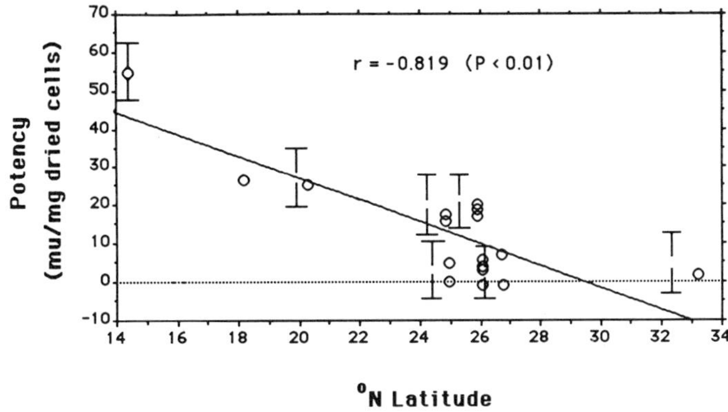

FIGURE 10. Potency (μ/mg dried cells) vs. latitude for all clones of *Gambierdiscus toxicus* examined in the genetic study by Bomber et al.[15] Seven clones are shown with their 95% confidence intervals generated by the *T* method and based upon an analysis of variance. Intervals that do not overlap are significantly different. (From Bomber et al., *J. Phycol.*, 25, 617, 1989. With permission.)

structure/composition of maitotoxin may be found, as were variations in the assemblage of toxins in *Alexandrium* spp.[19,186-190] Regardless, these data do not exclude the use of cell potency as a chemosystematic tool. Considering that the point of harvest in Bomber et al.[15] was the same among clones and was based on kinetics rather than biomass, the potency differences observed probably reflect content and/or compositional differences among clones due to genetic variation. Both total content and/or compositional differences appear to have a heritable component of variation, which can be compared once the environmental and developmental effects on phenotypic variability have been removed.[15]

Bomber et al.[15] also determined that the clonal potencies decreased with increasing latitude (Figure 10). This correlates with the incidence of the ciguatera disease[190] with which *G. toxicus* is associated.[192] Although populations of *G. toxicus* are as abundant in the Florida Keys as the Caribbean,[9,67,130,167,193] few cases of ciguatera are reported from the Florida Keys. These data suggest that Caribbean clones are inherently more toxic than those isolated from other areas. Differences in any character along a latitudinal gradient typically suggests that natural selection has an influence.[107] It is interesting that Maranda et al.[184] observed a similar trend for *Alexandrium*, but potency increased with increasing latitude in this case (Figure 11). These studies are two of only a handful that reveal how the variation of toxigenesis in a microorganism can dramatically affect human populations. The genetic variation of the progenitors discovered in these studies[15,194] could account for the concomitant latitudinal differences in the incidences of the diseases.

A high level of potency variation within a collection site (4 to 10 times) was encountered in the study by Bomber et al.[15] However, this was not as large as that between sites (up to 30 times). Babinchak et al.[182] also found within site variation among clones of *G. toxicus* collected from Marathon Key, Florida. The reader will recall the earlier discussion of the variation in isozyme banding patterns uncovered using electrophoresis. For example, Hayhome and Pfiester[74] found that there could be genetic variation among dinoflagellates within a site, but far greater variation existed with increased geographic distance between populations.

The reader may well be confused by now, and this reflects the status of research with dinoflagellate toxigenesis. In review, one study with *G. toxicus* suggests that total toxicity can be used genetically.[15] However, studies with *Alexandrium* spp. suggest that total toxicity cannot be used for clonal comparisons.[13] Within studies of *Alexandrium* spp., some studies suggest that toxin composition is a conservative character and can be used for clonal comparisons,[74,180] but

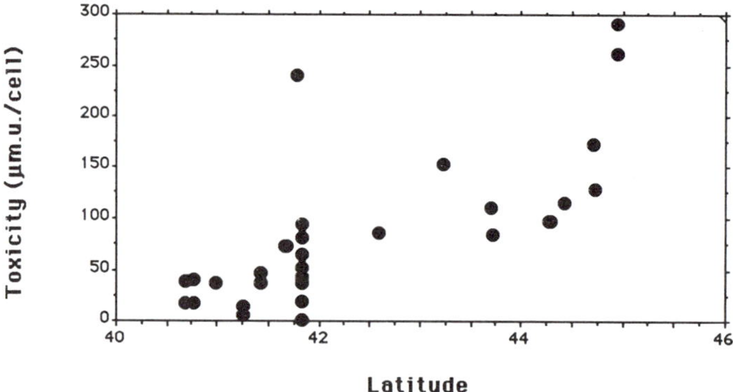

FIGURE 11. Toxicity values of isolates of *Alexandrium tamarense* a function of their latitude of origin. (From Maranda et al., *Est. Coast Shelf Sci.*, 21, 401, 1985. With permission.)

yet another implies utmost caution should be used in this regard.[181] In the author's opinion, such confusion should not reflect on the expertise of the aforementioned researchers. Rather, the confusion can probably be "blamed" on microorganismal genetic plasticity or other features of adaptation. In short, dinoflagellates must mutate in order to adapt to their ever-changing environments. Consider that, above this natural variation, further mutations undoubtedly occur in laboratory cultures.

Nevertheless, toxin content and profiles still offer an attractive way of evaluating population genetics of microalgae. Limitations of these methods should of course always be considered. However, the plasticity and range of variation within these characters provide a means of easily measuring differences. The wide variability in toxin production is evidence for the compounds being secondary metabolities, as such profound mutations influencing the quantity of primary metabolites produced would probably prove lethal. However, the following section on physiology contains information that supports roles for toxins as primary metabolites. Finally, although toxins have roles in causing human disease, they also have high biomedical value. Therefore, population geneticists using toxicology can serve the biomedical community while simultaneously testing hypotheses regarding evolutionary theory.

III. PHYSIOLOGY

A. BIOSYNTHESIS

Shimizu and his group have pioneered studies of saxitoxin biosynthesis in *Alexandrium* spp.[195,196] Determining the biosynthetic pathway has been a formidable task, primarily because these autotrophic algae do not readily take up exogenous, labeled compounds in tracer studies. However, Shimizu et al.[197] demonstrated that *A. tamarense* will take up [2-13^{C}] glycine. Using this and other tracers, Shimizu et al.[197] determined that saxitoxin is derived from acetate and methionine. They proposed a Claisen-type condensation of an acetate unit or its derivative to the amino group bearing the α-carbon of arginine or its equivalent. Thus, its synthesis was more complex than simple conversion of arginine, as previously thought.[196]

That acetate is involved in toxigenesis is further supported by Anderson's work.[13] He reported that the arginine content mirrors the toxin content. When the net toxin production was stimulated by phosphate limitation or low-temperature stress, arginine increased as well. Thus, this indicates that saxitoxin production could be an arginine "shunt", but raises the question of how other dinoflagellates deal with arginine accumulation. It will be interesting to monitor arginine accumulation in nontoxic dinoflagellates in future experiments, and possibly to search for molecules in these species that are similar to saxitoxin but have little or no toxicity.

A logical starting point in the study of polyether biosynthesis in dinoflagellates would be a review of the bacterial literature. However, although there are many more articles published on bacterial than dinoflagellate polyethers, the bacterial literature is still deficient. For example, there are few articles published regarding the physiology and nutritional requirements of Actinomycetes for producing polyethers. This, it turns out, is probably due to the high market potential of polyethers, which encourages researchers to keep culture parameters trade secrets. Many fermentation processes are patented;[140] consider that sales of the bacterial polyether monensin has a market potential of over 100 million dollars.[140]

Nevertheless, some studies have led to forming models for the biosynthesis of these compounds. Cane et al.[198] suggest that there are two basic structural prototypes (APPA and PAPA) that define the stereochemistry along the backbone of at least 30 polyether structures. The polyene backbones are thought to arise from the carboxylic acids acetate, propionate (the A and P in APPA and PAPA), and butyrate. These polyenes are oxidized and undergo cyclization to become polyethers.[199] This hypothesis is supported by work by Cane et al.,[200] who demonstrated that [2-$^{2}H_2$, 2-^{13}C] propionate was incorporated into erythromycins A and B (macrolides) in cultures of *Streptomyces erythreus*.

Although the polyketide route of synthesis is gaining wide support, some authors dispute its simplicity. For example, Hutchinson and Sherman[201] suggest that if erythromycin A is assembled from malonate analogs of acetate, propionate, or butyrate, their corresponding chiral centers in the C2-C4 subunits should have the same configurations. However, their data indicate that the stereochemistry of erythromycin is inconsistent with the "equivalent configurations" hypothesis and hence the polyketide pathway. Hutchinson and Sherman[196] go on to say that the biosynthesis of polyethers is more complex or that there are significant postsynthesis alterations of the products.

Many researchers are still convinced that there is a large degree of stereochemical uniformity that exists between the putative polyene precursors for each polyether throughout a series. In fact, the stereochemistry has led Cane et al.[198] to suggest that there is a common genetic basis influencing the production of polyethers among bacterial species. O'Hagen[199] went one step further in suggesting that polyethers and related macrolides also share a common genetic basis. This hypothesis is supported by work with dinoflagellate algae, which shows that both a polyether (okadaic acid) and a macrolide-containing macrocycle (Prorocentrolide) can occur in the same organism (*Prorocentrum lima*).[42] Shimizu et al.[202] and Thompson et al.[203,204] have suggested that dinoflagellate polyethers are also derived from the polyketide pathway, beginning with dicarboxylic acid precursors. Therefore, new studies of polyether synthesis in dinoflagellates may benefit greatly from finding ways to manipulate the carboxylic acid cycle.

Thompson et al.[203] also encountered difficulty in feeding labeled substrates to dinoflagellate cultures when they investigated brevetoxin synthesis in *Ptychodiscus brevis*. Nevertheless, in their work labeled acetate and methionine was taken up by *P. brevis* and incorporated into the brevetoxin molecule. These studies have profound implications regarding a strong phylogenetic link between polyether-producing bacteria and dinoflagellates.

B. ENVIRONMENTAL FACTORS AND BIOSYNTHESIS

Ideally, the course of a chemical study of an algal toxin would begin by using a simple bioassay to choose the best producer of toxin from a suite of clones. Secondly, this clone would be subjected to physiologic manipulation in order to enhance toxigenesis. In addition, monitoring toxigenesis within a batch culture would also ensue. These studies would then facilitate the purification of the chemical from crude extracts containing relatively large amounts of toxin. In fact, competing components can even be reduced by simply harvesting at the right time. For example, Tindall and Bomber (in preparation) have found that much of the lipid material interfering with the purification of maitotoxin from *Gambierdiscus toxicus* can be reduced. They accomplish this by harvesting the cells following maximum toxin accumulation, and this occurs prior to the onset of massive lipid accumulation.

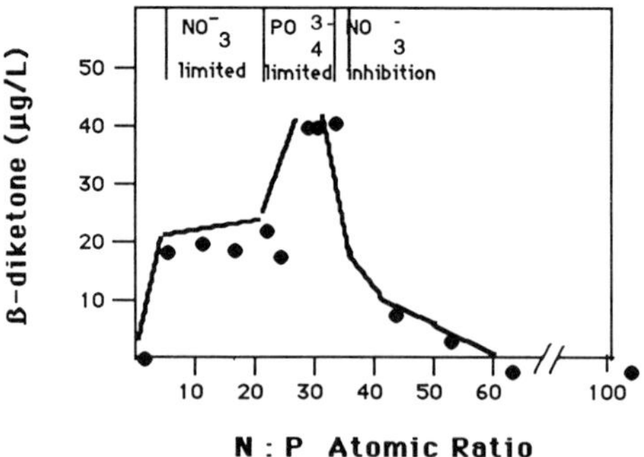

FIGURE 12. Influence of the initial N/P atomic ratio in the medium on the maximum ß-diketone concentration for *Prorocentrum minimum*. Final cell yields for all experiments were equivalent. (From Trick et al., *Can. J. Fish. Aquat. Sci.*, 41, 423, 1984. With permission.)

These aforementioned ideals have not been implemented in practice. Although few studies have actually dealt with *manipulating* toxigenesis in dinoflagellates, a number of studies have been able to at least *track* toxigenesis. These and other types of experiments began in the 1960s and continue presently.[204-206] In the cases of PSP (paralytic shellfish poisoning), NSP (neurotoxic shellfish poisoning), and ciguatera research, it seems that the rush to publish chemical structures has left a wake of phycologic "clean-up"; that is, only after chemical studies reach a *cul de sac* is the focus returned back to the progenitor organisms.

Trick et al.[43,165,207] have conducted admirable studies of ß-diketone and siderophore production in *Prorocentrum minimum* that provide a nice model for other new research with dinoflagellates. For example, Trick et al.[207] screened a number of species and clones for siderophore production and then manipulated its synthesis by varying a variety of culture parameters. Similar studies were later conducted with the same dinoflagellate and its production of the antibacterial norcarotenoid ß-diketone.[166] Environmental factors examined for their effects upon production of the antibiotic included iron concentration, light intensity, temperature, and salinity. Nitrogen to phosphorous atomic ratios were also found to have dramatic effects on production (Figure 12). The analysis of chemical structures conducted in relation to this work was conducted in tandem with the physiologic studies.[165]

Studies by Proctor et al.[208] determined that saxitoxin yield was inversely correlated with growth rate for *A. catenella* under continuous light. Ogata et al.[11] detected a similar trend, with toxigenesis declining with increasing growth rates. In later work, Ogata et al.[12] could find no clear correlation between the inherent growth rate and toxicity of clones of *A. tamarense*, although the least toxic clone examined had the fastest growth rate. However, Anderson[13] determined that in semicontinuous cultures under most conditions that he investigated, growth rate and net toxin production were directly proportional. Nevertheless, in the same study by Anderson, phosphate depletion caused a decrease in growth rate but an increase in toxin production. Hall[189] and Boyer et al.[180] also reported rather dramatic increases in the total toxin production in *Alexandrium* when grown in phosphate-limited cultures. The physiologic studies by Proctor et al.[208] and Ogata et al.[11] may simply reflect that harvesting took place in late log or stationary-phase growth, where phosphate stress is most certainly taking place. In addition, Prakash[204] found that toxin yield is a function of cell density, which may also reflect increased toxigenesis during phosphate reduction. Boyer et al.[180] state that their observed increase in toxin content under phosphate depletion could not be totally explained by changes in the average cell volume.

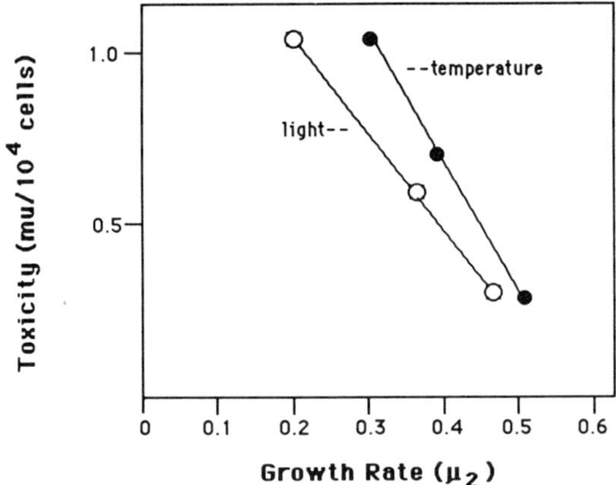

FIGURE 13. Relationship between toxicity and growth rates measured at different light intensities and water temperatures for *Alexandrium tamarense*. (From Ogata et al., *Mar. Biol.*, 95, 217, 1987. With permission.)

Anderson[13] and Anderson et al.[209] suggest that the effect of phosphate limitation is due to an increased availability of arginine in the cell, presumably to reduced demand from competing (phosphate-dependent?) pathways. The study by Anderson et al.[209] on the dynamics and physiology of saxitoxin in *Alexandrium* spp. is probably the most comprehensive study in this area to date. The observed dramatic increase in toxin production under phosphate limitation in continuous cultures was noted even after the cells stopped dividing. Consequently, the authors are the first to demonstrate that growth rate and rates of toxin production are not necessarily coupled, although they can be under certain conditions. These dynamics help explain the conflicting results found among reports regarding growth rate and toxigenesis.

The roles of other environmental parameters in toxigenesis of *Alexandrium* have also been explored. The effects of nitrogen stress on toxigenesis in *A. tamarensis* were examined by Boyer et al.[180] and Anderson et al.[209,210] Boyer et al.[180] reported a gradual reduction in toxin content during nitrogen-limited stationary-phase growth. Interestingly, Anderson et al.[209] report that nitrogen limitation, as well as CO_2 depletion, both affect pathways involved in toxigenesis before those needed for cell division.

White[211] found that the paralytic toxin content in *G. excavatum* increased with increasing salinity up to 37 ‰. Ogata et al.[11] show that the maximum toxicity is negatively correlated with the optimum temperature and light for growth (Figure 13). Overall, a more stressful condition (reduced growth rate) appears to enhance toxigenesis. Perhaps this phenomenon can also account for the high toxin content found in dinoflagellate cysts.[212,213]

An interesting study by Kodama et al.[214] revealed that smaller cells (20 to 30 μm) were less toxic than larger cells (30 to 40 and 40 to 95 μm) of *A. tamarense* and *A. catenella*. The smaller cells represent a newly divided subpopulation. Cells within this subpopulation are more metabolically active than older cells. Consequently, they may not yet be as phosphate deficient as are the older cells. Alternatively, the difference in toxicity could simply be explained by the younger cells not having had enough time to accumulate toxin.

Studies with *Alexandrium* suggest that saxitoxin may have a role in primary metabolism. Mickelson and Yentsch[14] and Anderson and Cheng[8] have conducted studies that suggest saxitoxin may be restricted to specific sties, being produced in the nucleus or on the nuclear membrane. In addition, saxitoxin accumulates in the dinoflagellate beginning in the log phase[13,180,181,209,210] and, as stated earlier, has a probable role as an arginine "shunt".[13,209] The results of these studies are not consistent with the pattern of secondary metabolite production.[1] Secondary metabolites typically do not begin accumulating until the stationary phase and are

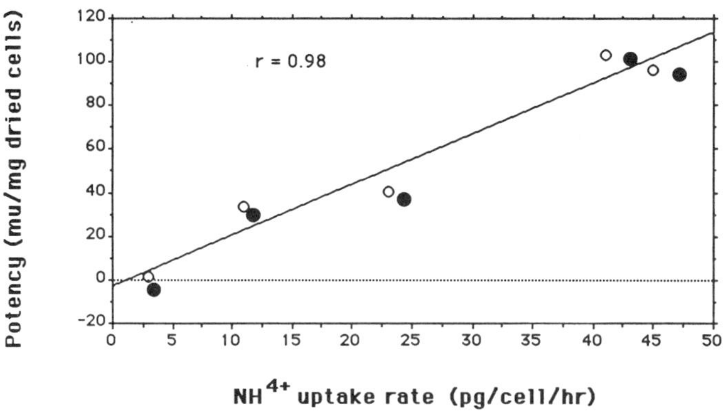

FIGURE 14. Total potency (μ/mg dried cells) of *Gambierdiscus toxicus* vs. its uptake rate of ammonium.

usually synthesized throughout the cytoplasm. Interestingly, Tindall and Bomber (unpublished) found that maitotoxin is also produced in the log phase. Work by Campbell et al.[94] suggests that polyether production in *G. toxicus* may also be localized, being primarily restricted to the cell wall. A number of interesting studies with antibodies have emerged from the Hawaiian research group from which the Campbell study emerged.[215]

Perhaps lessons regarding polyether toxigenesis can also be learned by examining the production in bacteria. For example, Stark et al.[216] found that iron had a dramatic effect on the production of the polyether monensin in *Streptomyces cinnamonensis*. The addition of ferric sulfate effected a three-fold increase in the production of monensin, and the addition of manganese chloride had a similar effect. These experiments suggest that monensin help balance trace metal chemistry in the bacterial cytoplasm. This work inspired experiments by Bomber et al.,[232] who have recently determined that the total toxicity in *G. toxicus* is positively correlated with ammonium ion uptake rates (Figure 14). These studies suggest that it is possible that the toxin(s) in *G. toxicus* facilitates the transport of ammonium ion across the dinoflagellate's cell membrane. The association between ammonium uptake rates and maitotoxin production may be an artifact of the density of a culture. For instance, Bomber et al.[232] found that as the density (cells/ml) of a culture of *Gambierdiscus toxicus* increases, the relative rate of uptake of a given nutrient increases. This is consistent with studies of nutrient uptake kinetics in other algae.[217] These factors may explain why the pattern of maitotoxin production and the density of a culture were found to be similar to the ammonium uptake/toxin content curves. Theoretically, this phenomenon has an evolutionary basis; that is, in a eutrophic environment, the faster a cell can capitalize a limiting nutrient, the better chance it has of surviving its competitors, at least in the short term. The opposite would probably be true in an oligotrophic environment.

The work mentioned above by Bomber et al. (unpublished) suggests that toxins produced by *G. toxicus* may actually have a role in primary metabolism. The positive correlation observed by Bomber et al.[15] between reproductive rate, time in culture, and potency in *G. toxicus* is also curious. Does the toxin(s) assist in helping the cultures acclimate to a new environment? Meeson and Faust[218] and Faust et al.[219] speculate that as *Prorocentrum* spp. adapted to new light-quality environments, their efficiency in converting photosynthetic products into new cells increased. Perhaps the work with *G. toxicus* reflects a similar trend. The clones of *G. toxicus* examined may slowly be improving their ability to convert and partition the products, some of which may be toxins.

In Bomber et al.[15,112] the observed correlation between reproduction rate and potency, coupled with an apparent effect of light-source type on potency, all suggest that the process of photosynthesis and toxin production may be linked. Apparently potency and the amount of chlorophyll *a* and c_2 per cell are negatively correlated. Considering that the most toxic clone

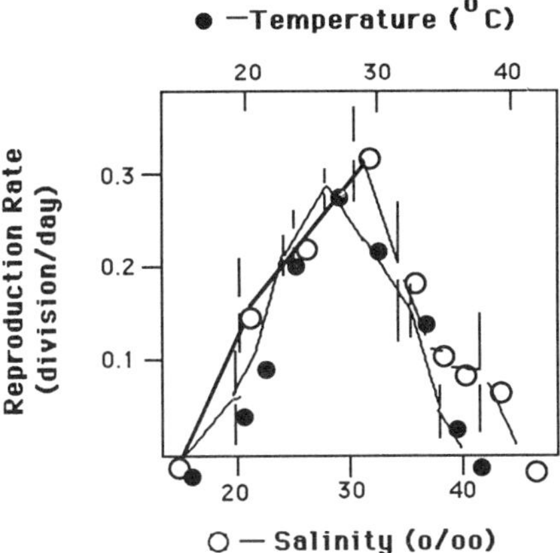

FIGURE 15. Reproduction rate (division/day) of *Prorocentrum lima* vs. temperature and salinity. Each point is the mean of four replicates and the bars are one standard deviation. (From Morton, S. L. and Norris, D. R., in *Toxic Marine Phytoplankton Blooms*, Elsevier, New York, in press. With permission.)

tested by Bomber et al.[112] (175) had the lowest level of chlorophylls per cell, but the highest amount of toxin per cell, studies with light and potency could yield exciting information regarding the role of maitotoxin in *G. toxicus*.

Although only a handful of studies examine toxigenesis in the ciguatera dinoflagellates,[15,130,220,221] several studies have made headway in understanding their biochemical composition and physiologic requirements.[130,167,221-224] Studies exploring the "symbiosis" between dinoflagellate epiphytes and their hosts are interesting,[130,225,226] and suggest that macroalgal metabolites have a significant effect upon epiphytic growth. This is probably due to the chelating abilities of the algal extracts.[225] At least three studies suggest that epiphytic dinoflagellates have rather restrictive growth requirements in terms of light intensity, light quality, and temperature/salinity[125,223,224] (Figure 15). However, the study by Bomber et al.[125] indicates that toxigenesis is possible over a wide range of conditions. Future work quantifying toxigenesis under different conditions will undoubtedly be exciting and also helpful in future purification of known and as-yet unknown toxins. The development of stains for toxins or immunofluorescent probes will help studies of toxigenesis progress more rapidly. These techniques can be coupled with flow cytometry,[227] and real-time monitoring of toxigenesis can be accomplished.

IV. DISCUSSION

A priori, the author had hoped that compiling over 200 references dealing with toxigenesis would have perhaps helped to resolve at least one enigmatic question. For example, are toxins produced *de novo*? Not a single study, nor can collective studies, unequivocally attest to this. Do toxins have an evolutionary role? That is, do they provide some benefit to the progenitors either physiologically or ecologically that would help them to survive or even dominate? Studies showing detailed molecular mechanisms revealing a certifiable physiologic role are nonexistent. Most studies to date can only imply that such roles exist from indirect evidence. Are toxins secondary or primary metabolites? There is evidence to support both cases. Until there are studies with pure toxins that show effects on competing organisms, allelochemical hypothesis are also speculative. Even then, how often are pure toxins produced exogenously, or, do they even need to be? After all, although selective forces begin at the individual level, they deal with entire populations. An older cell that lyses and releases an allelochemical had previously divided, and its genes regulating toxigenesis endure. Its lysis helps ensure the survival of remaining, toxin-producing genes in the population.

What can be gleaned from this review is that, fortunately, toxigenesis can be manipulated. This knowledge can help provide sufficient quantities of molecular probes from dinoflagellates for pharmacologic work. Secondly, there is good evidence to show that both qualitative and quantitative genetic variation in DNA exists within and among populations of dinoflagellates. Thus, assuming *de novo* synthesis of toxins, it is reasonable that the studies showing toxicity variation among isolates can be attributed to genetic causes. These genetic differences interfere with, yet stimulate, mankind's activities. Consequently, dinoflagellates afford us yet another, albeit unique, glimpse at how the destiny of mankind and microorganisms are inextricably linked.

ACKNOWLEDGMENTS

This chapter is dedicated to Dr. Dean Norris. His work with *Dinophysis, Ornithocercus*, red tides, and ciguatera, and his many students are a true legacy. Thanks to Drs. Donald Miller and Donald Tindall for making this possible. Deanna Hasenstab is greatly appreciated for countless hours spent in the library. Kevin Aikman and Melody Pearce helped watch the "bugs" so that I could write. Particularly helpful reviews were conducted by Dr. Donald Anderson, Kevin Aikman, and Steven Morton. Financial support from the U.S. Army Medical Research and Development Command, contract DAMD17-87-C-7002, is greatfully acknowledged. The views, findings, and opinions expressed herein are those of the author and should not be construed as those of the Department of the Army.

REFERENCES

1. **Martin, J. F. and Demain, A. L.,** Control of antibiotic biosynthesis, *Microbiol. Rev.*, 44, 230, 1980.
2. **Balandrin, M. F., Klocke, J. A., Wurtele, E. S., and Bollinger, W. H.,** Natural plant chemicals: sources of industrial and medicinal materials, *Science*, 228, 1154, 1985.
3. **Loeblich, A. R., III**, Dinoflagellate evolution: speculation and evidence, *J. Protozool.*, 23, 13, 1976.
4. **Yentsch, C. M., Lewis, C. M., and Yentsch, C. S.,** Biological resting in the dinoflagellate *Gonyaulax excavata*, *Bioscience*, 30, 251, 1980.
5. **Wall, D.,** Biological problems concerning fossilizable dinoflagellates, *Geo. Sci. Man. 3*, 1, 1971.
6. **Wall, D. and Dale, B.,** Modern dinoflagellate cysts and evolution of the Peridiniales, *Micropaleontology*, 14, 265, 1968.
7. **Freeberg, L. R., Marshall, A., and Heyl, M.,** Interrelationships of *Gymnodinium breve* (Florida Red Tide) within the phytoplankton community, in *Toxic Dinoflagellate Blooms*, Taylor, D. L., and Seliger, H. H., Eds., Elsevier, New York, 1979, 139.
8. **Anderson, D. M. and Cheng, T. P-O.,** Intracellular localization of saxitoxins in the dinoflagellate *Gonyaulax tamarensis, J. Phycol.*, 24, 17, 1988.
9. **Bomber, J. W.,** Ecology, Genetic Variability and Physiology of the Ciguatera-Causing Dinoflagellate *Gambierdiscus toxicus* Adachi and Fukuyo, Ph.D. thesis, Florida Institute of Technology, Melbourne, FL, 1987.
10. **Durand, M., Squiban, A., Viso, A.-C., and Pesando, D.,** Production and toxicity of *Gambierdiscus toxicus*. Effects of its toxins (maitotoxin and ciguatoxin) on some marine organisms, *Proc. Fifth Intl. Coral Reef Cong.*, Tahiti, 4, 483, 1985.
11. **Ogata, T., Ishimaru, T., and Kodama, M.,** Effect of water temperature and light intensity on growth rate and toxin production in *Protogonyaulax tamarensis, Mar. Biol.*, 95, 217, 1987.
12. **Ogata, T., Kodama, M., and Ishimaru, T.,** Toxin production in the dinoflagellate *Protogonyaulax tamarensis, Toxicon*, 9, 923, 1987.
13. **Anderson, D. M.,** Dynamics and physiology of saxitoxin production in *Alexandrium* spp., in *Toxic Marine Phytoplankton Blooms*, Graneli, E., Sundstrom, B., Edler, L., and Anderson, D. M., Eds., Elsevier, New York, in press.

14. **Mickelson, C. and Yentsch, C. M.,** Toxicity and nucleic acid content of *Gonyaulax excavata*, in *Toxic Dinoflagellate Blooms*, Taylor, F. and Seliger, H., Eds., Elsevier, New York, 1979, 131.
15. **Bomber, J. W., Tindall, D. R., and Miller, D. M.,** Genetic variability in toxin potencies among seventeen clones of *Gambierdiscus toxicus* (Dinophyceae), *J. Phycol.*, 25, 617, 1989.
16. **Taylor, F. J. R.,** The toxigenic gonyaulacoid dinoflagellates, in *Toxic Dinoflagellate Blooms*, Taylor, D. L. and Seliger, H. H., Eds., 1979, 47.
17. **Burke, J. M., Marchisotto, J., McLaughlin, J. J. A., and Provasoli, L.,** Analysis of the toxin produced by *Gonyaulax catenella* in axenic culture, *Ann. N.Y. Acad. Sci.*, 90, 837, 1960.
18. **Kodama, M., Ogata, T., Fukuyo, Y., Ishimaru, T., Wisessang, S., Saitanu, K., Panichyakarn, U., and Piyakarnchana, T.,** *Protogonyaulax cohorticula*, a toxic dinoflagellate found in the Gulf of Thailand, *Toxicon*, 26, 707, 1988.
19. **Hall, S., Neve, R. A., Reichardt, P. B., and Swisher, G. A.,** Chemical analysis of paralytic shellfish poisoning in Alaska, in *Toxic Dinoflagellate Blooms*, Taylor, D. L. and Seliger, H. H., Eds., Elsevier, New York, 1979, 345.
20. **Kobayashi, J., Ishibashi, M., Nakamura, H., and Ohizumi, Y.,** Amphidinolide-A, a novel antineoplastic macrolide from the marine dinoflagellate *Amphidinium* sp., *Tetrahedron Lett.*, 27, 5755, 1986.
21. **Yasumoto, T., Seino, N., Murakami, Y., and Murata, M.,** Toxins produced by benthic dinoflagellates, *Biol. Bull.*, 172, 128, 1987.
22. **McLaughlin, J. J. A. and Provasoli, L.,** Nutritional requirements and toxicity of two marine *Amphidinium*, *J. Protozool.*, 4(Suppl 7), 1957.
23. **Pincemin, B. C.,** Telemediateurs chimiques et equilibre biologique oceanique, 3e partie: etude in vitro de relations entre populations phytoplanctoniques, *Rev. Intern. Oceanogr. Med.*, 22-23, 165, 1971.
24. **Nakajima, I., Oshima, Y., and Yasumoto, T.,** Toxicity of benthic dinoflagellates in Okinawa, *Bull. Jpn. Soc. Sci. Fish.*, 47, 1029, 1981.
25. **Murata, M., Shimitani, B., Sugitani, H., Oshima, Y., and Yasumoto, T.,** Isolation and structural elucidation of the causative toxin of diarrhetic shellfish poisoning, *Bull. Jpn. Soc. Sci. Fish.*, 48, 549, 1982.
26. **Yokoyama, A., Murata, M., Oshima, Y., Iwashitaand, T., and Yasumoto, T.,** Some chemical properties of maitotoxin, a putative calcium channel agonist isolated from a marine dinoflagellate, *J. Biochem.*, 104, 184, 1988.
27. **Legrand, A. M., Cruchet, P., Bagnis, R., Murata, M., and Yasumoto, T.,** Chromatographic and spectral evidence for the presence of multiple ciguatera toxins, in *Toxic Marine Phytoplankton Blooms*, Graneli, E., Sundstrom, B., Edler, L., and Anderson, D. M., Eds., Elsevier, New York, in press.
28. **Nagai, H., Satake, M., and Yasumoto, T.,** Screening of marine phytoplankton for antifungal substances, in *Toxic Marine Phytoplankton Blooms*, Graneli, E., Sundstrom, B., Edler, L., and Anderson, D. M., Eds., Elsevier, New York, in press.
29. **Murakami, M., Makabe, K., Yamaguchi, K., and Konosu, S.,** Gonidomin A, a novel polyether macrolide from the dinoflagellate *Goniodoma pseudogoniaulax*, *Tetrahedron Lett.*, 29, 1149, 1988.
30. **Sievers, A. M.,** Comparative toxicity of *Gonyaulax monilata* and *Gymnodinium breve* to annelids, crustaceans, molluscs, and a fish, *J. Protozool.*, 16, 401, 1969.
31. **Walker, L. M. and Steidinger, K. A.,** Sexual reproduction in the toxic dinoflagellate *Gonyaulax monilata*, *J. Phycol.*, 15, 312, 1979.
32. **Schradie, J. and Bliss, C. A.,** The cultivation and toxicity of *Gonyaulax polyhedra*, *Lloydia*, 25, 214, 1962.
33. **Morey-Gaines, G.,** *Gymnodinium catenatum* Graham (Dinophyceae): morphology and affinities with armored forms, *Phycologia*, 21, 154, 1982.
34. **Tindall, D. R., Dickey, R. W., Carlson, R. D., and Morey-Gaines, G.,** Ciguatoxigenic dinoflagellates from the Caribbean, in *Seafood Toxins*, Ragelis, E. P., Ed., The American Chemical Society, Washington, D.C., 1984, 225.
35. **Abbott, B. C. and Ballantine, D.,** The toxin from *Gymnodinium veneficum* Ballantine, *J. Mar. Biol. Assoc. U.K.*, 36, 169, 1957.
36. **Norris, D. R., Bomber, J. W., and Balech, E.,** Benthic dinoflagellates associated with ciguatera from the Florida Keys. I. *Ostreopsis heptagona* sp. nov., in *Toxic Dinoflagellates*, Anderson, D. M., White, A. W., and Baden, D. G., Eds., Elsevier, New York, 1985, 39.
37. **Hashimoto, Y.,** Glenodinine, an ichthyotoxic substance produced by a dinoflagellate, *Peridinium polonicum*, *Bull. Jpn. Soc. Sci. Fish*, 34, 528, 1968.
38. **Steidinger, K. A. and Baden, D. G.,** Toxic marine dinoflagellates, in *Dinoflagellates*, Spector, D. L., Ed., Academic Press, Orlando, FL, 1984, 201.
39. **Tindall, D. R., Miller, D. M., and Bomber, J. W.,** Culture and toxicity of dinoflagellates from ciguatera endemic regions of the world, *Proc. Ninth World Cong. on Animal, Plant and Microbial Toxins, Toxicon*, in press.
40. **Dickey, R. W., Bobzin, S. C., Faulkner, D. J., Bencsath, F. A., and Andrzejewski, D.,** The identification of okadaic acid from a Caribbean dinoflagellate *Prorocentrum concavum*, *Toxicon*, in press.

41. **Murakami, Y., Oshima, Y., and Yasumoto, T.,** Identification of okadaic acid as a toxic component of a marine dinoflagellate *Prorocentrum lima, Bull. Jpn. Soc. Sci. Fish.*, 48, 68, 1982.
42. **Torigoe, K., Murata, M., and Yasumoto, T.,** Prorocentrolide, a toxic nitrogenous macrocycle from a marine dinoflagellate *Prorocentrum lima, J. Am. Chem. Soc.*, 110, 7876, 1988.
43. **Shimizu, Y.,** Dinoflagellate toxins, in *Marine Natural Products: Chemical and Biological Perspectives*, Vol. I, Scheuer, P. J., Ed., Academic Press, New York, 1978, 1.
44. **Trick, C. G., Harrison, P. J., and Anderson, R. J.,** Extracellular secondary metabolite production by the marine dinoflagellate *Prorocentrum minimum* in culture, *Can. J. Fish. Aquat. Sci.*, 38, 864, 1981.
45. **Gauthier, M. J., Bernard, P., and et Aubert, M.,** Modification de la fonction antibiotique de deux diatomees marines, *Asterionella japonica* (Cleve) et *Chaetoceros lauderi* (Ralfs), par le dinoflagelle *Prorocentrum micans* (Ehrenberg), *J. Exp. Mar. Biol. Ecol.*, 33, 37, 1978.
46. **Uchida, T.,** Excretion of a diatom-inhibiting substance by *Prorocentrum micans* Ehrenberg, *Jpn. J. Ecol.*, 27, 1, 1977.
47. **Lin, Y.-Y., Risk, M., Ray, S. M., Van Engen, D., Clardy, J., Golick, J., James, J. C., and Nakanishi, K.,** Isolation and structure of brevetoxin B from the "red tide" dinoflagellate *Ptychodiscus brevis* (*Gymnodinium breve*), *J. Am. Chem. Soc.*, 103, 6773, 1981.
48. **Harada, T., Oshima, Y., Kamiya, H., and Yasumoto, T.,** Confirmation of paralytic shellfish toxins in the dinoflagellate *Pyrodinium bahamense* var. compressa and bivalves in Palau, *Bull. Jpn. Soc. Sci. Fish.*, 48, 821, 1982.
49. **Steidinger, K. A.,** A re-evaluation of toxic dinoflagellate biology and ecology, in *Progress in Phycological Research, Vol. 2.*, Round, F. E. and Chapman, D. J., Eds., Elsevier, New York, 1983, 147.
50. **Beam, C. A. and Himes, M.,** Dinoflagellate genetics, in *Dinoflagellates*, Spector, D. L., Ed., Academic Press, Orlando, FL, 1984, 263.
51. **Loeblich, A. R., III,** Dinoflagellate physiology and biochemistry, in *Dinoflagellates*, Spector, D. L., Ed., Academic Press, Orlando, FL, 1984, 300.
52. **Adachi, R. and Fukuyo, Y.,** The thecal structure of a marine toxic dinoflagellate *Gambierdiscus toxicus* gen. et sp. nov. collected in a ciguatera endemic area, 45, 67, 1979.
53. **Fukuyo, Y.,** Taxonomical study on benthic dinoflagellates collected in coral reefs, *Bull. Jpn. Soc. Sci. Fish.*, 47, 967, 1981.
54. **Norris, D. R. and Berner, L. D., Jr.,** Thecal morphology of selected species of *Dinophysis* (Dinoflagellata) from the Gulf of Mexico, *Contrib. Mar. Sci.*, 15, 145, 1970.
55. **Balech, E.,** The genus *Alexandrium* or *Gonyaulax* of the tamarensis group, in *Toxic Dinoflagellates,* Anderson, D. M., White, A. W., and Baden, D. G., Eds., Elsevier, New York, 1985, 33.
56. **Taylor, F. J. R.,** On dinoflagellate evolution, *Bio Systems*, 13, 68, 1980.
57. **Steidinger, K. A. and Cox, E. R.,** Free-living dinoflagellates, in *Phytoflagellates*, Cox, E. R., Ed., Elsevier, New York, 1980, 407.
58. **Dodge, J. D.,** Dinoflagellate taxonomy, in *Dinoflagellates,* Spector, D. L., Ed., Academic Press, Orlando, FL, 1984, 17.
59. **Netzel, H. and Durr, G.,** Dinoflagellate cell cortex, in Spector, D.L., Ed., *Dinoflagellates*, Academic Press, Orlando, FL, 1984, 43.
60. **Shimizu, Y., Alam, M., Oshima, Y., Buckley, L. J., and Fallon, W. E.,** Chemistry and distribution of deleterious dinoflagellate toxins, in *Marine Natural Products Chemistry*, Faulkner, D. J. and Fenical, W. H., Eds., Plenum Press, New York, 1977, 261.
61. **Pfiester, L. A. and Anderson, D. M.,** Dinoflagellate reproduction, in *The Biology of the Dinoflagellates,* Taylor, F. J. R., Ed., Blackwell Scientific Publishers, Palo Alto, CA, 1984, 610.
62. **Beam, C. A. and Himes, M.,** Sexual isolation and genetic diversification among some strains of *Crypthecodinium cohnii*-like dinoflagellates. Evidence of speciation, *J. Protozool*, 4, 532, 1977.
63. **Beam, C. A. and Himes, M.,** Distribution of members of the *Crypthecodinium cohnii* (Dinophyceae) species complex, *J. Protozool.*, 29, 8, 1982.
64. **Beam, C. A. and Himes, M.,** Evidence of sexual fusion and recombination in the dinoflagellate *Crypthecodinium (Gyrodinium) cohnii*, *Nature*, 250, 435, 1974.
65. **Beam, C. A., Himes, M., Himelfarb, J., Link, C., and Shaw, K.,** Genetic evidence of unusual meiosis in the dinoflagellate *Crypthecodinium cohnii*, *Genetics*, 87, 19, 1977.
66. **Destombe, C. and Cambella, A.,** Mating-type determination, gametic recognition and reproductive success in *Alexandrium excavatum* (Gonyaulacales, Pyrrophyta), a toxic red-tide dinoflagellate, unpublished manuscript.
67. **Bomber, J. W., Morton, S. L., Babinchak, J. A., Norris, D. R., and Morton, J. G.,** Epiphytic dinoflagellates of drift algae — Another toxigenic community in the ciguatera food chain, *Bull. Mar. Sci.*, 43, 204, 1988.
68. **Murphy, L. S.,** Biochemical taxonomy of marine phytoplankton by electrophoresis of enzymes. II. Loss of heterozygosity in clonal cultures of the centric diatoms *Skeletonema costatum* and *Thalassiosira pseudonana*, *J. Phycol.*, 14, 247, 1978.

69. **Brand, L. E.,** Genetic variability in reproduction rates in marine phytoplankton populations, *Evolution*, 35, 1117, 1981.
70. **Taylor, F. J. R.,** A description of the benthic dinoflagellate associated with maitotoxin and ciguatoxin, including observations on Hawaiian material, in *Toxic Dinoflagellate Blooms,* Taylor, F. and Seliger, H., Eds., Elsevier, New York, 1979, 71.
71. **Baden, D. G. and Tomas, C. R.,** Variations in major toxin composition for six clones of *Ptychodiscus brevis, Toxicon,* 26, 961, 1988.
72. **Klein, T. M., Wolf, E. D., Wu, R., and Sanford, J. C.,** High velocity microprojectiles for delivering nucleic acids into living cells, *Nature*, 327,70, 1987.
73. **Hayhome, B. A., Whitten, D. J., Harkins, K. R., and Pfiester, L. A.,** Intraspecific variation in the dinoflagellate *Peridinium volzii, J. Phycol.*, 23, 573, 1987.
74. **Hayhome, B. A. and Pfiester, L. A.,** Electrophoretic analysis of soluble enzymes in five freshwater dinoflagellate species, *Am. J. Bot.*, 8, 1165, 1983.
75. **Watson, D. A. and Loeblich, A. R., III,** The application of electrophoresis to the systematics of the marine dinoflagellate genus *Heterocapsa, Biochem. Sys. & Ecol.,* 11, 67, 1983.
76. **Cembella, A. D. and Taylor, F. J. R.,** Biochemical variability within the *Protogonyaulax tamarensis/catenella* species complex, in *Toxic Dinoflagellates,* Anderson, D. M., White, A. W., and Baden, D. G., Eds., Elsevier, New York, 1985, 55.
77. **Cembella, A. D. and Taylor, F. J. R.,** Electrophoretic variability within the *Protogonyaulax tamarensis/ catenella* species complex: pyridine linked dehydrogenases, *Biochem. Sys. Ecol.*, 3, 311, 1986.
78. **Whitten, D. J. and Hayhome, B. A.,** Comparative electrophoretic analysis of two binucleate dinoflagellates. *J. Phycol.*, 22, 348, 1986.
79. **Sako, Y., Uchida, A., and Ishida, Y.,** Electrophoretic analysis of isozymes in red tide dinoflagellates (*Gymnodinium nagasakiense, Protogonyaulax catenella*, and *Peridinium bipes*), in *Red Tides: Biology, Environmental Science and Toxicology*, Okaichi, T., Anderson, D. M., and Nemoto, T., Eds., Elsevier, New York, 1989, 325.
80. **Cembella, A. D., Taylor, F. J. R., and Therriault, J.-C.,** Cladistic analysis of electrophoretic variants within the toxic dinoflagellate genus *Protogonyaulax, Bot. Mar.*, 39, 39, 1988.
81. **Sako, Y., Machida, S., Toda, H., and Ishida, Y.,** Purification and characterization of calmodulin (Ca^{2+} binding protein) from *Crypthecodinium cohnii* and *Peridinium bipes*, in *Red Tides: Biology, Environmental Science and Toxicology*, Elsevier, New York, 1989, 337.
82. **Avise, J. C.,** Systematic value of electrophoretic data, *Syst. Zool.*, 23, 465, 1974.
83. **Schmidt, R. J. and Loeblich, A. R., III,** A discussion of the systematics of toxic *Gonyaulax* spp. containing paralytic shellfish poison, in *Toxic Dinoflagellate Blooms*, Taylor, D. L. and Seliger, H. H., Eds., Elsevier, New York, 1979, 83.
84. **Lewontin, R. C.,** Population genetics, *Ann. Rev. Gen.,* 19, 81, 1985.
85. **Taylor, F. J. R.,** The taxonomy and relationship of red tide dinoflagellates, in *Toxic Dinoflagellates,* Anderson, D. M., White, A. W., and Baden, D. G., Eds., Elsevier, New York, 1985, 11.
86. **Taylor, F. J. R.,** Toxic dinoflagellates: taxonomic and biogeographic aspects with emphasis on *Protogonyaulax*, in *Seafood Toxins,* Ragelis, E. P., Ed., The American Chemical Society, Washington, D.C., 1984, 77.
87. **Sako, Y., Kim, C. H., and Ishida, Y.,** Isozyme and cross analysis of mating population in *Protogonyaulax catenella/tamarensis* species complex, in *Toxic Marine Phytoplankton Blooms,* Graneli, E., Sundstrom, B., Edler, L., and Anderson, D. M., Eds., Elsevier, Amsterdam, in press.
88. **Spector, D. L.,** Dinoflagellate nuclei, in *Dinoflagellates*, Spector, D. L., Ed., Academic Press, Orlando, FL, 1984, 107.
89. **Yentsch, C. M., Mague, F. C., Horan, P. K., and Muirhead, K.,** Flow cytometric DNA determinations of individual cells of the dinoflagellate *Gonyaulax tamarensis var. excavata, J. Exp. Mar. Biol. Ecol.*, 67, 175, 1983.
90. **Steele, R. E. and Rae, P. M. M.,** Comparison of DNA's of *Crypthecodinium cohnii*-like dinoflagellates from widespread locations, *J. Protozool.*, 27, 479, 1980.
91. **Fliermans, C. B. and Schmidt, E. L.,** Immunofluorescence for autecological study of a unicellular bluegreen alga, *J. Phycol.*, 13, 364, 1977.
92. **Campbell, L., Carpenter, E. J., and Iacono, V. J.,** Identification and enumeration of marine chroococcoid cyanobacteria by immunofluorescence, *App. Environ. Microbiol.*, 46, 553, 1983.
93. **Tayeh, M. A. and Madigan, M. T.,** ELISA analysis of malate dehydrogenases from nonsulphur purple phototrophic bacteria, *EEMS Microbiol. Lett.*, 55, 151, 1988.
94. **Campbell, B., Nakagawa, L. K., Kobayashi, M. N., and Hokama, Y.,** *Gambierdiscus toxicus* in gut contents of the surgeonfish *Ctenochaetus strigosus* (Herbivore) and its relationship to toxicity, *Toxicon*, 25, 1125, 1987.
95. **Baden, D. G., Mende, T. J., Walling, J., and Schultz, D. R.,** Specific antibodies directed against toxins of *Ptychodiscus brevis* (Florida's red tide dinoflagellate), *Toxicon*, 22, 783, 1984.

96. **Baden, D. G., Mende, T. J., and Block, R. E.,** Two similar toxins isolated from *Gymnodinium breve*, in *Toxic Dinoflagellate Blooms*, Taylor, D. L. and Seliger, H. H., Eds., Elsevier, New York, 1979, 327.
97. **Spinrad, R. W. and Yentsch, C. M.,** Observations on the intra- and interspecific single cell optical variability of marine phytoplankton, *Appl. Optics*, 26, 357, 1987.
98. **Yentsch, C. M.,** Detection, enumeration and quantification of cell properties by automated analysis, in *Red Tides: Biology, Environmental Science, and Toxicology*, Okaichi, T., Anderson, D. M., and Nemoto, T., Eds., Elsevier, New York, 1989, 221.
99. **Gallagher, J. C. and Alberte, R. S.,** Photosynthetic and cellular photoadaptive characteristics of three ecotypes of the marine diatom *Skeletonema costatum* (Grev.) Cleve, *J. Exp. Mar. Biol. Ecol.*, 94, 233, 1985.
100. **Wood, A. M.,** Molecular biology, single cell analysis and quantitative genetics: new evolutionary genetic approaches in phytoplankton ecology, in *Immunological Approaches to Estuarine, Coastal and Oceanographic Questions,* Yentsch, C. M. and Mague, F., Eds., Springer Verlag, New York, in press.
101. **Guillard, R. R. L., Kilham, P., and Jackson, T. A.,** Kinetics of silicon-limited growth in the marine diatom *Thalassiosira pseudonana* Hasle and Heimdal (=Cyclotella nana Hustedt), *J. Phycol.*, 9, 233, 1973.
102. **Titman, D.,** Ecological competition between algae: experimental confirmation of resource-based competition theory, *Science,* 192, 463, 1976.
103. **Guillard, R. R. L. and Ryther, J. H.,** Studies of marine planktonic diatoms. I. *Cyclotella nana* Hustedt, and *Detonula confervacea* (Cleve) Gran, *Can. J. Microbiol.*, 8, 229, 1962.
104. **Gavis, J., Guillard, R. R. L., and Woodward, B. L.,** Cupric ion activity and the growth of phytoplankton clones isolated from different marine environments, *J. Mar. Res.*, 39, 315, 1981.
105. **Brand, L. E., Sunda, W. G., and Guillard, R. R. L.,** Limitation of marine phytoplankton reproductive rates by zinc, manganese and iron, *Limnol. Oceanogr.*, 28, 1182, 1983.
106. **Eppley, R. W., Rogers, J. N., and McCarthy, J. J.,** Half-saturation 'constants' for uptake of nitrate and ammonium by marine phytoplankton, *Limnol. Oceanogr.*, 14, 912, 1969.
107. **Falconer, D. S.,** *Introduction to Quantitative Genetics, 2nd ed.*, Longman, New York, 1981.
108. **Simmonds, N. W.,** *Principles of Crop Improvement*, Longman, New York, 1979.
109. **Brand, L. E.,** Low genetic variability in reproduction rates in populations of *Prorocentrum micans* Ehrenb. (Dinophyceae) over Georges Bank, *J. Exp. Mar. Biol. Ecol.*, 88, 55, 1985.
110. **Brand, L. E., Guillard, R. R. L., and Murphy, L. S.,** A method for the rapid and precise determination of acclimated phytoplankton reproduction rates, *J. Plankton Res.*, 3, 193, 1981.
111. **Brand, L. E., Murphy, L. S., Guillard, R. R. L., and Lee, H.-T.,** Genetic variability and differentiation in the temperature niche component of the diatom *Thalassiosira pseudonana*, *Mar. Biol.*, 62, 103, 1981.
112. **Bomber, J. W., Tindall, D. R., Venable, W., and Miller, D. M.,** Pigment composition and low-light response of 14 clones of *Gambierdiscus toxicus*, in *Toxic Phytoplankton Blooms*, Graneli, E., Sundstron, B., Edler, L., and Anderson, D. M., Eds., Elsevier, New York, 1990, 263.
113. **Arnold, S. J.,** Morphology, performance and fitness, *Am. Zool.*, 23, 347, 1983.
114. **Wood, A. M., Lande, R., and Fryxell, G. A.,** Quantitative genetic analysis of morphological variation in an Antarctic diatom grown at two light intensities, *J. Phycol.*, 23, 42, 1987.
115. **Lande, R.,** Natural selection and random genetic drift in phenotypic evolution, *Evolution*, 30, 314, 1976.
116. **Lande, R.**, Statistical tests for natural selection on quantitative characters, *Evolution*, 31, 442, 1976.
117. **Wright, S.,** Evolution in Mendelian populations, *Genetics*, 16, 97, 1931.
118. **Pianka, E. R.,** On r and k selection, *Am. Naturalist*, 592, 1970.
119. **MacArthur, R. H. and Wilson, E. O.,** *The Theory of Island Biogeography*, Princeton University Press, Princeton, NJ, 1967.
120. **Beseda, E. G.,** Study of the Morphology, Toxicity and Sterol Composition of Marine Tropical Benthic Dinoflagellates: Family Ostreopsidaceae, M.S. thesis, University of Houston, 1982.
121. **Loeblich, A. R., III and Indelicato, S. R.,** Thecal analysis of the tropical benthic dinoflagellate *Gambierdiscus toxicus*, *Mar. Fish. Rev.*, 48, 38, 1986.
122. **Wood, A. M., Horan, P. K., Muirhead, K., Phinne, D. A., Yentsch, C. M., and Waterbury, J. B.,** Discrimination between types of pigments in marine *Synechococcus* sp. by scanning spectroscopy, epifluorescence microscopy and flow cytometry, *Limnol. Oceanogr.*, 30, 1303, 1986.
123. **Withers, N.,** Dinoflagellate sterols, in *Marine Natural Products: Chemical and Biological Perspectives, Vol. V*, Scheuer, P.J., Ed., Academic Press, New York, 1983, 87.
124. **Keller, M. D., Selvin, R. C., Claus, W., and Guillard, R. R. L.,** Media for the culture of oceanic ultraphytoplankton, *J. Phycol.*, 23, 633, 1987.
125. **Bomber, J. W., Guillard, R. R. L., and Nelson, W. G.,** Roles of temperature, salinity and light in seasonality, growth and toxicity of ciguatera-causing *Gambierdiscus toxicus* Adachi et Fukuyo (Dinophyceae), *J. Exp. Mar. Biol. Ecol.*, 115, 53, 1988.
126. **Sokal, R. R. and Rohlf, F. J.,** *Biometry, 2nd Ed.*, W.H. Freeman, New York, 1981.
127. **Kodama, M., Ogata, T., and Sato, S.,** Bacterial production of saxitoxin, *Agric. Biol. Chem.*, 52, 1075, 1988.

128. **Tosteson, T. R., Ballantine, D. L., Tosteson, Hensley, V., and Bardales, A. T.,** Associated bacterial flora, growth and toxicity of cultured benthic dinoflagellates *Ostreopsis lenticularis* and *Gambierdiscus toxicus*, *App. Environ. Microbiol.*, 55, 137, 1989.
129. **Sousa E Silva, E.,** Endonuclear bacteria in two species of dinoflagellates, *Protistologica,* 14, 113, 1978.
130. **Carlson, R. D., Morey-Gaines, G., Tindall, D. R., and Dickey, R. W.,** Ecology of toxic dinoflagellates from the Caribbean Sea. Effects of macroalgal extracts on growth in culture, in *Seafood Toxins,* Ragelis, E. P., Ed., The American Chemical Society, Washington, D.C., 1984, 271.
131. **Durand, M., Squiban, A., Ribier, R., Bagnis, R. ,and Puiseux-Dao, S.,** Pseudonuclear vesicles in the toxic dinoflagellate *Gambierdiscus toxicus*, *Biol. Cell,* 56, 171, 1986.
132. **Tosteson, T. R., Ballantine, D. L., Tosteson, C. G., Bardales, A. T., Durst, H. D., and Higerd, T. B.,** Comparative toxicity of *Gambierdiscus toxicus*, *Ostreopsis* cf. *lenticularis*, and associated microflora, *Mar. Fish. Rev.*, 48, 57, 1986.
133. **Westley, J. W., Blount, J. F, Evans, R.H., Jr., and Liu, C.-M.,** C-17 epimers of deoxy-(o-8)-salinomycin from *Streptomyces albus*, (ATCC 218387), *J. Antibiot.*, 30, 610, 1977.
134. **Carmichael, W. W.,** Algal toxins, *Adv. Bot. Res.*, 12, 47, 1986.
135. **Prosser, B. La-T. and Palleroni, N. J.,** Taxonomy of the polyether antibiotic-producing organisms, in *Polyether Antibiotics: Naturally Occurring Acid Ionophores, Vol. 1, Biology,* Westley, J. W., Ed., Marcel Dekker, New York, 1982, 21.
136. **Schulman, L. S., Roszell, L. E., Mende, T. J., and Baden, D.,** A new polyether from Florida's red tide dinoflagellate *Ptychodiscus brevis*, in *Toxic Marine Phytoplankton Blooms*, Graneli, E., Sundstrom, B., Edler, L., and Anderson, D. M., Eds., Elsevier, New York, in press.
137. **Seto, H., Mizoue, K., Otake, N., Gachon, P., Kergomard, A., and Westley, J. W.,** The revised structure of alborixin, *J. Antibiot.*, 32, 970, 1979.
138. **Tachibana, K., Scheuer, P. J., Tsukitani, Y., Kituchi, H., Engen, D. V., Clardy, J., Gopichand, Y., and Schimitz, F. J.,** Okadaic acid, a cytotoxic polyether from two marine sponges of the genus *Halichondria*, *J. Am. Chem. Soc.*, 103, 2469, 1981.
139. **Moore, R. E., Helfrich, P., and Patterson, G. M. L.,** The deadly seaweed of Hana, *Oceanus*, 25, 54, 1982.
140. **Westley, J. W.,** Notation and classification, in *Polyether Antibiotics: Naturally Occurring Acid Ionophores, Vol. 1, Biology,* Westley, J. W., Ed., Marcel Dekker, New York, 1982, 1.
141. **Freudenthal, A. R. and Jijina, J. L.,** Potential hazards of *Dinophysis* to consumers and shellfisheries, *J. Shellfish Res.*, 7, 695, 1988.
142. **Kodama, I., Kondo, N., and Shibata, S.,** Electromechanical effects of okadaic acid isolated from black sponge in guinea-pig ventricular muscles, *J. Physiol.*, 378, 359, 1986.
143. **Shibata, S., Ishida,Y., Kitano, H., Ohizumi, Y., Habon, J., Tsukitani, Y., and Kikuchi, H.,** Contractile effects of okadaic acid, a novel ionophore-like substance from black sponge on isolated smooth muscles under the condition of calcium deficiency, *J. Pharmacol. Exp. Ther.*, 223, 135, 1982.
144. **Sze, H.,** Nigericin-stimulated ATPase activity in microsomal vesicles of tobacco callus, *Proc. Natl. Acad. Sci. USA*, 77, 5904, 1980.
145. **Estrada-O., S., Rightmire, B., and Lardy, H. A.,** Specific inhibition of ion transport in mitochondria by the monensins, *Antimicrob. Agents Chemother.*, 1967, 279, 1968.
146. **Pressman, B. C.,** Biological applications of ionophores, *Ann. Rev. Biochem.*, 45, 501, 1976.
147. **Pressman, B. C.,** Ionophorous antibiotics as models for biological transport, *Fed. Proc.*, 27, 1283, 1968.
148. **Liu, C-M.,** Microbial aspects of polyether antibiotics: activity, production and biosynthesis, in *Polyether Antibiotics: Naturally Occurring Acid Ionophores, Vol. 1, Biology,* Westley, J.W., Ed., Marcel Dekker, New York, 1982, 43.
149. **Taylor, R. W., Kauffman, R. F., and Pfeiffer, D. R.,** Cation complexation and transport by carboxylic acid ionophores, in *Polyether Antibiotics: Naturally Occurring Acid Ionophores, Vol. 1, Biology,* Westley, J.W., Ed., Marcel Dekker, New York, 1982, 103.
150. **Gachon, P., Kergomard, A., Staron, T., and Esteve, C.,** Grisorixin, an ionophorous antibiotic of the nigericin group. 1. Fermentation, isolation, biological properties and structure, *J. Antibiot.*, 28, 345, 1975.
151. **Liu, C-M., Hermann, T. E., Prosser, B. La T., Palleroni, N. J., Westley, J. W., and Miller, P.A.,** X-14766A, a halogen containing polyether antibiotic produced by *Streptomyces malachito-fuscus* subsp. *downeyi*. Discovery, fermentation, biological properties and taxonomy of the producing culture, *J. Antibiot.*, 34, 133, 1981.
152. **Harold, F. M. and Baarda, J. R.,** Effects of nigericin and monensin on cation permeability of *Streptococcus faecalis* and metabolic capabilities of potassium-depleted cells, *J. Bacteriol.*, 95, 816, 1968.
153. **Harned, R. L., Hidy, P. H., Corum, C. J., and Jones, K. L.,** Nigericin, a new crystalline antibiotic from an unidentified *Streptomyces*, *Antibiot. Chemother.*, 1, 594, 1951.
154. **Lubin, M.,** Intracellular potassium and control of protein synthesis, *Fed. Proc.*, 23, 994, 1964.
155. **Ragelis, E.,** Ciguatera seafood poisoning: overview, in *Seafood Toxins*, Ragelis, E., Ed., American Chemical Society Symposium Series, Book 262, Washington D.C., 1984, 25.

156. **Scheuer, P. J., Takahashi, W., Tsutsumi, W., and Yoshida, T.,** Ciguatoxin: isolation and chemical nature, *Science*, 155, 1267, 1967.
157. **Tindall, D. R. and Miller, D. M.,** Purification of maitotoxin from the dinoflagellate, *Gambierdiscus toxicus* using high pressure liquid chromatography, in *Toxic Dinoflagellates,* Anderson, D. M., White, A. W., and Baden, D. G., Eds., Elsevier, New York, 1985, 321.
158. **Gillespie, N., Lewis, R., Burke, J., and Holmes, M.,** The significance of the absence of ciguatoxin in a wild population of *Gambierdiscus toxicus, Proc. Fifth Intl. Coral Reef Cong.*, Tahiti, 4, 437, 1985.
159. **Bomber, J. W., Norris, D. R., and Mitchell, L. E.,** Benthic dinoflagellates associated with ciguatera from the Florida Keys. II. Temporal, spatial and substrate heterogeneity of *Prorocentrum lima,* in *Toxic Dinoflagellates*, Anderson, D. M., White, A. W., and Baden, D. G., Eds., Elsevier, New York, 1985, 45.
160. **Hokama, Y.,** A rapid, simplified enzyme immunoassay stick test for the detection of ciguatoxin and related polyethers from fish tissue, *Toxicon,* 23, 939, 1985.
161. **Uda, T., Itoh, Y., Nishimura, M., Usagawa, T., Murata, M., and Yasumoto, T.,** Enzyme immunoassay using monoclonal antibody specific for diarrhetic shellfish poisons, in Natori, S., Hashimoto, K., and Ueno, Y., Eds., *Mycotoxins and Phycotoxins*, Elsevier, Amsterdam, 1988, 335.
162. **Barbier, M.,** Marine chemical ecology: the roles of chemical communication and chemical pollution, in *Marine Natural Products, Chemical and Biological Perspectives, Vol. IV*, Scheuer, P. J., Ed., Academic Press, New York, 1981, 148.
163. **Paul, V. J. and Fenical, W.,** Isolation of halimedatrial: chemical defence adaptation in the calcareous reef-building alga *Halimeda, Science*, 221, 747, 1983.
164. **Hansen, P. J.,** The red tide dinoflagellate *Alexandrium tamarense*: effects on behavior and growth of a tintinnid ciliate, in *Toxic Marine Phytoplankton Blooms*, Graneli, E., Sundstrom, B., Edler, L., and Anderson, D. M., Eds., Elsevier, New York, in press.
165. **Trick, C. G., Anderson, R. J., and Harrison, P. J.,** Environmental factors influencing the production of an antibacterial metabolite from a marine dinoflagellate *Prorocentrum minimum, Can. J. Fish. Aquat. Sci.*, 41, 423, 1984.
166. **Andersen, R. J., LeBlanc, J. J., and Sum, F.W.,** 1-(2,6,6-trimethyl-4-hydroxycyclohexenyl)-1,3-butanedi-one, an extracellular metabolite from the dinoflagellate *Prorocentrum minimum, J. Org. Chem.*, 45, 1169, 1980.
167. **Carlson, R. D.,** Distribution, Periodicity, and Culture of Benthic/Epiphytic Dinoflagellates in a Ciguatera Endemic Region of the Caribbean, Ph.D. thesis, Southern Illinois University, Carbondale, IL, 1984.
168. **Hardin, G.,** The competitive exclusion principle, *Science*, 131, 1292, 1960.
169. **Bomber, J. W., Tindall, D. R., and Norris, D. R.,** Allelopathy in an epiphytic community, *J. Phycol.*, 25(Suppl.), 14, 1989.
170. **Miller, D. M. and Tindall, D. R.,** Physiological effects of HPLC-purified maitotoxin from a dinoflagellate *Gambierdiscus toxicus*, in *Toxic Dinoflagellates*, Anderson, D. M., White, A. W., and Baden, D. G., Eds., Elsevier, 1985, 375.
171. **Yasumoto, T., Nakajima, I., Bagnis, R., and Adachi, R.,** Finding of a dinoflagellate as a likely culprit of Ciguatera, *Bull. Jpn. Soc. Sci. Fish.*, 43, 1021, 1977.
172. **Schantz, E. J., Mold, J. D., Stanger, D. W., Shavel, J., Riel, F. J., Bowden, J. P., Lynch, J. M., Wyler, R. S., Riegel, B., and Sommer, H.,** Paralytic shellfish poison. VI. A procedure for isolation and purification of the poison from toxic clams and mussels, *J. Am. Chem. Soc.*, 79, 5230, 1957.
173. **Steidinger, K. A., Burklew, M. A., and Ingle, R. M.,** The effect of *Gymnodinium breve* toxin on estuarine animals, in *Marine Pharmacognosy*, Martin, D. F. and Padilla, G. M., Eds., Academic Press, New York, 1973, 179.
174. **Yentsch, C. M. and Mague, F. C.,** Evidence of an apparent annual rhythm in the toxic red tide dinoflagellate *Gonyaulax excavata, Int. J. Chronobiol.*, 7, 77, 1980.
175. **Sweeney, B. M.,** Circadian rhythmicity in dinoflagellates, in *Dinoflagellates*, Spector, D. L., Ed., Academic Press, Orlando, FL, 1984, 343.
176. **White, A. W.,** High toxin content in the dinoflagellate *Gonyaulax excavata* in nature, *Toxicon,* 24, 605, 1986.
177. **Cembella, A. D., Therriault, J.-C., and Beland, P.,** Toxicity of cultured isolates and natural populations of *Protogonyaulax tamarensis* from the St. Lawrence Estuary, *J. Shellfish Res.*, 7, 611, 1988.
178. **Ballantine, D. L., Tosteson, T. R., and Bardales, A. T.,** Population dynamics and toxicity of natural populations of benthic dinoflagellates in southwestern Puerto Rico, *J. Exp. Mar. Biol. Ecol.*, 119, 201, 1988.
179. **White, A. W. and Maranda, L.,** Paralytic toxins in the dinoflagellate *Gonyaulax excavata* and in shellfish, *J. Fish. Res. Bd. Can.*, 35, 397, 1978.
180. **Boyer, G. L., Sullivan, J. J., Andersen, R. J., Harrison, P. J., and Taylor, F. J. R.,** Effects of nutrient limitation on toxin production and composition in the marine dinoflagellate *Protogonyaulax tamarensis, Mar. Biol.*, 96, 123, 1987.
181. **Boczar, B. A., Beitler, M. K., Liston, J., Sullivan, J. J., and Cattolico, R. A.,** Paralytic shellfish toxins in *Protogonyaulax tamarensis* and *Protogonyaulax catenella* in axenic culture, *Plant Physiol.*, 88, 1285, 1988.

182. **Babinchak, J. A., Jollow, D. J., Voegtline, M. S., and Higerd, T. B.**, Toxin production by *Gambierdiscus toxicus* isolated from the Florida Keys, *Mar. Fish. Rev.*, 48:53, 1986.
183. **Durand-Clement, M.**, Study of production and toxicity of cultured *Gambierdiscus toxicus*, *Biol. Bull.*, 172, 108, 1987.
184. **Tindall, D .R., Miller, D. M., and Tindall, P. M.**, Toxicity of *Ostreopsis lenticularis* from the British and U.S. Virgin Islands, in *Toxic Marine Phytoplankton*, Greneli, E., Sundstrom, B., Edler, L., and Anderson, D. M., Eds., Elsevier, Amsterdam, in press.
185. **Dickey, R. W., Miller, D. M., and Tindall, D. R.**, A water soluble toxin from a dinoflagellate, *Gambierdiscus toxicus*, in *Seafood Toxins*, Ragelis, E. P., Ed., The American Chemical Society, Washington, D.C., 1984, 257.
186. **Yentsch, C. M., Dale, B., and Hurst, J. W.**, Coexistence of toxic and non-toxic dinoflagellates resembling *Gonyaulax tamarensis* in New England Coastal Waters (NW Atlantic), *J. Phycol.*, 14, 330, 1978.
187. **Alam, M. I., Hsu, C. P., and Shimizu, Y.**, Comparison of toxins in three isolates of *Gonyaulax tamarensis* (Dinophyceae), *J. Phycol.*, 15, 106, 1979.
188. **Oshima, Y., Hayakawa, T., Hashimoto, M., Kotaki, Y., and Yasumoto, T.**, Classification of *Protogonyaulax tamarensis* from Northern Japan into 3 strains by toxin composition, *Bull. Jpn. Soc. Sci. Fish.*, 48, 851, 1982.
189. **Hall, S.**, Toxins and Toxicity of *Protogonyaulax* from the Northeast Pacific, Ph.D. thesis, University of Alaska, Fairbanks, AL, 1982.
190. **Cembella, A. D., Sullivan, J. J., Boyer, G. L., Taylor, F. J. R., and Andersen, R. J.**, Variation in paralytic shellfish toxin composition within the *Protogonyaulax tamarensis/catenella* species complex; red tide dinoflagellates, *Biochem. System. Ecol.*, 15, 171, 1987.
191. **Lewis, N. D.**, Ciguatera in the Pacific: incidence and implications for marine resource development, in *Seafood Toxins*, Ragelis, E.P., Ed., The American Chemical Society, Washington, D.C., 1984, 289.
192. **Ohizumi, Y.**, Pharmacological actions of the marine toxins ciguatoxin and maitotoxin isolated from poisonous fish, *Biol. Bull.*, 172, 132, 1987.
193. **Carlson, R. D. and Tindall, D. R.**, Distribution and periodicity of toxic dinoflagellates in the Virgin Islands, in *Toxic Dinoflagellates*, Anderson, D. M., White, A. W. and Baden, D. G., Eds., Elsevier, New York, 1985, 171.
194. **Maranda, L., Anderson, D. M., and Shimizu, Y.**, Comparison of toxicity between populations of *Gonyaulax tamarensis* of Eastern North American Waters, *Est. Coast. Shelf Sci.*, 21, 401, 1985.
195. **Shimizu, Y.**, Recent progress in marine toxin research, *Pure Appl. Chem.*, 54, 1973, 1982.
196. **Shimizu, Y., Gupta, S., Norte, M., Hori, A., Genenah, G., and Kobayashi, M.**, Biosynthesis of paralytic shellfish toxins, in *Toxic Dinoflagellates*, Anderson, D. M., White, A. W., and Baden, D. G., Eds., Elsevier, New York, 1985,
197. **Shimizu, Y., Norte, M., Hori, A., Genenah, A., and Kobayashi, M.**, Biosynthesis of saxitoxin analogs: the unexpected pathway, *J. Am. Chem. Soc.*, 106, 6433, 1982.
198. **Cane, D. E., Celmer, W. D., and Westley, J. W.**, Unified stereochemical model of polyether antibiotic structure and biogenesis, *J. Am. Chem. Soc.*, 105, 3594, 1983.
199. **O'Hagen, D.**, Structural and stereochemical homology between the macrolide and polyether antibiotics, *Tetrahedron*, 44, 1691, 1988.
200. **Cane, D. E., Liang, T. C., Taylor, P. B., Chang, C., and Yang, C. C.**, Macrolide biosynthesis. 3. Stereochemistry of the chain-elongation steps of erythromycin biosynthesis, *J. Am. Chem. Soc.*, 108, 4957, 1986.
201. **Hutchinson, C. R., Sherman, M. M., Vederas, J. C., and Nakashima, T. T.**, Biosynthesis of macrolides. 5. Regiochemistry of the labelling of lasalocid A by ^{13}C, ^{18}O-labelled precursors, *J. Am. Chem. Soc.*, 103, 5953, 1981.
202. **Shimizu, Y., Gupta, S., and Krishna Prasad, A. V.**, Biosynthesis of dinoflagellate toxins, in *Toxic Marine Phytoplankton Blooms*, Graneli, E., Sundstrom, B., Edler, L., and Anderson, D. M., Eds., Elsevier, New York, in press.
203. **Thompson, J. E., Murphy, P. T., Bergquist, P. R., and Evans, E. A.**, *Biochem. Syst. Ecol.*, 15, 595, 1987.
204. **Prakash, A.**, Growth and toxicity of a marine dinoflagellate, *Gonyaulax tamarensis*, *J. Fish. Res. Bd. Can.*, 24, 1589, 1967.
205. **Kim, Y. S. and Martin, D. F.**, Effects of salinity on synthesis of DNA, acidic polysaccharide and ichthyotoxin in *Gymnodinium breve*, *Phytochem.*, 13, 533, 1974.
206. **MacIsaac, J. J., Grunseich, G. S., Glover, H. E., and Yentsch, C. M.**, Light and nutrient limitation in *G. excavata*. Nitrogen and carbon trace results, in *Toxic Dinoflagellate Blooms*, Taylor, D. L. and Seliger, H. H., Eds., Elsevier, New York, 1979, 107.
207. **Trick, C. G., Andersen, R. J., Price, N. M., Gillam, A., and Harrison, P. J.**, Examination of hydroxamate-siderophore production by neritic eukaryotic marine phytoplankton, *Mar. Biol.*, 75, 9, 1983.
208. **Proctor, N. H., Chan, S. L., and Trevor, A. J.**, Production of toxin by cultures of *Gonyaulax catenella*, *Toxicon*, 13, 1, 1975.
209. **Anderson, D. M., Kulis, D. M., Sullivan, J. J., Hall, S., and Lee, C.**, Dynamics of physiology of saxitoxin production by the dinoflagellate *Alexandrium* spp., unpublished manuscript.

210. **Anderson, D. M., Kulis, D. M., Sullivan, J. J., and Hall, S.,** Toxin composition variations in one isolate of the dinoflagellate *Alexandrium fundyense*, unpublished manuscript.
211. **White, A. W.,** Salinity effects on growth and toxin content of *Gonyaulax excavata*, a marine dinoflagellate causing paralytic shellfish poisoning, *J. Phycol.*, 14, 475, 1978.
212. **Dale, B., Yentsch, C. M., and Hurst, J. W.,** Toxicity in resting cysts of the red-tide dinoflagellate *Gonyaulax excavata* from deeper water coastal sediments, *Science*, 201, 1224, 1978.
213. **Cembella, A. D., Destombe, C., and Turgeon, J.,** Toxin composition of alternative life history stages of *Alexandrium*, as determined by high-performance liquid chromatography, in *Toxic Marine Phytoplankton Blooms*, Graneli, E., Sundstrom, B., Edler, L., and Anderson, D. M., Eds., Elsevier, New York, in press.
214. **Kodama, M., Fukuyo, Y., Ogata, T., Igarashi, T., Kamiya, H., and Matsuura, F.,** Comparison of toxicities of *Protogonyaulax* cells of various sizes, *Bull. Jpn. Soc. Sci. Fish.*, 48, 567, 1982.
215. **Hokama, Y., Honda, S., Kobayashi, M., Nakagawa, L., Kurihara, J., and Miyahara, J.,** Monoclonal antibodies in the detection of ciguatoxin (CTX) and related polyethers in contaminated fish tissue, in *Progress in Venom and Toxin Research,* Gopalakrish-Nakone, P. and Tan, C. K., Eds., National University of Singapore, 1987, 384.
216. **Stark, W. M., Knox, N. G., and Westhead, J. E.,** Monensin, a new biologically active compound. II. Fermentation studies, *Antimicrob. Agents Chemother.*, 1967, 353, 1968.
217. **Dortch, Q.,** Effect of growth conditions in accumulation of internal nitrate, ammonia, amino acids and protein in three marine diatoms, *J. Exp. Mar. Biol. Ecol.*, 61, 243, 1982.
218. **Meeson, B. W. and Faust, M. A.**, Response of *Prorocentrum minimum* (Dinophyceae) to different spectral qualities and irradiances: growth and photosynthesis, in *Marine Biology of Polar Regions and Effects of Stress on Marine Organisms*, Gray, J. S. and Christiansen, M. E., John Wiley, 1985, 445.
219. **Faust, M. A., Sager, J. C., and Meeson, B. W.,** Response of *Prorocentrum mariae-lebouriae* (Dinophyceae) to light of different spectral qualities and irradiances: growth and pigmentation, *J. Phycol.*, 18, 349, 1982.
220. **Bergmann, J. S. and Alam, M.,** On the toxicity of the ciguatera producing dinoflagellate, *Gambierdiscus toxicus* Adachi and Fukuyo isolated from the Florida Keys, *J. Environ. Sci. Health*, A16, 493, 1981.
221. **Durand-Clement, M.,** A study of toxin production by *Gambierdiscus toxicus* in culture, *Toxicon*, 24, 1153, 1986.
222. **Miller, D. M., Tindall, D. R., and Venable, C. W.,** NMR spectroscopy of components isolated from *Gambierdiscus toxicus*, in *Toxic Marine Phytoplankton Blooms*, Graneli, E., Sundstrom, B., Edler, L., and Anderson, D. M., Eds., Elsevier, New York, in press.
223. **Morton, S. L. and Norris, D. R.,** Role of temperature, salinity and light on the seasonality of *Prorocentrum lima* (Ehrenberg) Dodge, in *Toxic Marine Phytoplankton Blooms*, Graneli, E., Sundstrom, B., Edler, L., and Anderson, D. M., Eds., Elsevier, New York, in press.
224. **Aikman, K. E. and Tindall, D. R.,** The effect of light intensity and acclimation on the physiology and growth of the toxic dinoflagellate *Prorocentrum concavum*, *J. Phycol.*, 25(Suppl.), 17, 1989.
225. **Bomber, J. W., Rubio, M. G., and Norris, D. R.,** Epiphytism of dinoflagellates associated with the disease ciguatera: substrate specificity and nutrition, *Phycologia*, 28, 360, 1989.
226. **Saint-Martin, K., Durand-Clement, M., and Bourdeau, P.,** Contribution a l'etude des rapports entre les macroalgues et *Gambierdiscus toxicus* (Dinophyceae), agent casual de la ciguatera, *Cryptogamie, Algologie*, 9, 195, 1988.
227. **Yentsch, C. M.,** Flow cytometric analysis of cellular saxitoxin in the dinoflagellate *Gonyaulax tamarensis* var. *excavata*, *Toxicon*, 19, 611, 1981.
228. **Tindall, D. R.,** unpublished data.
229. **Bomber, J. W. and Tinder, D. R.,** unpublished results.
230. **Tindall, D. R. and Bomber, J. W.,** in preparation.
231. **Babinchak, J. A.,** personal communication.
232. **Bomber, J. W., et al.,** unpublished data.

INDEX

F

G

H

I

L

Q

R

S

T

U

V

W

X

Y